Freedom to Practise

The development of patient-centred nursing

Alison Binnie MA RGN RM Dip.N
Nurse Practitioner, Vascular Unit, The John Radcliffe Hospital,
Oxford, UK

and

Angie Titchen MCSP, MSc DPhil(Oxon)
Senior Research and Development Fellow, RCN Institute,
Oxford, UK

Edited by **Judith Lathlean** BSc(Econ) MA DPhil(Oxon)
Independent Health Care Research Consultant and Visiting Professor,
University of Reading, UK

With a foreword by **Marie Manthey**

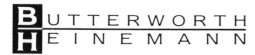
BUTTERWORTH
HEINEMANN

OXFORD AUCKLAND BOSTON JOHANNESBURG MELBOURNE NEW DELHI

Butterworth-Heinemann
Linacre House, Jordan Hill, Oxford OX2 8DP
225 Wildwood Avenue, Woburn, MA 01801-2041
A division of Reed Educational and Professional Publishing Ltd

A member of the Reed Elsevier plc group

First published 1999
Reprinted 2001

British Library Cataloguing in Publication Data
A catalogue record for this book is available from the British Library

Library of Congress in Publication Data
A catalogue record for this book is available from the Library of Congress

ISBN 0 7506 4075 8

Composition by Genesis Typesetting, Rochester, Kent
Printed and bound in Great Britain by Biddles Ltd, *www.biddles.co.uk*

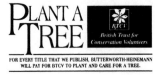

Contents

List of Stories   xi

Foreword by Marie Manthey   xiii

Acknowledgements   xv

Part One   **1**

Introduction   **3**
   The research and development project   **3**
   The structure of the book   **4**

1. **Background issues**   **6**
   Practice issues   **9**
     Traditional nursing   9
     Individualized nursing   12
     Patient-centred nursing   16
   Research issues   **21**

2. **Origins and context of the study**   **27**
   Practice background   **27**
     The contemporary scene   30
   The research questions   **30**
   Choice of methodology   **31**
   Key influences on the development of the action research strategy **33**

3. **The research strategy**   **37**
   The action research design   **37**
     Exploratory work   39
     The observational study   40

The action spirals   40
   Spiral 1: Moving from team nursing to primary nursing   42
   Spiral 2: Alison's clinical role in the ward   42
   Spiral 3: New nursing roles   43
   Spiral 4: The Care Plan Project   44
   Spiral 5: Ward round behaviour   44
   Spiral 6: Becoming a patient-centred practitioner   45
   Spiral 7: The changing role of the sister   45
   Spiral 8: The staff nurse support group   46
The research partnership   **46**
Data collection methods   **47**
   Participant observation   48
   Depth interviews   49
   Reflective conversations   50
   Documentary evidence   50
Practical research issues   **51**
   Access   51
   Participation   51
   Confidentiality   52
Bias   **53**
Data analysis and theory generation   **53**
   The exploratory case study   53
   The main study   53
Generalizing from this study   **56**

Part Two   **57**

4. The organizational journey   **59**
   Introduction   **59**
      Resource implications   59
   Decentralizing the system   **60**
      The 'ends' system   62
       'Doing the baths'   62
       Being 'in charge'   63
      Strategies for creating effective teams   64
       Establishing predictable continuity   65
       Devolving decision-making   66
        Devolving clinical decision-making 67
        Devolving managerial decision-making 68
       Restructuring communication channels   69
      The flattened hierarchy   71
       Responses to organizational change   71
       The rise and fall of the co-ordinator 72
       Teething troubles   75
       The ward runs itself   81
   Developing new roles   **82**
      Role ambiguity   83
      Strategies for clarifying roles   86
       Time out   86

Facilitating learning from experience   91
    Relating theory to practice   91
    Demonstrating new roles   92
Knowing what is expected   93
    Primary nurse in name only   94
    Practising confidently   96

5. **The cultural journey**   **99**
    Introduction   **99**
    Shaping ward life   **100**
        Doing what you are told   100
        Strategies for increasing participation and democracy 102
            Facilitating participation   102
            Encouraging experimentation   103
        The creative team   104
    Learning to work professionally   **105**
        Getting through the work   105
        Strategies for developing a professional work ethos 106
        Professional commitment   108
    Learning at work   **109**
        Missed learning opportunities   110
        Strategies for promoting curiosity, openness and debate 111
        The lively, critical community   114
    Caring for each other   **116**
        The sociable team   116
        Strategies for creating a climate of concern and support 118
        The caring team   120

6. **The leadership journey**   **123**
    Introduction   **123**
    Developing a clinical leadership role   **125**
        'I can't win'   125
        Strategies for redesigning the role   128
            Reshaping expectations   128
            Time management   130
            Structuring the clinical role effectively   131
            Delegation   133
        The new style sister   133
    Influencing and supervising practice   **137**
        Traditional ward teaching   137
        Strategies for facilitating learning from practice   139
            Enhancing role modelling by articulating expert
                clinical knowledge   139
            Guiding reflection and promoting independent thinking
                and action   140
        Calling nurses to account   141

New style supervision   141
'What I was trying to do here was ... '   142
'Tell me about ... '   143
'Not just an observer'   146

7. **The practice journey**   **149**
    Introduction   **149**
    Experiencing the challenge of nursing   **151**
    The daily grind   152
    Strategies for uncovering the potential of basic care   153
    Nursing is exciting   156
    Becoming a patient-centred nurse   **158**
    Passing acquaintances   159
    Strategies for developing skills for patient-centred nursing 162
        Being there in the background to give confidence   162
        Role modelling and articulating practice   163
        Thinking ahead, taking things further   164
    Skilled companions   165
        Therapeutic relationships   166
        Unpopular patients   175
        Family care   178
        The personal cost of patient-centred nursing   182
        Making a difference   185

8. **The doctor–nurse journey**   **189**
    Introduction   **189**
    Earning respect   **190**
    Reluctant handmaidens   191
    Strategies for promoting collaborative work   95
        Role modelling and coaching   196
        Informing doctors about changes in nursing   198
        Practical communication strategies   200
    Working as colleagues   201
    Ward round behaviour   **204**
    At the back of the crowd   205
    Strategies for influencing ward round behaviour   207
        Creating incentives   207
        Organizational strategies   208
        Role modelling and articulating practical strategies 209
        Enlisting the help of junior doctors   210
    Being there for the patient   210

Part Three   **215**

9. **Principles for practice development**   **217**
    Introduction   **217**
    Changing the practice philosophy   **217**
    Educating the heart as well as the head   218

The ward sister as clinical leader   221
Organizational support and leadership   222
The process of change in practice   **223**
Initiative and control   224
A 'horticultural model' of change   225
The change as a series of 'journeys'   226
Investing in professional development   **229**
Some reflections on action research   **231**
Summary of principles for practice development   **233**

References   **236**

Index   **247**

List of Stories

Passing the Buck 76
Overstepping the mark: Part 1 85
Overstepping the mark: Part 2 93
Expecting her to be Fierce 101
Three Sets of Keys 102
Removing the Charts 106
Camouflaged Task-Oriented Nursing 109
Ruth's Story 115
A Chain of Bad Feeling 121
'I let them all down' 132
'I was trained to be slick' 138
'Did you touch him?' 142
Saying the word 'cancer' 144
'I want to get into their heads' 145
The Two Daughters Story 146
Humping George About 153
Washing Ray 154
Making Things Familiar for Daphne 157
The Lavender Story 158
'He couldn't talk about dying' 159
'I'm not mad, am I?' 160
Giving a Gentle Push 162
'He doesn't want to sit down. He wants to walk in the corridor' 163
'She asked me what I was going to do' 165
Tim and the Orange 166
A Fear of Needles 169
The Reconciliation 172
All he could say was 'Yes' 173
Paul's Recipe 174
'I just basically got to know him' 176
'I just went straight over' 177
'Just arrange an appointment with my secretary' 177
Gerald and Agnes 178
'I asked the questions she couldn't ask' 180
'One might have pushed her out' 181
'Let them have a bit of dignity' 191

Janice and the Psychiatrist   197
'Face-saving'   198
'I pulled out all the stops'   201
'What did all that mean?'   212
'They're talking about me as if I'm not here'   212
'Excuse me'   213

Foreword

The beauty of nursing is that it is such a worthwhile activity. A nurse's interaction with a patient can, at any time, be the single most important thing happening to that person. In fact, in hospital nursing, that is often exactly true. Yet, traditional nursing, with its emphasis on technical tasks and ritual practices, has often resulted in impersonal interactions which make patients feel more like objects than people. In spite of efforts to modernize and humanize nursing practice, there are still many influences that continue to disrupt or devalue personalized, humane care.

In this book, Alison Binnie and Angie Titchen describe a project that successfully transformed a traditional, task-based care delivery system into a professional, patient-centred service. There was a sound intellectual underpinning to the project, but it was also firmly rooted in the reality of practice experience. It produced remarkable results for patients, staff and others involved with the change process. The beauty of nursing became visible and tangible for both those receiving and giving care. . . . It doesn't get much better than that in this life!

Reading about Alison and Angie's work was like renewing an acquaintance with an old friend. Although the setting was quite different from the ones I have worked in, I felt I knew the nurses, shared their experiences and celebrated their successes. Alison and Angie have produced a book of enormous importance. It documents very thoroughly a change process that transformed the behaviour of nurses, enabling them to provide more humane and personalized care for patients. The action research structure of their project has produced valuable insights which show how this transformation was achieved, and a wealth of information which will help others interested in improving care delivery.

There are several notable features of this book. One of the most important is the sheer comprehensiveness of the work: this is one of the most thorough expositions of a transformational culture change I have ever seen. It describes the change from every significant perspective and thus highlights the scope and complexity of the work involved in developing a professional practice unit. Through the action research, the authors have been able to document carefully the multiple dimensions of the project, including the emotional reactions of participants. Their richly detailed reporting will undoubtedly help others embarking on a similar change process. Of particular interest to me was the ambivalence in participants' responses. The transition from a 'worker' to a 'professional' ethos required a climate and culture change of great magnitude and it was a change that did not proceed in a straight line. Ambivalence and hesitation returned time and again as the project evolved from one phase to the next.

The importance of the leader's role in facilitating change is clearly demonstrated throughout the book. Of particular value is the description of specific strategies that Alison used to develop new patterns of thinking and behaviour in the staff. The use of reflection, asking open questions and articulating expectations about professional rather than task based practice are precisely the techniques that leaders can use in any setting to facilitate transformational change. Another valuable strategy was the use of 'away days'. Although not common practice, and often seemingly impossible to arrange and afford (from a staffing perspective), the payoff in terms of increased staff morale and motivation is almost always priceless. When Alison figured out how (both politically and financially) to release nurses for time away together, she found the development work was fast-forwarded to such a degree that the investment was never questioned.

The chapter describing the 'practice journey' wraps up the whole project's ultimate impact on practice. In the introduction to this chapter the authors make an important point, namely, that changing the organization, culture and leadership style on a unit does not necessarily ensure patient-centred practice – it merely creates an environment conducive to its development. Key leadership strategies are described in this chapter, showing how they can be applied in the real world of patient care and how they can have a real effect upon a nurse's ability to practise in a creative and therapeutic way. The authors' liberal use of patient/nurse stories demonstrates how learning took place and how this unit found solutions to common problems, such as the 'difficult patient'. Finally, this chapter deals with the stresses and strains of working in a professional practice setting – again in ways that readers will be able to relate to and compare with their own experience.

The authors' concentration on core issues, rather than situational features, gives this study the quality of universal applicability. The challenges of role and culture change, leadership impact and practice development are handled in ways that minimize situational differences. Clinical leaders can apply the study findings on any patient care unit . . . in the UK, the USA, or elsewhere. Whether the title is Ward Sister, Nurse Manager, or Head Nurse, the leadership role always carries the component of 'leading the practice', which presents a challenge in time use for those with managerially complex roles. Many of the techniques that Alison used are not time-consuming, but they do require the discipline of focussing attention on clinical practice. Although role expectations differ from one hospital to another, and from one country to another, the way Alison led the development of clinical nursing is applicable to any setting.

In this comprehensive account of a journey into professional practice, the authors have dealt carefully with every major aspect of the transformational process. With scholarly thoroughness, each dimension has been covered from a theoretical point of view, as well as from the experiential perspective. Within the context of my thirty plus years of experience in this particular field, I have never read a more thorough, more interesting, or more practical discussion of the practice development process. This should be a seminal work, upon which future research and development initiatives can build to create environments where nurses are genuinely free to practise.

Marie Manthey

Acknowledgements

This book has been a long time in the making. The practice development work it reports began in 1989, the writing began in 1993. The whole venture turned out to be a much bigger undertaking than either of us anticipated. Many people helped us along the way.

Many patients, relatives and hospital staff participated in the study and we are especially grateful to the Medical Unit nurses who lived through the project with us, learning with us and sharing their experiences so openly.

Susan Pembrey, in her role as Clinical Practice Development Nurse for Oxfordshire, laid the foundations upon which our work was built. As the first Director of the National Institute for Nursing, she was also instrumental in setting up our project and subsequently, as mentor and friend, she always believed in the value of our work.

As Chief Nurse, Jacqueline Flindell brought the vision of a practice-led service to Oxfordshire. She and her successor, Malcolm Ross, created an organizational structure and climate in which our work was able to flourish.

Funding for our project came from The King's Fund and the National Institute for Nursing, Oxford. Alison Kitson, currently Director of the Royal College of Nursing Institute, formally supervised our research and we have appreciated her wisdom, patience and understanding.

Our families, friends and other colleagues, too many to mention by name, have given us invaluable support in the background.

A.B. and A.T.

Part One

Introduction

During the 1970s, the values underpinning the British hospital nursing system began to be widely questioned within the nursing profession. Values inherited from the Victorian era, which placed nursing in subservience to medicine and patients in the role of passive recipients of care from both professions, were rejected as untenable in a society increasingly concerned about the rights of both women and consumers. Thus, the work routines and the social relationships that constituted the old order in hospital ward life began to be eroded.

The demise of the old order has been followed by a period of uncertainty and instability. New ideas from theorists, educators, managers, and occasionally from practitioners themselves, have been taken up by ward nurses, with varying degrees of enthusiasm, in attempts to reform ward life and to create a nursing service that reflects modern values. Some thoughtful, comprehensive and apparently successful practice development work has been reported, but it has usually been associated with isolated and relatively small-scale initiatives. Overall, there still appears to be a wide gulf between the way many nurses actually practise and the way their education and socialization has led them to believe they should practise.

A key factor persistently undermining the emergence of a modern style of ward nursing, with the clarity and robustness of its predecessor, seems to be a widespread failure to appreciate the complexity of ward life and the fundamental nature of the reform required to revitalize it. This underestimate of the challenges facing ward nurses is reinforced by a strong tendency, both within and beyond the profession, to undervalue nursing practice. Investment in practice reform has consequently been grossly inadequate and, when compared with investment in both educational and managerial reforms, it looks trivial.

THE RESEARCH AND DEVELOPMENT PROJECT

The action research project reported in this book arose out of the challenge to develop a genuinely 'patient-centred' nursing service in a busy and somewhat demoralized medical unit, where an outmoded traditional approach to professional life and practice was still much in evidence. It was a collaborative venture, supported by the John Radcliffe Hospital and the National Institute for Nursing in Oxford. Research funding came from the Institute and included a substantial grant from the King's Fund. The project was initiated in 1989 by Alison Binnie, then newly appointed as a senior sister in the John Radcliffe Medical Unit. Angie Titchen, who had a background in physiotherapy education and research, joined the staff of the Institute to become Alison's research partner.

The project had a dual purpose. It was established to support a major change in the style of nursing practised in the medical wards. At the same time, it was designed to provide a means of investigating and analysing the complex process of developing nursing practice in a busy hospital setting. It addressed fundamental questions about the problems of managing and leading a modern hospital nursing service. It resulted in a detailed, theorized account of the nature of patient-centred nursing and captured the ways in which this kind of care was experienced by patients, relatives and staff.

The project findings should be helpful to practising nurses in most hospital specialties. They will also be relevant to policy-makers, purchasers, managers and educators who are responsible for supporting the development and delivery of high quality health care.

THE STRUCTURE OF THE BOOK

The book is based upon an earlier, full report of the project (Binnie and Titchen, 1998). It is structured in three parts. The first part sets the scene for the research and places the practice development work in context, both locally and nationally. Chapter 1 includes an analysis of the history of practice development and some of the associated research issues. It should be helpful to those who are understandably confused by the various 'bandwagons' that have excited clinical nurses in recent years. A discussion of the philosophical and methodological issues that informed the work is presented in Chapter 2, and the way in which the research was conducted is described in Chapter 3.

The second and most substantial part of the book (Chapters 4–8) provides an account of the development of nursing in one busy medical ward, over a three year period. Each chapter presents a different aspect of the practice development 'journey', against which other nurses should be able to 'map' their own efforts to develop a patient-centred style of practice. The analysis of data from the early days of the project should enable nurses to identify, in their own clinical settings, what may remain of dysfunctional traditional values, attitudes and practices. Similarly, those who are trying to introduce change are likely to recognize many of the difficulties encountered in the project ward as comparable with their own. At a practical level, the change strategies found to be effective during the project may work for others, helping them out of blind alleys or to avoid some obstacles altogether. Data reported from the latter stages of the project provide a detailed picture of a patient-centred style of nursing and of the ward life that supported it. For those who have little experience of this kind of practice, it offers a vision of what can be achieved for both patients and nurses, as a result of sustained investment and commitment at ward level.

The final part – Chapter 9 – provides a broad overview of the practice development process, which may be helpful to those who, from a distance, find it difficult to understand why new ideas about ward practice have so often been taken up only slowly, hesitantly and with limited success, in spite of their promise and in spite of encouragement from official bodies and professional leaders. The concluding chapter also draws together the common themes that emerged from the study and highlights the lessons that were learned. It includes a number of principles for practice development, which will hopefully serve as a useful guide for nurses wishing to make their practice more patient-centred.

Finally, a comment about the writing style. We were both very much involved in the project, as participants as well as researchers, and so, as is common in action research, we have reported our work in the first person.

Chapter 1

Background issues

The task of providing a twenty-four hour nursing service for patients presents hospital nurses with a major organizational challenge. Over the years, the various approaches to the problem, and the solutions that have been found, have inevitably reflected the aims and values of nursing at the time and of the contemporary society in general.

Currently in vogue in the UK is an organizational system known as primary nursing. It was developed in the USA in the 1960s, as a response to both the frustrations that were being experienced with the existing method of work organization and the growing demands, both within and outside the profession, for a more humane and personalized service (Manthey, 1980). Different views have been expressed in the literature about whether primary nursing is purely a work organization method, or whether it is a broader concept also embracing a philosophy of care. Essentially, however, primary nursing is designed to free staff nurses who provide bedside care for patients from the tight constraints that characterized the traditional, bureaucratically managed service. Instead, it offers them a professional structure in which they are given personal responsibility for managing the nursing of their own patients.

In the UK, in the early 1970s, it became evident that the established nursing system was failing to meet the demands of the modern health service and to satisfy new recruits to the profession. Since then, nurse management structures have been reorganized several times and new legislation has led to a massive programme of educational reform. Change in the practice sphere has been less dramatic, more cautious and more uncertain. Yet it is in this arena that reform is arguably most urgent, for practice is the front-line – both the reason for the profession's existence and the product by which it is judged.

Over the last couple of decades, attempts have been made to clarify the aims of modern practice. According to a Royal College of Nursing document on standards of care,

'The nursing care of each patient should be individually planned, the plan being based on an assessment of individual needs.' (RCN, 1981, p. 9)

This statement about 'good nursing' is a relatively early example of an explicit commitment to the ideal of a personalized service for patients. Nowadays, a glance at virtually any nursing philosophy statement, quality programme or nursing curriculum will reveal a familiar rhetoric expressing a firm belief that the focus of the practising nurse's work should be the personal concerns, wishes and needs of the individual patient. The emergence of this personal, or 'patient-centred', philosophy, underpinning most recent developments in nursing theory, policy and practice, can be seen, essentially, as mirroring the respect for the individual that is valued, if not always achieved, by present-day society.

Failure to translate the widely accepted patient-centred philosophy into practical reality is still common in British hospitals. An Audit Commission survey, for example, found that *'a third of respondents who had been in hospital in the previous 12 months complained about the rigid timetable of the ward, being woken early and . . . one in five said the nurses had been "too busy to attend to their individual needs"* (Audit Commission, 1992). Furthermore, the same publication reported that, *'On the majority of wards in the . . . sample, the methods used to organise care prevent nurses from giving continuous, personalised care to patients'* (p. 15). This picture persists despite the efforts of many nurse leaders to encourage change and despite the publication of an enormous amount of promotional material in the popular nursing press.

In the late 1970s and early 1980s, there was a major campaign to introduce the nursing process into everyday ward life. The nursing process is not a method of work allocation, but a way of making decisions about how patients are nursed. By guiding practising nurses through a logical problem-solving cycle, it is designed to equip them to approach each patient's problems afresh and to create a plan of nursing care tailor-made for the individual. Each element of the plan is written down, so that it is communicated to all the nurses involved in a patient's care. The arrival of the nursing process, another import from the USA, was probably more influential than anything else in raising ward nurses' awareness of the limitations of their existing system and in popularizing the patient-centred philosophy. Its success in actually changing practice, however, was nowhere near as great as was hoped (de la Cuesta, 1983). It appears that the key to its disappointing performance, as a catalyst for practice change, was the failure to link it with a complementary change in work organization. Asking individual nurses to draw up personalized care plans for patients, in traditionally organized wards where individual nurses had no formal authority to instruct others to follow their plans, seems, in retrospect, like a recipe for inevitable failure. Carried along on the tide of enthusiasm generated by a good idea, it seems that few nurses involved in the nursing process movement stopped to examine critically its implications for other aspects of practice life.

The more recent primary nursing movement threatens, possibly, to be heading along a similar path. On the positive side, it can be regarded as the long-overdue organizational reform that could bring the nursing process to life. Primary nurses, with real authority to manage their patients' nursing, could use the nursing process, in the thoughtful, creative way that was intended, to plan truly individualized care. In this way, as many authors have suggested, quality of care *could* be improved and nurses' job satisfaction *could* be increased. However, research studies carried out over the last twenty years have failed to demonstrate conclusively whether or how primary nursing affects these and a range of other variables.

Taking a more cautious view, on the other hand, it has to be acknowledged that introducing primary nursing into British hospitals, where the legacy of traditional practice is still a powerful influence, implies a radical shake-up of the whole system. At the heart of the change is a major decentralization of decision-making (Manthey, 1980). Staff nurses becoming primary nurses leave behind the safety of ward routines, the sister's rules and standardized procedures and are expected to act as adult professionals, thinking issues through for themselves, weighing options and making decisions with patients that may be complex and even risky. If this transition is to be handled safely and effectively, it is obvious that nurses must be properly prepared for their new roles, that managers, from sisters upwards, must adopt a wholly new stance and style to support more independent practitioners, and that relationships with other disciplines, particularly medicine, must be reconsidered and renegotiated. These are big changes; introducing primary nursing is not simply a matter of attaching nurses' names to groups of patients and then carrying on in much the same way as before.

While primary nursing is logically an attractive option for those who see personalizing care as a key element in improving quality, it cannot be regarded as an easy option. One might even question whether it is a responsible option, unless there is investment in making it work and substantial change in the wider hospital organization to accommodate it. Given the scale of change that a serious introduction of primary nursing would involve for many hospitals at the present time, it would be reasonable to explore the possibility of any other work organization system that might allow nurses more personal contact with their patients; one that might help them to develop the skills of professional work without at once rushing them into a system they are not ready to handle.

A type of team nursing has emerged in many British hospital wards as just such a compromise. It is arguably the most appropriate step for many wards in this country and yet it seems to be developing almost unnoticed. It is quite different from American team nursing and being a British product, rather than an American import, may in itself be something to commend it. Nothing substantial appears to have been published on the subject since 1985 (Waters, 1985) and there is no team nursing bandwagon. Yet, quietly it seems, this is what many practitioners are opting for: 49 per cent of the Audit Commission's (1992) sample described their method of work allocation as team nursing and 71 per cent of ward sisters questioned in another study claimed to be using some aspects of team nursing (Thomas and Bond, 1990). It is clear, however, from both these studies and contact with many practising nurses around the country, that interpretations of the term 'team nursing' vary considerably.

The question of how best to organize a twenty-four hour nursing service in a modern British hospital is, thus, not easily resolved. The traditional system is recognized as incompatible with contemporary demands for a personal service, but its heritage is deeply rooted in hospital culture and is not easy to leave behind. Primary nursing appears, on the surface, to be the obvious answer, but there is confusion in the literature about what it is and whether it is effective and, in the real world, practitioners have been slow to adopt it. Team nursing seems to be a more popular alternative among ward nurses, but there is even greater confusion about what this system is and what values it embodies, and research exploring the way it works in this country is non-existent. The purpose of the research which forms the basis of this book has been to illuminate some of the detail of this rather muddled picture and, thereby, to contribute some clarity to the debate about why and how to change the organization and practice of ward nursing.

To provide a general background to the study, the rest of this chapter addresses, in more detail, the nursing practice issues in question and the research issues that lie behind the choice of methodology.

PRACTICE ISSUES

The question that ought logically to precede any discussion about *how* to organize a twenty-four hour nursing service is: what *kind* of nursing service is required? In other words, what values should the service aim to reflect in its practice; where should its attention be particularly focussed; and what characteristics will distinguish the style of nursing that is practised? Only when it is clear what end-product and what processes are required, can a judgement be made about the appropriate means of achieving them.

The literature of the last couple of decades presents an array of new ideas about the delivery of hospital nursing and a variety of new terms describing new approaches to practice. While any one of these may be fairly easily explored in some depth, how or whether they all relate to each other, and what implications they have for the management of the service as a whole, are much harder to discern.

Three distinct *styles* of practice can be identified from the literature, that is, three general approaches to practice that reflect different values and different philosophical and social influences. These styles of practice, which we have labelled *traditional nursing*, *individualized nursing* and *patient-centred nursing*, can be regarded as three ideal end-products towards which the service has aimed during different periods in its recent history. Commitment within a service to any one particular style of practice will influence how its nurses define nursing work and will determine the focus of their practice. In turn, the way that nurses perceive their work inclines them to adopt a particular method of work organization, i.e. one likely to help them to deal with what they focus upon in their daily work and to achieve the style of practice to which they are committed.

Where there is a comfortable match, a congruence within the service, between style, focus and organizational method, then it is likely that the service will run fairly smoothly towards achieving its aims. Where there is a mismatch, however, there is likely to be tension and confusion. Perhaps a service aspires to new ideals, but its practitioners have not fully intern!lized them and the focus of their daily work and its organization remain unchanged. Alternatively, a new organizational method may be foisted upon practitioners whose beliefs, commitment and focus have not moved.

The three styles of practice are explored briefly below, with particular attention being paid to issues that are contentious or unclear.

Traditional nursing

The term 'traditional practice' is used to describe a style of nursing that had become widespread and well rooted in British hospitals by the middle of this century. It describes the established order that, in recent years, has been increasingly challenged by new ideas, coming often from the other side of the Atlantic. However, it represents the style of practice in which many nurses at work today trained and its influence is still very much alive in many hospital wards.

Traditional practice was itself the product of two distinct, and in some respects conflicting, nursing traditions which can be represented by the two figures most influential in shaping modern hospital nursing, Florence Nightingale and Mrs Bedford-Fenwick. For Nightingale, nursing was a vocation, literally a calling to the service of God. Christian devotion to the care of the sick was a tradition formerly carried out by religious orders and Nightingale's great achievement was to bring this Christian tradition into the secular hospital world and, thus, to create the foundations for nursing as a respectable occupation for lay women. Mrs Bedford-Fenwick valued the good influence of Christian principles in hospital wards, but her strongest motive was to establish nursing as a self-regulating profession. Nightingale opposed Bedford-Fenwick's campaign for registration because she believed that the primary importance it gave to educational qualifications, and the emphasis it placed upon recognition and status, undermined the essence of nursing as a Christian vocation.

Bradshaw (1994) criticized contemporary nursing historians for neglecting the fundamentally important influence that Nightingale's spiritual motivation had on establishing the caring tradition of modern nursing. In addition, she suggested that the holistic focus of the Christian approach to caring and healing, as promoted by Nightingale, has been largely overlooked. Modern historians (such as Davies, 1980; Baly, 1980; Dingwall *et al.*, 1988) have been more inclined to highlight the battle for registration and formal professional status, presenting it as a struggle to free nurses from an oppressive religious ideology that kept women in subservient, self-effacing roles. A balanced reading of both perspectives might suggest that, in fact, there was a light and a dark side to both the vocational and the professionalizing traditions and that the style of practice that became established by the middle of this century was a product of each accommodating the other, in the various aspects of nursing life, with varying degrees of success.

Thus, the two traditions can be seen as leaving both helpful and handicapping legacies. From Miss Nightingale, nursing inherited its commitment to humane, holistic caring – an ethos that has continued to inspire and motivate individual nurses throughout this century. But it carried with it the discipline, obedience and self-denial of the religious life which, when translated into the secular world, inhibited the development of a strong, assertive, professional practice, with its own distinct identity. Mrs Bedford-Fenwick's campaign resulted in British nurses being the first in the world to achieve legal professional status and it established a professional structure with a level of independence, in areas such as educational control and conduct and disciplinary matters, which is still the envy of nurses in many other countries. However, Mrs Bedford-Fenwick shifted the focus of nursing away from the spiritual and towards the scientific and, as 'scientific' in hospitals at that time referred to medical science, nursing education became focussed more upon disease and treatment than upon care of the suffering person.

The style of nursing that emerged under these influences emphasized the service of medicine as a means of helping patients and was essentially concerned with the dutiful completion of a hierarchy of practical tasks. The adoption from industry of the production-line model of work organization was therefore a logical move. By allocating different nursing tasks to different nurses according to grade, the system ensured that key tasks were performed, by appropriately skilled nurses, in the shortest possible time. The system was undoubtedly reliable and efficient and it allowed for tight central control of a largely unskilled workforce. But its rigid timetabling and narrow focus limited the scope of nursing, so that nurses came to see their work in terms of doing 'the washes', 'the temperatures', 'the medicines' etc. and, when these tasks were completed, 'the work' was done. The fact that the system also severely limited opportunities for nurses and patients to talk at any length to each other, simply reinforced the scientific medical view, at that time, that personal involvement with patients was unhealthy and unprofessional.

Menzies' (1970) classic study of hospital nursing, carried out in the late 1950s, provides a vivid and insightful picture of the traditional style of practice. She described the system as functioning as an organizational defence against stress and anxiety. The task-focussed work patterns protected nurses from close contact with their patients' distress and suffering and the depersonalization and categorization of both staff and patients kept relationships formal and unemotional (nurses were identified by grade and uniform, and patients by disease or bed number). The system also protected nurses from the stresses associated with responsibility and decision-making, for the number of decisions to be made by an individual nurse was minimized by the strict routines and standard procedures governing almost every aspect of nursing work. Personal responsibility was avoided by checking and counter-checking or by passing responsibility up through the nursing hierarchy to senior, 'more responsible' figures.

Menzies noted that, in spite of the protectiveness of the system, stress was far from absent among the nurses working within it. She observed that, while nurses were shielded from much immediate stress, this was at the expense of challenges and experiences which would, in the longer term, help them develop a greater capacity to handle the stresses of responsibility and involvement. Menzies concluded that the traditional system was dysfunctional for both patients and nurses, in that it denied patients the comfort and support of sustained, caring relationships and nurses the satisfaction of seeing patients progress in a way they could easily connect with their own efforts. She added,

'The poignancy of the situation is increased by the expressed aims of nursing at the present time, i.e. to nurse the whole patient as a person. The nurse is instructed to do that, it is usually what she wants to do, but the functioning of the nursing service makes it impossible.' (p. 31)

Menzies recognized that there were no simple solutions to the problems of the nursing service and that any change would take time to achieve. She suggested that,

'The ultimate solution must be a restructuring of the system of work organization and nurse-training. . .For example, one might try systems of ward organization which give nurses more continuous and intensive contact with patients; this would require new techniques for dealing with the stress that would arise initially.' (Menzies, 1960, p. 16)

She saw the most hopeful approach to such far-reaching change as being through the building, refining and dissemination of a 'working model'.

Menzies presented this challenge to the nursing profession over thirty years ago. Since then, some working models of a more personal style of practice have emerged in the UK, most notably those from Burford and Beeson (Pearson, 1988) and Tameside (Wright, 1990), with accounts of how other centres have taken up or developed the ideas appearing in the popular nursing press. However, in spite of this encouragement, the pace of change as a whole has been very slow. As the Audit Commission (1992) noted,

> *'The methods of allocation practised on the majority of wards prevent the development of stable patient–nurse relationships. Patients often do not know which nurse is looking after them. The feeling that all the nurses are in some sense responsible creates uncertainty in their minds about which nurse to approach about serious worries or concerns.'* (p. 16)

The less desirable aspects of the traditional style of practice and its impersonal, task-focussed, method of work organization are still influential in many hospital wards. Reform of practice and a reformulation of the caring ethos of nursing, in some form appropriate for our modern world, seem long overdue.

Individualized nursing

The style of practice we have called individualized nursing had its roots in the American nurses' struggle for professional status. It began to emerge in the 1950s as a result of two parallel developments – the rapid growth of academic nursing and deepening dissatisfaction with the existing 'functional', or task-focussed, pattern of care.

A major concern of the professional movement was to make university education available to nurses and to begin to establish nursing as a credible scientific discipline in its own right, distinct from medicine (Glaser, 1966). Nursing initially gained access to American universities through departments of education and it entered the academic world at a time when American education generally was profoundly influenced by the pragmatist philosophy of John Dewey (Morgenbesser, 1987). Early pioneers of nursing higher education and research in American universities, most notably Annie Goodrich, reflected the pragmatists' optimistic faith in science and Dewey's instrumental view of knowledge as a tool for solving practical problems. The pragmatist concern, to counter the mechanical approach of traditional objective science with an appreciation of subjective human experience, was also attractive to nurses who were beginning to recognize the dehumanizing effects of the hospital system.

During the 1950s and 1960s, American nursing research in the universities began to flourish. In contrast, the practice arena was bedevilled by manpower shortages and a dilution of the trained workforce, which both undermined the quality of care and confused and threatened the process of professionalizing nursing practice (Strauss, 1966). There was an urgent need to clarify the role of the professional nurse and to address the problems of a style of hospital practice which was increasingly being recognized as failing to satisfy both patients and nurses (Brown, 1966). Nurse leaders, responding to this challenge, tried to define the essence of nursing in terms that sounded modern and professional. New models or theories of nursing were developed which, in an attempt to move away from a purely medical model, drew upon other disciplines. Keen to present the concern of nursing as working with patients as individual people, much of the new theory started from a holistic standpoint and incorporated ideas from human relations psychology. However, deeply anxious to be scientifically credible, many of the theorists produced models that were essentially based on approaches, such as systems theory or developmental theory, which belong firmly in the realm of conventional science. The mixed motives driving the new breed of nurse theorists may, at least in part, explain why so much of their work lacks internal consistency and why, as a consequence, it has been so difficult to apply in practice (Webb, 1986; Bradshaw, 1994).

An important feature of the early theorists' work was the notion that nursing practice is a dynamic process rather than a fixed set of procedures, and that the nursing problems of individual patients require individualized solutions. The steps of this 'nursing process' were defined by Yura and Walsh, in 1967, as those of the formal problem-solving described in the education literature of the pragmatist era. The presentation of practical nursing as a process akin to the process of research had a scientific ring to it that was immediately attractive in the contemporary climate (Henderson, 1982). The idea of creating an individualized plan of care was initially developed as an educational tool to help nursing students to think systematically about their work, but soon its translation into practice, though ultimately quite problematic (Shea, 1984), was promoted with great zeal.

The desire to individualize patient care and the new focus on producing a personal, written care plan for each patient inevitably influenced the way nurses organized their work. However, the path American nurses took, as they moved away from task allocation, was also influenced by the severe shortages of registered nurses in the 1950s and the large numbers of practical nurses and aides employed in hospitals as a result. A system of team nursing was developed which spread rapidly through the country. Under the task system, nurses were allocated their work from a central point and worked mostly alone. The idea of team nursing was to group two or three nurses, with a registered nurse team leader, and to give them responsibility for planning and delivering the care of a specific group of patients. The team leader was expected to assess the individual needs of patients, allocate work to her team members, according to ability, and then be available herself to supervise the team and to undertake more highly skilled work. Team nursing became very popular, probably because it provided a way of supervising the work of less skilled staff, but, in other respects, its interpretation in practice was a disappointment to those who originally promoted the system (Brown, 1966; Kron, 1987). The registered nurse's role became increasingly supervisory and technical. Within the teams, work was still allocated on a task basis, only now for a smaller group of patients, and care plans, designed to individualize care, became yet another task completed in a routine manner. The ideal of genuinely individualized care was still a long way off.

University education for nurses was established much later in Britain and research casting a critical eye at the actual practice of nursing did not begin to appear until the early 1970s (see the RCN Study of Nursing Care Series, e.g. Lelean, 1973; Wright, 1974; Jones, 1975). This research brought into sharp focus the fundamental problem with the traditional system, namely, that if a particular patient needed care that did not exactly match what was on offer from the routine task rounds, it was often omitted. Nobody was seen as responsible for care outside the prescribed routine and the system was not flexible enough to accommodate it. In addition, individual nurses did not have authority to adapt standard protocols to the differing needs of individual patients. The outcome of this rigid system, as the research demonstrated, was not just omission of the fine niceties of care; it could amount to totally inappropriate, or even dangerous, practice.

Exposure of this problem opened up the debate, still not properly resolved, about how nurses working with large groups of patients, within the constraints of an institutional setting, could best address the particular needs of each individual without compromising the efficiency of the whole. Academics and policy-makers turned to the apparently more advanced nurses in America for solutions. The nursing process, promising a practical way of individualizing patient care, was adopted enthusiastically and uncritically and, within only four years, was firmly embedded in the training syllabus for general nurses (GNC, 1977). Hospitals were put under great pressure to introduce the nursing process and, consequently, its implementation was, on the whole, top-down, rushed and inadequately supported by in-service education. Emphasis was placed more upon producing the visible, written care plan than on changing the way patients were nursed. The high-profile campaign to promote the nursing process did much to raise awareness amongst ordinary nurses of the shortcomings of the traditional system and it seems to have established the notion of individualized care as an ideal that modern nursing should aspire to. However, as in North America, the success of care planning in practice was very limited indeed (de la Cuesta, 1983).

Nursing models were imported from the USA as well, but it has been mostly educationalists who have promoted them. Their reception in practice has been lukewarm. The most widely used model in Britain is the Roper, Logan and Tierney (1980) development of earlier American work (Henderson, 1966). It has provided many practising nurses with an accessible and useful framework for gathering information about their patients which is a step away from the traditional medical model, but it falls a long way short of its holistic intentions. Its 'activities of living' structure encourages a compartmentalized view of the person and reinforces the traditional bias towards physical aspects of caring. Few practising nurses use a model for anything more than its assessment framework and it is not too difficult to bolt on an 'activities of living' framework to what is, essentially, a fairly traditional style of practice.

Changes in methods of work organization in British nursing have not mirrored the American experience quite so closely, perhaps because of differences in the labour market and the British tradition of relying heavily upon a student workforce. However, developments have followed a broadly similar pattern. Patient allocation (i.e. each individual nurse being responsible for the total care of a specific group of patients, for the duration of a shift) was promoted as the organizational method that should replace task allocation (Pembrey, 1975; Berry and Metcalf, 1986). But this system, though different in theory from American team nursing, became in practice very like it.

Pembrey's (1980) study made an important early contribution to the work organization debate. It highlighted the principle that individualized care depends upon individual nurses being allocated personal responsibility for the nursing care of specific patients. Pembrey considered it to be the ward sister's responsibility to assess the particular needs of each patient, to prescribe appropriate nursing care, to delegate the total care of each patient to an individual nurse and then, in due course, to receive feedback on the effectiveness of the care by calling each nurse to account for her work. Of the fifty ward sisters that Pembrey observed, only nine were seen to complete this cycle of management activities associated with patient allocation and required to achieve individualized nursing.

Patient allocation was being discussed in the UK, as an alternative to task allocation, as early as the mid-1950s (RCN, 1956; Jenkinson, 1958) and, later, the Briggs Report recommended a more 'patient-orientated' form of ward organization to counter the tendency, inherent in the task system, to *reduce the patients to a series of functions*'(DHSS, 1972, p. 122). However, it was not until the nursing process was being promoted that the idea of patient allocation really became popular (Norton, 1981), though, as Pembrey's study suggests, it was rarely practised in the pure form demonstrated by her nine successful ward sisters. More commonly, a ward was divided geographically in half and two or three nurses shared the care of the patients in each half of the ward, often still organizing their work in terms of tasks. It is here that the boundaries between what was called patient allocation in Britain and team nursing in North America become blurred. In practice, whatever the intention, the common interpretation of both systems involved the allocation of a small group of nurses to a relatively large group of patients, for the duration of a shift. The most senior nurse in the group, formally or informally, acted as team leader, supervising the others and allocating the work between them, usually on a task basis and following, perhaps a little more loosely than in the past, an established ward routine. A sister/head nurse, or deputy, remained in overall charge of the shift, taking responsibility for major decisions, co-ordinating ward activity as a whole and channelling communications between individual nurses and members of other disciplines visiting the wards.

The shift to the American style of team nursing or to patient allocation, in however modified a form, reduced the number of patients nurses had to relate to each day and allowed them a little more flexibility in the organization of care. Thus, more personal contact was possible and there was more space to accommodate individual needs. Nonetheless, the system still limited opportunities to develop caring relationships and to deliver truly individualized care. The allocation of a nurse, or group of nurses, to a specific group of patients was only *for the duration of a shift*. On their next shift, the nurses might be working with a different group of patients. In many wards, an attempt was made to encourage continuity by allocating nurses to the same patients for several consecutive shifts, but duty rotas were not designed with this continu)ty in mind, so nurses could never be sure whether they would personally be able to follow up tomorrow what they had begun today. The absence of *predictable* continuity inevitably inhibits the development of depth and closeness in caring relationships. It is often clearly inappropriate to become intimately involved with a patient's problems and to begin offering emotional support, if it is likely that the next day the nurse may be working with other patients and only able to offer a passing greeting. An underlying assumption is maintained that it is what nurses do that matters, not who they are, and therefore nurses of equivalent grade and ability are interchangeable and continuity of a personal relationship is unimportant.

In the traditional, task-orientated system, a degree of continuity and predictability was maintained for patients by the rigidity of ward routines and the standardization of nursing procedures. Patients knew what to expect because everything was always done the same way. It was anticipated, with individualized nursing, that continuity and predictability would be maintained through the care plan. However, the good intentions, both to individualize care and to maintain continuity, were frequently undermined because the work organization system failed to allocate individual nurses authority for planning and managing a patient's nursing beyond the duration of one shift.

Many of the problems nurses deal with cannot be solved in the space of an eight hour shift. Managing a wound, teaching a new diabetic how to manage insulin therapy, or helping an amputee to adjust to his loss and rehabilitate, are obvious examples of nursing work that needs to be planned and co-ordinated over a much longer time span. In this kind of work, there is potential for considerable creativity, with the nurse working alongside the patient to develop helping strategies uniquely designed to meet his particular situation. But being creative, to achieve what is best for a particular patient, may mean being unconventional and perhaps taking risks. To embark upon such a plan, a nurse needs the authority to see it through, to monitor it, modify it and take responsibility for its outcome. The work organization methods described so far do not give individual nurses, other than the ward sister, this kind of authority. When one nurse goes off duty, another takes her place with equal authority to make or change decisions about how a patient is nursed during the next shift. With no authority to instruct other nurses beyond their own shift and no guarantee that others will not change what they prescribe, the incentive for nurses to be creative is low and the risk high. It is easier and safer to prescribe standard care that others are unlikely to challenge or misinterpret. Thus, as a result of the nurses' limited authority, patients are denied the highly individualized care the system intended them to have and they can never be sure when, or by whom, their care will be changed.

In the literature, the term individualized care is often used interchangeably with patient-centred care (Abdellah *et al.*, 1960; Levine, 1991). Indeed, it was the intention of individualized nursing to place the needs of each patient, rather than a series of practical tasks, at the centre of nurses' attention. However, we have chosen to make a distinction between the terms. We have used 'individualized nursing' to refer to the style of care that represents a first attempt to establish nursing practice as independent of medicine, depicted in its own theoretical models and achieved through its own special process. But we have suggested that, because its methods of work organization limit the development of relationships and stifle creativity, this style of practice has never become truly patient-centred.

Patient-centred nursing

Patient-centred nursing is a style of practice that demonstrates a respect for the patient as a person. The acknowledgement and valuing of each patient's own way of perceiving and experiencing what is happening to him are fundamental to this way of nursing. Its aim is to transform patients' experiences of illness, taking them, for example, from pain to comfort, from fear to confidence, from distress to coping, from loss to adjustment. This kind of nursing is a therapy in its own right; indeed, some authors have called it 'therapeutic nursing' (McMahon and Pearson, 1991). The role of the patient-centred nurse is *to be there*, offering personal support and practical expertise, but letting patients follow the path of their own choosing, in their own way. This style of nursing reflects the influence of existentialist philosophy and the humanistic psychology that grew from it. It is also in tune with the individualism of modern society.

Existentialism embraces the ideas of a rather disparate group of philosophers, including Kierkegaard and Nietzche and, later, Husserl, Heidegger and Sartre. The common focus of their work was the analysis of the nature of human existence, which they saw as a process of becoming, rather than a fixed state of being. In other words, they rejected the determinism of earlier Western thinking which portrayed man as merely a product of heredity, environmental factors and childhood experiences (Graham, 1986). Existentialists emphasized people's ability to rise above these influences, to transcend mundane reality and to realize their true human potential. They were interested, above all, in human freedom and concerned to show people that they were free to choose '*not only what to do on a specific occasion, but what to value and how to live*' (Warnock, 1970, p. 2).

The term 'humanistic psychology' was first used in 1958 by John Cohen, a British psychologist who fiercely opposed the approach of the '*ratomorphic robotic psychology*' of the past (Graham, 1986, p. 66). It subsequently became highly influential, in many spheres, through the work of American psychologists, notably Carl Rogers, Abraham Maslow and Rollo May. In the European existentialism, these psychologists found a philosophical basis for the scientific study of human behaviour that accommodated subjective experience and acknowledged the uniqueness and unpredictability of each human being. The American interpretation of existentialism reflects a more optimistic view of human nature and the human condition than does the European original, but it shares the same concern with everyday human experience and the possibility of free choice and personal growth. Perhaps the most influential therapeutic application of this psychology has been that of Carl Rogers. He believed in the individual's inherent capacity and tendency for psychological growth.

'*It is the urge which is evident in all organic and human life – to expand, extend, become autonomous, develop, mature. . .This tendency may become deeply buried under layer after layer of encrusted psychological defences; it may be hidden behind elaborate facades which deny its existence; but it is my belief that it exists in every individual, and awaits only the proper conditions to be released and expressed.*' (Rogers, 1967, p. 35)

The aim of Rogers' psychotherapy is to provide a relationship for the client in which the proper conditions for promoting psychological growth are present. The key characteristics of this 'helping relationship' are an openness and genuineness on the part of the therapist, a valuing of the client as a person, regardless of how he presents himself, and an empathetic understanding of the client's world, an attempt to see it through his eyes. This kind of relationship can provide the client with the security and confidence he needs to examine his perceptions of himself and his world and to reorganize them in a healthier way. As Rogers put it,

'*When these conditions are achieved, I become a companion to my client, accompanying him in the frightening search for himself, which he now feels free to undertake.*' (Rogers, 1967, p. 33)

It is significant that in this psychotherapy, and the style of counselling modelled upon it, the therapist does not set him or herself up as an expert who offers solutions for the client, but rather uses his expertise to enable the client to find his own solutions. This stance reflects the existentialist commitment to freedom, choice, personal responsibility and psychological growth.

Nurse theorists influenced by existentialism and humanistic psychology have emphasized the importance of addressing the patient's personal experience and describe the therapeutic potential of the nurse–patient relationship (e.g. Travelbee, 1971; Paterson and Zderad, 1976; Watson, 1985). Instead of nurses doing things to or for patients, the emphasis shifts to nurses becoming involved with patients to help them deal with what they are facing. The patient's status changes from passive recipient, or object, of nursing care to active partner engaged in improving his own situation.

It is the presence of the therapeutic nurse–patient relationship that lies at the heart of a patient-centred style of nursing. With this kind of practice, a nurse's starting point for caring is making real human contact with patients and addressing their perceptions and concerns. It means avoiding over-hasty categorization of patients and avoiding assumptions about what they are experiencing. It means, instead, being ready to listen and watch with an open mind and attending to issues that patients present as readily as to those that arise from their medical problems. By working *with* patients, and making a commitment to see problems through with them, nurses can fine-tune the practical and emotional support they offer.

The emphasis on relationship in patient-centred nursing transforms how nurses perceive practical bedside care. Building and sustaining a relationship means spending time with the other person and sharing experiences. Practical nursing affords a unique opportunity of often very intimate time together and the sharing of very personal difficulties and successes. In skilled hands, the opportunities presented by everyday bedside caring become the medium through which a patient's experience of illness can be transformed; they b%come a medium for promoting personal growth and healing. Patient-centred nurses, recognizing their unusually privileged access to patients and the potential it offers, do not regard practical caring as menial work and are not in a hurry to give it away to untrained or junior personnel.

The aims of individualized nursing to be systematic and scientific are not abandoned by patient-centred nurses. Problem-solving, through individualized assessment and care planning, is still part of their repertoire and has its place, but its importance is diminished. It becomes just one strategy for delivering therapeutic nursing. For a patient-centred nurse, scientific methods are the servants of a healing art which involves, most importantly, being emotionally and physically present with patients in their suffering and accompanying them as a 'skilled companion' on their journey through an illness (Campbell, 1984).

Making patients' personal experiences of health and illness the main focus of their work helps nurses to clarify the distinct nature of their contribution to health care and, in particular, to clarify the ways in which nursing is different from, but complementary to, medicine (Benner and Wrubel, 1989). Patient-centred nurses will still make observations, collect specimens and administer drugs to help doctors in their main task of diagnosing and treating disease, but this forms only a small and relatively simple part of nursing work. With this style of practice, the nurse's major concern is understanding what disease means for patients and helping them and their families to cope with its consequences. The patient-centred nurse offers practical skill and a trained presence to help patients face what is happening to them and to move forward in their own way, adjusting to loss or disability, regaining strength and independence, or accepting death. This work can be complex and demanding. It requires intelligence, creativity and patient, sensitive attention to detail. For the nurse, it can be immensely rewarding. For the patient, it can make the difference between being sent home as a mended body or a healed person.

Achieving a patient-centred style of nursing consistently in a hospital ward is dependent not only upon the presence of skilled and committed nurses, but also upon having an organizational system that does not interrupt their relationships with patients any more than is absolutely necessary. In some UK hospitals during the last decade, a form of team nursing has been developing which offers nurses the continuity they need to make and sustain close relationships with their patients. This form of team nursing is different from the classic American team nursing and the British patient allocation described earlier. It appears not to be described or examined in any detail in the literature, but there are many nurses who use it in practice.

With this kind of team nursing, each team, made up of perhaps five or six nurses, is responsible for the care of a small group of patients *throughout their time in the ward.* The duty rota for each team of nurses is organized to ensure that there is always at least one member of the team on duty every shift. That nurse provides the total nursing care for his or her patients whilst on duty and knows that, when next on duty, he or she will work with the same patients. Patients know that they will only be cared for by the small number of team nurses and they can be told who will be looking after them when. The small caseload size and the predictable continuity built into this system make the development of close, stable relationships a possibility. However, it appears that responsibility for clinical decision-making remains much as it was with patient allocation, changing from shift to shift, though now from one team nurse to the next. The scope for individual nurses to initiate highly personalized strategies of care in response to the insights they gain through continuing relationships with their patients is, therefore, still likely to be limited.

The method of work organization that offers both predictable continuity of care and continuing personal authority for clinical decision-making is primary nursing. There is a considerable amount of literature on primary nursing, most of it either describing the concept and its aims or reporting experiences of introducing it in practice. Within this material, definitions of primary nursing vary, ranging, as one reviewer put it, '*from the sphere of organizational systems to philosophies of care and on into the realms of Utopia*' (Macdonald, 1988). Whilst sympathetic towards the view of writers, such as Hegevary (1982), who have broadened the definition of primary nursing to encompass a philosophy of care, we have chosen to use the term, like Manthey (1980) the acknowledged founder of primary nursing, in a purely organizational sense. It is true that primary nursing as an organizational system is most appropriately, and probably most effectively, employed where nurses share '*a view of nursing as professional patient-centred practice*' (Hegevary, 1982). However, it cannot be assumed that because certain organizational features exist in a nursing service, a particular philosophical commitment is also present. Linking organization and philosophy in the one definition risks encouraging that assumption. It is more helpful to recognize clearly both the value and the limitations of an organizational system and, then, to focus separately upon the beliefs, attitudes, abilities and behaviours of nurses, which will ultimately determine the impact the system has on patient care (Shukla, 1981).

Primary nursing, as an organizational system, was designed specifically to promote patient-centred practice and to counter the problems arising from fragmented care, complex communication channels and shared responsibility which beleaguered the American hospital nursing system during the 1950s

(Manthey, 1980). The system simply involves devolving responsibility for the total nursing management of a small group of patients to an individual staff nurse. As primary nurses, staff nurses provide most of their patients' nursing care whenever they are on duty and leave clear directions for other nurses in their absence. The system makes it possible for nurses to work closely and continuously with a small number of patients, throughout their hospital stay, and it clarifies for the patients precisely who is in charge of their nursing. No other method of organizing hospital nursing allows the individual nurse this amount of freedom to practise as a professional.

The major structural change that occurs when primary nursing is introduced to a ward is a clear, formal devolution of authority for clinical nursing decision-making. Authority to make decisions about a patient's nursing is no longer vested centrally in the sister or nurse in charge of the shift, nor shared vaguely between team members but, instead, rests squarely with the individual primary nurse. Whilst in itself clear-cut and simple, this one structural change, if it is taken seriously, has far-reaching implications. It shakes the foundations of traditional practice and demands review and often fundamental change of every aspect of ward life.

Primary nurses are not bound by the rules and routines of traditional practice. They are free to decide, with their own patients, how best the individuals should be nursed. This freedom may be liberating for nurses, but it also carries a heavy burden of responsibility (Johns, 1990; Goulding and Hunt, 1991). Abandoning safe routines means having to think for yourself, weigh up options, make choices and then justify to others the decision you have made. Practice life becomes more challenging, but also more uncertain, more risky and more emotionally demanding (Dewing, 1991). This is the price to be paid for a patient-centred nursing service.

The literature is clear that getting results from a primary nursing system, that is, seeing a patient-centred service emerge, depends to a great extent upon the style and quality of management, both in the ward and in the hospital as a whole (Manthey *et al.*, 1970; Zander, 1977; Shukla, 1982; McMahon, 1991). If primary nurses are to realize their potential as practitioners, they need support, understanding and encouragement. Their educational base may require strengthening and they need easy, comfortable access to senior practitioners who can advise them. The traditional rule of fear in nursing management no longer serves a useful purpose. If staff nurses are competent enough to be entrusted with complex professional decisions, they deserve to be respected and supported as adult colleagues, not treated as juniors at the bottom of the hierarchy. Manthey (1980) describes her motivation, in developing the primary nursing system, as the *'rehumanisation of hospital care'* and she reminds us that *'patients cannot receive humane and thoughtful care from staff members who have been treated in a dehumanised fashion by their managers'* (p. xvii). Elsewhere, she emphasizes the crucial significance of the right kind of managerial climate:

'The first requirement for the successful application of the primary nursing concept is an atmosphere in which individuals feel free to learn, to risk, to make mistakes, and to grow. The philosophy of the nursing department and its leaders must demonstrate this trust and give support to nurses whose attempts at comprehensive patient care lead to unorthodox activities.' (Manthey *et al.*, 1970, p. 74)

Making this cultural change to support primary nursing is one of the least understood aspects of practice development. It appears that there are many nurses whose efforts to practise in a patient-centred way are being thwarted by managers who may mean well, but whose style is mistrustful and controlling.

Making the patient the central focus of nursing is by no means a new idea. Florence Nightingale's (1859) *Notes on Nursing* portray good practice as characterized by minute attention to very personal detail, in both the observation of the individual patient and in the management of his or her comfort and well-being. But from what she wrote, it is clear that Nightingale was describing something nearer to an ideal than to what she had commonly observed in homes and hospital wards. The thread of patient-centredness continued to run through nursing texts published during the first half of this century (e.g. see Pearce, 1937) but in practice, during that period, the expansion of the hospital system, the rapid growth of scientific medicine and the influence of industrial models of efficiency, all served to marginalize the patient as a person, and nursing became the impersonal and ritualized activity described as the traditional style of practice (Menzies, 1970; Chapman, 1983; Walsh and Ford, 1989).

The struggle to develop the personal focus of caring in nursing, and to kindle the spark of creativity that can transform routine ward work into a healing art, is a struggle that has been embraced by many modern nurses. But the obstacles to success are many and the process of this particular change is slow and complex. Our own experiences of managing change in hospital wards have given us rich insights into the processes of growth and transformation that have to occur before a nursing team is able to offer a genuinely patient-centred service. The research venture described in this book was undertaken with the intention of making what we have learned accessible to others who are also engaged in the process of developing a patient-centred nursing service.

Research issues

Systematic investigation of the practice of nursing, by nurses, is a relatively new development in the profession's history. It followed naturally from the growth of higher education for nurses and the establishment of university departments of nursing. These prerequisites for formal research activity did not begin to emerge until the 1960s in Britain, though some years earlier in North America. Arriving much later in the university world than the established professions, nursing has been under pressure to prove itself as a credible academic discipline, particularly in the eyes of medical colleagues, looking on sceptically from the position of a well-respected scientific tradition. It seems likely that this pressure has been one of the key factors influencing novice nurse researchers in their approach to theoretical and methodological issues. In the USA, where economic imperatives took a high profile in the health care field earlier than in the UK, managerial demands for analysis of efficiency and cost-effectiveness undoubtedly also shaped the way academic nurses formulated their research questions. In recent years, the same influence has been increasingly evident in the British nursing research world.

Experimental research, by measuring the influence of one variable upon others, is designed to evaluate the effectiveness of specific interventions. It aims to produce results upon which judgements about predictable outcomes in particular situations can be based. The experiment is regarded by many in the orthodox scientific community as *the* scientific method, or the 'gold standard' for research, so that knowledge which has not been tested under experimental conditions is not granted the status of 'scientific knowledge'. In the world of management, experimental science is also highly valued because its results provide evidence of what works and what does not, and it can therefore inform decisions about business development and allocation of resources. However, conducting meaningful experimental research requires certain preconditions, namely, a detailed understanding of all the variables at work in the situation under investigation and stable conditions in which the different variables can be reliably controlled and manipulated. These preconditions are often not present in new fields of research generally and in the field of social research in particular.

Nursing practice is a relatively new area for systematic study and many of its concerns are of a social, rather than biological, nature. The wisdom of resisting temptation or pressure to engage, prematurely or inappropriately, in experimental work has been appreciated in some quarters of the academic nursing world (e.g. McFarlane, 1977; Kidd and Morrison, 1988; Holmes, 1990). Elsewhere, broad and balanced thinking about the methodological challenges presented by research in nursing practice has been less evident. The study of the practice of primary nursing provides a good example of an area where nurse researchers have been over-hasty in their use of the experimental method and have produced disappointing results as a consequence.

Reports of research asking questions about primary nursing have been appearing in the literature since the mid-1970s, initially from the USA and then later from the UK and elsewhere. Giovannetti (1986) undertook a comprehensive review of empirical works published before 1984, some 29 in all. The major thrust of this research effort was to demonstrate the efficacy of primary nursing. All the investigators used conventional experimental research designs to compare wards using primary nursing with wards employing other work organization methods, or to compare wards before and after the introduction of primary nursing. They measured a range of outcomes which proponents of primary nursing claim can be improved by the system (e.g. quality of care, patient satisfaction, quality of records, job satisfaction). However, Giovannetti pointed out serious methodological problems which go some way towards explaining why, when taken together, the study findings have nothing conclusive to offer. Of particular concern (and indicating premature use of the experimental method) was the absence, in all the studies, of an operational definition of primary nursing and, with few exceptions, the lack of adequate validity and reliability testing of instruments used to measure criterion variables. These are serious criticisms since, as Giovannetti put it,

> *'If it is not known what is going to be measured, and it is not known whether the instruments really measure what is to be measured, intelligible inter-pretations of the research effort cannot be made.'* (p. 130)

Giovannetti suggested that it was not only the flaws in experimental design and instruments that limited this research but, more fundamentally, the choice of experimental methodology itself. The nature of a practice setting can make the management of a true experiment so problematic as to be inappropriate. She suggested that it would be wiser and more fruitful to explore other research strategies.

In spite of Giovannetti's widely referenced critique, primary nursing research since her review has continued in much the same mould. Two Canadian studies, for example, adopted a cross-over design to compare team and primary nursing. One reported an increase in the quality of care after the introduction of primary nursing (Wilson and Dawson, 1989), while the other found no significant differences between the two systems (McPhail et al., 1990). The different time-scales allowed before the impact of primary nursing was assessed (nine months and five months, respectively) may, in part, account for the contrasting results, but other influences could also have been present.

In the UK, Reed (1988) assessed quality of care and nurses' philosophy and job satisfaction in a ward practising primary nursing and in one that was not. Although the wards were alike in some respects, there were many factors other than method of work organization (not least the fact that the wards were situated in different health authorities) that could have accounted for differences. Manley (1989) conducted a before and after study in one half of an intensive care unit, using the other half as a control. No firm conclusions can be drawn because of the very small scale of the project, the influence of many factors that could not be controlled and the short time interval (only 1 month) between the introduction of primary nursing and the 'after' measures.

MacGuire (1989a; 1989b) undertook a well considered and more sophisticated study, of quasi-experimental design, in which a serious attempt was made to address the methodological weaknesses of earlier work, but she acknowledged that this was only partially successful (MacGuire, 1989c). The work very helpfully highlights the range and complexity of the changes associated with the introduction of primary nursing and it emphasizes the time required for nurses and other staff to adapt to these changes. It also provides an interesting analysis of nurses' experiences of the changes, which supports the view that primary nursing can provide nurses with a high level of job satisfaction (MacGuire and Botting, 1990). However, the work is particularly valuable for its presentation of the methodological difficulties associated with trying to evaluate the effects of primary nursing on quality of care (MacGuire, 1991). The conclusion drawn from a valiant attempt to battle with these difficulties was that,

> 'The changes involved in primary nursing are so great and potentially so far-reaching that the question 'Is primary nursing better than team nursing or task allocation?' is probably not the one we should be trying to answer.' (MacGuire, 1989c)

Bond et al. (1991) reported another British study which failed in its original aim to determine whether primary nursing made a difference to patient care, but which produced some interesting findings and some important methodological comment. No firm conclusion about the effectiveness of primary nursing per se can be drawn from their comparative case study because, although matched in some respects, there were a number of fundamental differences between the control and study wards, other than mode of work organization, which could have influenced the findings. However, the comparison is interesting, for it was surely no accident that the differences between the two wards all favoured the experimental ward practising primary nursing. The value system, leadership style and staffing levels of the experimental ward made primary nursing an appropriate choice of organizational method, and the good staff morale, sensible workload management and healthy interdisciplinary relationships will have contributed to effective use of the system and to positive service outcomes generally. In the control ward, institutional values, weaker leadership and lower staffing levels would have made the introduction of primary nursing problematic, and the hospital's morale and image problem, the absence of workload control and the less collaborative relationship between disciplines would have undermined its potential. Circumstances were clearly conspiring against the control ward, regardless of its choice of organizational system. The detailed reporting of this study shows the problems of attempting to compare what may at one level appear to be well-matched wards. It also shows the problem of trying to isolate the method of work organization from other factors that influence the work of a nursing team. In a subsequent publication, Thomas and Bond (1991) reviewed the methodological problems that have so consistently frustrated researchers' efforts to evaluate primary nursing. Like MacGuire, and Giovannetti before her, they concluded that different questions should be asked which, in turn, means exploring new methodologies.

In the substantial body of experimental and quasi-experimental research that now exists on the subject, primary nursing is singled out as the independent variable and comparisons are made, either between 'matched' control and experiment wards, or within the same wards before and after introducing primary nursing, or by combining both strategies in a cross-over design. A range of criteria are measured or described on the basis that, if significant differences are identified, all other things being equal, they can be causally attributed to primary nursing.

The assumption underlying all this research is that there can be a simple, direct, causal relationship between the work organization method in a ward and service outcomes. Furthermore, the research assumes that it is possible to isolate the work organization method from other factors in ward life and to change it while everything else remains constant. Researchers have interpreted the theoretical literature as suggesting that introducing primary nursing can 'cause' improvement in quality of care, or patient satisfaction, or whatever. They have then set out to prove or disprove these relationships by making comparisons between situations which they claimed were virtually the same, apart from the presence or absence of primary nursing. Any significant differences, they then argued, had to be attributable to primary nursing.

This kind of research seems to ignore Manthey's (1980) clear statement that,

> '*The quality of nursing service in a Primary Nursing system can be good or bad, comprehensive or incomplete, co-ordinated or spasmodic, individualized or standardized, creative or routine.*' (p. 31)

Manthey recognized that, as an organizational system, primary nursing is only a framework within which nurses work, and no more. The system provides nurses with *opportunities* to work closely, continuously and creatively with their patients, but it cannot guarantee that this is what the nurses will actually do. How nurses perform within the system and whether they are able to make the most of the opportunities it offers, will depend upon many factors, including the skills, beliefs and motivation of individual nurses, the commitment and co-operation of their team colleagues and the quality of support and leadership available from their seniors. Thus, the presence of a primary nursing system is only one of many interrelated variables that make a patient-centred style of practice achievable in a hospital ward.

Furthermore, it has to be remembered that, while primary nursing is in itself a relatively simple organizational concept to grasp, it is quite unlike most existing patterns of nursing work organization and its design was based upon values and goals very different from those that have influenced the functioning of hospital wards in the past. Introducing primary nursing to a ward challenges nurses to adopt new roles, to relate to patients and other disciplines in new ways and to think and work very differently. As Ferrin (1981) put it, *'primary nursing is relatively easy to understand but complex to successfully implement'* (p. 1).

The literature that describes primary nursing and experiences of using it in practice paints a picture 7hich does not match the somewhat simplistic assumptions underlying the body of experimental research. It describes the introduction of primary nursing as a highly complex organizational change and as a gradual process involving experimentation, adjustment and readjustment, rather than as a one-off event. Research that attempts to measure the impact of introducing primary nursing after just a few months fails to recognize the scale of the change that primary nursing sets in motion and the time and effort that are required to help nurses reap the benefits of the system. Studies with a cross-over design also fail to recognize that nurses learn and grow through the experience of this kind of change, so that, as practitioners, they are never quite the same again. For anyone who has really grappled with the responsibility of being a primary nurse, the idea that one could then switch back to being a team nurse, as if nothing had happened, is simply absurd.

Asking research questions of the type: 'Does primary nursing work?', 'Does primary nursing improve X, Y or Z?', is arguably inappropriate and somewhat naive. Primary nursing gives nurses the opportunity to work in new, more patient-centred ways. Studying whether nurses do work differently as primary nurses tells us nothing about the system, but only whether the particular nurses studied have been successful at using it or not. It is not surprising that the results of this kind of research are inconclusive; one would expect some nurses to make a greater success of the system than others. A more promising line of enquiry would seem to be to start by acknowledging that, *logically*, improvements in certain aspects of ward life are possible when a primary nursing system is used. Investigation would then focus upon what factors contribute to its success or failure. In other words, instead of asking *whether* primary nursing works, one would be asking *how* can it be made to work.

Pearson (1992) reported an important research venture which departed from the orthodox experimental design. In Burford Community Hospital, he set out to initiate, guide and study the process of changing nursing practice from a traditional style to a patient-centred style. He wanted to find out whether the new ideology being promoted by nursing's academic elite could be introduced into an 'ordinary' unit and to see what effects such a change would have on those involved. Primary nursing was introduced, but as an integral part of fundamental change affecting almost every aspect of the small hospital's life. Although Pearson did use some 'before and after' measures in an attempt to quantify the changes that were made, he used an action research framework to guide the main part of the study and most of his data were qualitative. It is this rich descriptive material that provides the most convincing evidence that real changes were achieved. Furthermore, Pearson's analysis of it provides valuable insights into how the new style of practice was achieved and how the transition was experienced by participants.

Pearson's focus upon the process of change and his open exploration of its impact were much more fruitful than the experimental approach, given the complexity of the context. The study reported in this book can be seen as building on the pioneering efforts of Pearson and his colleagues at Burford.

Chapter 2

Origins and context of the study

The practice and research issues addressed so far have provided a general back-cloth for the research study which forms the basis for this book. By considering its history, we have tried to show the complexity of the practice development field and some of the problems encountered by those who research it. In this chapter, we trace the origins of our own project, which included both practice development and research elements. The history of the project is important because it explains the context of the development work that was studied. It also explains how the research questions arose and the choice of methodology.

PRACTICE BACKGROUND

It was not by accident that the project emerged in Oxfordshire. It was a late product of a whole cycle of work undertaken within the Health Authority, beginning in the late 1970s. The focus of this work was to create a structure and a climate that would enable practitioners to set the agenda for the nursing service. Giving those who worked most closely with patients authority, status and a voice in the organization was considered a powerful way of serving the interests of patients.

The vision of a practice-led service originated from the Chief Nurse. She appointed like-minded senior staff and gave them the authority to invest in clinical nurses and to make changes in the way the service was run. One of the early products of this strategy was the Burford Nursing Development Unit, the cottage hospital that shed its very traditional style and, as one of the first centres in this country to use primary nursing, developed a patient-centred service for its local community (Alderman, 1983). Burford was the model for the national network of Nursing Development Units that was subsequently established.

The educational investment required to support practice development within the Authority was recognized early on. A special education team was set up, in addition to the usual pre- and post-registration teams, with a remit to provide courses and other educational activities specifically geared to helping nurses achieve change in their practice setting. The practice orientation, and the climate of support for innovation fostered by leaders of nursing in Oxfordshire, attracted able, creative practitioners and many of them have led influential changes (*Nursing Times*, 1989).

An important step in raising the status of nursing practice and practitioners in Oxfordshire was a flattening of the nursing management hierarchy, achieved in 1983 through the reorganization prompted by the Government's *Patients First* document (DHSS, 1977). In the interest of bringing decision-making nearer to the bedside, authority for managing clinical staff was fully devolved to senior ward sisters. The nursing officer tier of middle management was completely removed on the basis that a patient-centred service requires only three levels of management: a primary nurse to manage the care of individual patients, a ward sister to manage teams of nurses, and a director of nursing to manage the nursing service.

Following the principle that a ship needs only one captain, each ward had only one ward sister, but wards were paired or grouped and one of the ward sister posts in each pair or group of wards was reserved for a more experienced figure who took on the role of senior sister. Senior sisters had full responsibility for running their own wards, but they were also expected to provide professional leadership to steer the development of the other ward/s in their department. In addition, senior sisters formed the senior nurse group that advised the director of nursing on running the service.

This simple structure had two major advantages. First, management decisions, placed in the hands of senior sisters, were always informed by recent first-hand experience of practice, which meant that the perspective and priorities of nursing management became much more closely rooted in the daily reality of caring for patients. Second, all ward sisters had real authority to manage their own clinical areas, without interference from another tier of management. Many sisters experienced this structure as liberating and used their new authority to test out their own ideas for improving their service to patients and, in this way, valuable practice initiatives were born.

The structure and climate of nursing in Oxfordshire has favoured the development of a patient-centred service for many years, but structure and climate alone do not guarantee the service product. It is the individual leaders in each ward or department who ultimately have the most significant influence upon how patients are nursed. There has thus been a conscious strategy in the Health Authority of identifying, recruiting, or 'growing' clinical leaders, placing them in key positions whenever opportunities have arisen and supporting them as much as possible.

Alison Binnie was recruited to the Health Authority in 1984, as one of the new 'breed' of senior sisters. Within one of the main hospitals, she became clinical leader for a unit of three surgical wards and ward sister for one of them. Having inherited conventional nursing teams, which consisted of only a small proportion of registered nurses, she set up a controversial skill-mix project. She showed that it was possible, within the existing budget, to run the wards with a high proportion of registered nurses, but with fewer 'pairs of hands' (Binnie, 1987). Her rationale for this initiative was based upon the fact that providing a personalized service for acutely ill patients requires frequent, skilled assessment and decision-making at the bedside. Only registered nurses are educated and licensed to carry this level of professional responsibility. Furthermore, she argued that registered nurses are good value for money, because they can work flexibly and can combine a range of highly skilled and more simple activities together, in one patient contact. Formal evaluation of this project was fairly crude, but it did suggest that there was some improvement in the quality of care following the change in skill-mix (Binnie, 1987). The general consensus locally was that the initiative was successful and gradually, as opportunities arose, the skill-mix on all the acute wards in the Health Authority's hospitals was adjusted in the same way.

With more appropriately designed nursing teams in the Surgical Unit, Alison went on to review the organization of ward nursing and the roles and responsibilities of different grades of staff. Impressed by the work at the Burford Nursing Development Unit, she wanted to translate its approach to patient-centred nursing into a form manageable in busy, acute wards. The result was one of the first primary nursing systems to be established, in an acute hospital setting, in the UK (Binnie, 1989). The work attracted a lot of publicity and Alison was often called upon to share her experiences of primary nursing with others. She was conscious of having learned a great deal about the complexity of developing nursing practice and recognized that creating a genuinely patient-centred service required much more than just organizational change. However, this complexity was difficult to articulate. The detail of the change process that Alison and her staff had lived through had not been formally captured and recorded. Many of her own change strategies and her responses to problems had been intuitive and it was impossible, in retrospect, to analyse with any accuracy what she had done, and what had been effective and what had not. It was frustration at not being able to make her knowledge and experience accessible and useful for other practitioners that provided Alison with the stimulus to initiate this research study.

In 1988, Alison had sabbatical leave to study for a master's degree. She undertook an ethnographic study of 'The working lives of staff nurses' in the general medical wards within her own hospital. These wards had been able to change their skill-mix when student nurses had become supernumerary and they were staffed almost entirely by qualified nurses. However, Alison found that their style of nursing had remained essentially traditional. The nursing work was task-focussed and routinized and, though busy coping with a heavy workload, the nurses were bored, frustrated and dissatisfied with the way they cared for patients (Binnie, 1988).

When Alison returned from leave, she took up a post as a senior sister, based in one of these medical wards and responsible for the clinical leadership in a unit of two wards. Because of her experience in the Surgical Unit, she also negotiated an informal role as adviser on practice development to the sisters in the other medical wards. She was thus faced, for the second time, with the task of helping ward nurses to make the difficult journey from traditional nursing to patient-centred nursing. In addition, she had the new challenge of indirectly influencing practice in other wards by working with their ward sisters. Alison was determined that, this time, the development processes would be captured and analysed in such a way that they could be helpfully communicated to other practitioners. She approached the then newly established Institute of Nursing, in Oxford, and proposed setting up a collaborative venture which would both support and study the development work in the medical wards. Angie Titchen was appointed by the Institute, to work full-time as Alison's research partner. She brought experience of research and education in physiotherapy, and her commitment to patient-centred practice and student-centred learning enabled her to identify comfortably with the goals of nursing development work in Oxford.

The contemporary scene

During the life of the project, the context for the development work changed considerably. The Health Service reforms, associated with the shift to a market economy, precipitated dramatic organizational and cultural change in hospitals throughout the country. In Oxfordshire, the transformation of the Health Authority into a purchasing body meant that the Nursing Department at District level, which had been both a driving force and a political ally behind practice development, disappeared. The focus of nursing leadership shifted from the District to individual Trusts. The Trusts inevitably brought a new style of management and new priorities, and nurses, like everyone else, had to review their commitments and their aspirations in the light of the new corporate agendas.

As in most Trusts, the devolution of service management to clinical teams, rather than through functional hierarchies, was a central strand in the early work of the Oxford Radcliffe Trust. The directorate system (in Oxford, and some other Trusts, directorates are called 'clinical centres' and they have sub-units called 'service delivery units' or 'SDUs') was potentially a threat to the values embedded in the senior sister structure, but it also presented opportunities. The senior sisters did not want to lose their managerial authority to business managers in the new system, so it was important for them to work within it. They could also see the advantages within the SDUs of having, for the first time, formal working relationships with doctors, outside the clinical arena. However, they did not want to abandon their clinical positions to become full-time business managers themselves, as had many senior nurses elsewhere. The senior sisters negotiated a compromise: they took on the roles of SDU managers, but without giving up their wards and their commitment to spend a substantial proportion of their time in nursing practice. Within the SDUs, they work alongside clinical directors, usually medical consultants who have also not given up their practice. The doctor and nurse managing the SDU are supported in their business responsibilities by a business manager attached to the clinical centre. Particularly in the larger SDUs, sharing SDU work with other clinical staff serves the dual purpose of involving others in service management and of lightening the workload of the core SDU management team.

During the course of this project, Alison took on the role of SDU manager for the general medical service. There were tensions between this responsibility and her clinical commitments, but she found them outweighed by the advantages of being directly involved in decisions which affected the medical service and of being able to bring an authoritative clinical perspective to management discussions.

THE RESEARCH QUESTIONS

The origins of the research questions go back to the beginning of the project and Alison's concern to try to answer the questions being posed by the practitioners she met all over the country. She found that practitioners could see the potential of primary nursing as an organizational system. They appreciated that, logically, if nurses were able to work continuously with the same patients and were given the authority to manage their care, then they would have the *opportunity* to deliver truly patient-centred nursing. Thus, they were not asking, 'Does primary nursing work?'; they wanted to know *how* to introduce the system into wards with a traditional or individualized style of practice, and they wanted to know *how* to get the best out of the system for both patients and staff. From these practitioners' questions, our key research question was formulated:

How can primary nursing be used to develop a twenty-four hour patient-centred nursing service, in an acute hospital ward?

The question 'how?', or 'in what way?', implied a search for a process – a process that was effective in achieving the aim of patient-centred nursing. Three subsidiary research questions about this process helped to focus our work:

1 What are the different aspects and stages of this developmental process?
2 What difficulties are encountered during the process of development?
3 What strategies are effective in overcoming these difficulties and in moving the development along?

Because of Alison's involvement in practice and her remit to develop a patient-centred service, we wanted to seek answers to the questions by actually engaging in the process of development and tracing its progress. By capturing and drawing on the experiences and insights of those involved in the process with us, we hoped to devise development strategies appropriate for the context and to test their effectiveness. By recording and analysing the development work, rather than just doing it, we wanted to generate a theoretical account of the process, and people's experiences of it, which other nurses would be able to relate to their own situations. Thus, in summary, in seeking to answer the research questions, the specific aims of the project were:

1 To improve the quality of nursing care in the study wards by developing a patient-centred style of practice.
2 To analyse and interpret the experiences of those directly involved in, or affected by, the changes in nursing practice.
3 To develop a detailed understanding of how the transition from a traditional style of nursing to a patient-centred style can be achieved.
4 To make the insights generated by the research accessible to other nurses.

CHOICE OF METHODOLOGY

The project questions and aims committed us, at the same time, to achieving a concrete social change and to pursuing a rigorous intellectual enquiry. This dual task located the work in the field of action research.

Action research is generally agreed to have emerged after the Second World War, when social scientists became concerned that traditional science was not contributing significantly to resolving the urgent social problems of the day. Kurt Lewin is said to have introduced the term 'action research' when he was engaged in a number of community projects in post-war America. He saw the involvement of the researcher in the social situation, and his action upon it, as a means of achieving social change, as well as a means of generating theory about social issues (Lewin, 1946). In their account of the origins of action research, Susman and Evered (1978) also acknowledge the contributions of the Tavistock Institute of Human Relations, in Britain, and John Collier (1945), again in North America. Coming from different backgrounds to Lewin, both the Tavistock group and Collier also recognized, at about the same time, the value of collaboration between social scientists and practitioners in the field, as a means of exploring and addressing difficult social issues.

Since this early work, action research has been used in a variety of settings, including industry, hospitals, social engineering programmes, mainstream education and, more recently, in nursing (e.g. Lathlean and Farnish, 1984; Fretwell, 1985; Smith, 1986; Hunt, 1987; FitzGerald, 1989a; Webb, 1989; Wilson-Barnett et al., 1990; Armitage et al., 1991; Batehup, 1991; Pearson, 1992; Meyer, 1993; Nolan and Grant, 1993; Owen, 1993). This body of work shows action research to be a valuable method for challenging, examining and changing established practices and, at the same time, for involving practitioners in both using and generating theory. But the studies also illustrate the limitations of the approach and some of the difficulties associated with it. They show that action research is unlikely to follow a well-ordered plan or to deliver quick results. It is a complex and largely unpredictable venture, demanding a high level of personal involvement and commitment from the researcher. It is dependent upon successful collaboration with participants and involves a degree of risk for both researcher and participants – things may go wrong or there may be unanticipated consequences from the project. Meyer (1993) provides a particularly honest and insightful account of some of these problems. Furthermore, it is fair to say that action research is still not widely accepted as a credible 'scientific' method. This may, in part, be due to the fact that it is a qualitative approach, which means that its findings are not necessarily widely generalizable. Generalization depends upon readers recognizing the relevance of findings for their own situations.

Fundamentally, action research is a strategy which brings about social change through action, developing and improving practice and, at the same time, generating and testing theory. However, action research has become a very broad church and it means different things to different people. Interpretations of action research could be placed on a continuum. At one end lies the open approach of reflective practice, described by Schon (1983), in which the practitioner theorizes practice by reflecting upon events and experiences in the practice setting. At the other end lies a highly structured approach, ideologically linked to the critical theory tradition, where action research must involve a group of practitioners researching their own practice by adhering to a design with tightly defined characteristics (Carr and Kemmis, 1986; Kemmis and McTaggart, 1988). Between these extreme positions lies the pragmatic approach of those who focus upon studying practical issues and solving practical problems, without ideological bias (e.g. Brown and McIntyre, 1981).

Exploring the philosophical and epistemological issues that lie behind the different interpretations of action research is not a venture for the fainthearted: they are enormously complex. An attempt to pick a way through this intellectual minefield is presented elsewhere by Titchen (1993) and Hart and Bond (1995). Here, we dip into these esoteric realms only in so far as they influenced, or now illuminate, our particular action research strategy.

KEY INFLUENCES ON THE DEVELOPMENT OF THE ACTION RESEARCH STRATEGY

Arising logically from our initial questions and aims, and from the way the project was established, were four principles, which had to be satisfied in the design of our action research strategy. The strategy developed gradually as our appreciation of the philosophical and methodological issues grew.

Principle 1:

We wished to capture and present an account of the perceptions and experiences of participants in the project.

This material would serve three purposes:

- It would enable other nurses to relate the project findings to their own experiences of practice development.
- It would allow us, and our readers, to assess the impact of the changes made in the wards.
- It would inform our change strategy.

In approaching this aspect of the study, we drew upon the phenomenological research tradition. Two distinct strands of this tradition were developed – by Schutz (1967), on the one hand, and by Heidegger (1962) and Benner (1985) on the other. Broadly, however, phenomenological research attempts to describe and understand everyday life as seen through the eyes of the actors involved; it attempts to reveal people's 'lived experience'. It aims to discover the meaning particular situations hold for people and the way they construct their social reality. It requires qualitative research methods to capture data about what people do and say in particular settings, and about people's perceptions and interpretations of their world.

To record these data as accurately as possible, researchers have to be conscious of the values, assumptions, expectations and opinions that they bring with them into the situation. They need to be highly disciplined in acknowledging their preconceptions and, as it were, putting them on one side, so that they can attend to the research situation with a kind of open naivety. Schutz (1962) calls this discipline an attempt to 'bracket' one's own understandings, or to 'suspend belief', whilst Gadamer (1979) refers to this process as a 'suspension of prejudices'.

Data analysis in phenomenological research is an interpretive process. The researcher attempts to make sense of the data by developing theoretical concepts from the material and weaving them into an account which captures the essence of the participants' world, as they experienced it. If the account is valid, it should 'ring true' and be meaningful to the participants.

In this project, the phenomenological approach influenced the role that Angie adopted as the main data collector and it guided the way in which most of the data were collected, analysed and reported.

Principle 2:

We wished to adopt a collaborative change strategy.
We were committed to developing a patient-centred style of practice, but we wanted the nurses to be involved in determining how and at what pace the

changes required to achieve that broad aim were managed. We considered participation of all the nurses in steering the change process to be crucial because:

- We wanted to establish a lasting change that was owned by all the ward staff and that was not dependent for its survival upon our presence.
- The practice of patient-centred nursing is dependent upon the presence of competent, confident, self-respecting practitioners who can think independently. The development of these qualities in the nurses was likely to be enhanced by a change strategy that valued their views, gave them personal responsibility and acknowledged their individual contributions. (The reverse would be likely with a 'top-down' strategy that imposed changes.)
- Establishing a patient-centred style of nursing, as a sustainable and central ethos in ward practice, meant changing not only the perceptions and behaviours of individual nurses, but also the structural and cultural norms of ward life. Renegotiating the principles and the values that give shape and meaning to the social world of a particular group cannot take place without their participation.

Action researchers who draw upon critical theory stress the importance of the 'empowerment' and the 'emancipation' of the participants in the research venture. They recognize the value of interpretive social science (which includes phenomenological research) as a means of illuminating how things are, but they are critical of its failure to deal with how things might be changed (Carr and Kemmis, 1986). Within the critical theory tradition, groups of practitioners engage in a process of collaborative enquiry, open critical debate and reflection, and democratic decision-making. The aim of this process is to enable the group to explore not only their own understandings of their situation, but also the social conditions, such as ideology, traditions, customs and control structures, which influence how they see their world and how it operates. Ultimately, the group is 'enlightened' by the process and 'empowered', not only to change the way they think about their practice, but also to change the structures and conditions which constrain or limit their practice, or distort it away from values they cherish. Thus, they generate knowledge about how to transform practice.

The goals of critical social science, as presented in relation to the educational field by Carr and Kemmis (1986), matched our goals for ward nursing in many respects. Their view of action research influenced the design and conduct of the project significantly, particularly in relation to Alison's role, as head of the practitioner group, and in relation to the involvement of staff nurses in reflection, critical debate and decision-making. This influence has meant that the project can be placed somewhere near the critical social science end of the action research spectrum.

Principle 3:

We wanted to generate a theorized account of the change processes we experienced, identifying different stages of the development, problems that were encountered and strategies that were effective in moving the development along.

From her experience in the Surgical Unit, Alison knew that introducing primary nursing and using it to develop patient-centred practice was a highly complex process. The literature confirms this and points to some aspects of the process that need attention, such as educational preparation (Hegevary, 1982 FitzGerald, 1991), a supportive managerial climate (Manthey, 1980) and change in the ward sister role (Zander, 1977), but there appears to be no adequate account of the true complexity of these issues and of how they might be most effectively managed. Thus, Alison found that neither her own experience nor the literature in the field provided her with a means of articulating adequately the reality she knew. She realized that she had never fully analysed and given a name to much of what she and her staff had lived through in the past, so that now much of what they had learned was lost.

Throughout the project, we wanted to capture the detail of the development process in our data. In analysing the data, we hoped to develop concepts which would, as it were, label what we observed or experienced. By conceptualizing the stages of the development, the ways they were experienced, the problems that were encountered and the strategies that were used to overcome them, and by identifying the relationships between these aspects of the process, we hoped to 'map out' the process in a way that would be meaningful for others. This 'conceptual map' would be the theorized account of the process of developing patient-centred nursing.

Very broadly, the critical social science approach to the development work provided a mechanism for generating theory about how change of this kind can be managed effectively, while the phenomenological approach to the fieldwork conducted alongside the development provided a means of generating theory about the nature of this particular change process. However, we recognized from the literature that these two strands of the study need not run independently. Kemmis and McTaggart (1988) emphasize the value of exploratory work preceding and informing the initial planning and action of the action research process. Brown and McIntyre (1981) take this idea further and suggest that running an open, observational (i.e. phenomenological) study alongside the action provides data that can continue to inform the action and that can also be used to generate theory about the change process.

Principle 4:

We were committed to working in a partnership in which we both contributed to and took responsibility for the action and the research elements of the project.

The research partnership came about as a solution to a practical problem. Alison recognized at the outset of the project that it would be impossible for her to carry, single-handed, the full burden of responsibility for the development work, on the scale that was planned, and for a substantial research study. Angie's appointment meant that responsibility for these two strands of the work could be shared. Our individual roles and responsibilities within the partnership were determined, in part, by our positions within the organization and by our individual skills and interests, but they were also influenced by the strengths and weaknesses of the two types of action researcher role described in the literature.

Within nursing, action research undertaken by practitioners researching as 'insiders' in their own practice setting appears to have been very successful, in the sense of achieving the desired practice changes (e.g. FitzGerald, 1989a; Batehup, 1991; Pearson, 1992). The practitioner/researchers' formal authority within the practice setting, their commitment to the change agenda and their responsibility for its consequences must be significant advantages here. Indeed, Carr and Kemmis (1986) would go so far as to say they are crucial and, from a critical social science perspective, only 'insider' research is legitimate research. However, there may be considerable personal cost associated with engaging in action research while also fully committed to a practice role. There is a real risk of work overload and a risk that either practice or research, or both, may be compromised, leaving the practitioner/researcher feeling guilty and frustrated, as well as exhausted. These concerns supported Alison's view that it was unwise to initiate a major action research project, in a highly pressured nursing service, without some additional support from outside.

When the researcher is an 'outsider' to the practice setting, there is a division of labour which makes the project more manageable. The researcher may have a diagnostic function, collecting data, feeding back observations and making recommendations to the participants, while the practitioners 'inside' the setting are responsible for initiating, managing and evaluating change. Where both parties remain committed to the same change agenda and where the 'outside' researcher is able to support effective 'inside' practice change agents, then it seems that this kind of project can be successful (e.g. Lathlean and Farnish, 1984). On the other hand, major problems of differing expectations or agendas within the project can arise because responsibility for the 'action' and the 'research' are vested in different parties (e.g.Smith, 1986; Hunt, 1987).

From the start of the project, the main problems of Alison being a lone 'inside' researcher were avoided by Angie's appointment. However, Alison did not wish to give up all responsibility for the research to Angie. She would then have lost the advantages of being an 'inside' researcher and would have risked the tensions that can occur through putting the research entirely in the hands of an 'outsider'. To balance Alison's concern to have a foot in both camps, and recognizing that Angie brought facilitation skills that would be valuable in the development process, we explored ways of providing Angie with a role that brought her partly 'inside' ward life, but without losing all the freedom of her 'outside' status. Thus, in developing our action research partnership, we were guided by the literature to see the advantages of us both having responsibilities within the spheres of 'the action' and 'the research'.

In summary, our approach to studying and trying to improve ward practice was influenced by both the phenomenological and the critical social science traditions. In developing the research strategy, we had to address the challenge of combining these two perspectives within a single action research scheme while, at the same time, allowing each to be used to make its distinct contribution. Our working partnership, which gave us each a foot in both the action and research camps, helped us to handle the tricky juxtaposition of the openness of the phenomenologist and the committed position of the critical social scientist. The partnership also helped us to cope with the complexity and the considerable demands of managing a project that involved both a major practice innovation and substantial academic work.

Chapter 3

The research strategy

THE ACTION RESEARCH DESIGN

The design of an action research project classically follows the spiralling structure first described by Lewin (1946). Each turn of Lewin's spiral consists of a cycle of four steps: planning, action, observation and reflection. What is learned from reflection at the end of the first cycle informs the planning at the beginning of the next, and so on, as the work continues. Kemmis and McTaggart (1988) depict the action research spiral as shown in Figure 3.1.

Kemmis and McTaggart (1988) add to Lewin's spiral scheme a 'reconnaissance phase' to identify the 'thematic concerns' to be addressed when planning begins in the first action research cycle. They describe this phase as an initial period of reflection on the situation to be studied which serves as a way to get started on the action research spiral. We incorporated a similar introductory phase into our project in the shape of an exploratory study. As well as fulfilling its reconnaissance function, this early work also identified for Angie the practical problems associated with analysing large amounts of qualitative data and with the mechanics of generating theory in this kind of research (see Titchen and McIntyre, 1993; Titchen and Binnie, 1993a; 1993b).

McNiff (1988) found that managing and studying change in a practice setting is more complex than Lewin's spiral suggests. She pointed out that one might begin by focussing upon a central problem and by working through the steps of the spiral with participants, but that new issues would inevitably arise and have to be tackled separately, as new spirals of work. We had the same experience and came to see our project, not as following Lewin's single spiral, but as a kind of 'tree' of interrelated spirals (Figure 3.2). We also became concerned about the adequacy of the spiral structure for addressing our research questions fully. These concerns highlighted the need for a more thorough exploration of the philosophical basis of the research (the results of which have been reported in Chapter 2). Deeper philosophical insights led to an appreciation of the need to recognize the interplay in the project of critical social science ideas and phenomenology and, ultimately, to the integration of a continuous observational strand within our overall research scheme.

Unravelling the philosophical and methodological issues behind the practical conduct of action research was a major focus of Angie's early work. It involved wide reading, particularly in the field of educational research, where action

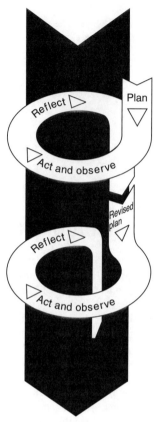

Figure 3.1 *The action research spiral (from Kemmis and McTaggart, 1988)* ©*(1988) Deakin University*

research has been most fully developed, and it involved networking and exchanging ideas with educationalists and nurses engaged in action research. Finally, it involved writing a series of methodological papers for publication (Titchen, 1993; Titchen and Binnie, 1993c; Titchen, 1994; Titchen, 1995a).

The overall research scheme is depicted in Figure 3.2. There were three elements of the scheme: the exploratory work, the action spirals and the observational study.

The fieldwork of the main study was extended beyond its initial allocation of time. The problem of time running out in an action research study is a common one, because the pace of the change being studied is determined by what actually happens in the practice setting, not by a predetermined research plan. To provide a complete picture of the transition to patient-centred nursing, it was crucial to obtain data from the study ward as the new style of practice was becoming established and as ward life was beginning to restabilize after the upheaval of enormous change. This case was made to the funding body, and an additional eight months of fieldwork was granted.

A further complication was the protracted and discontinuous period over which the final analysis and writing up occurred. It reflects our initial

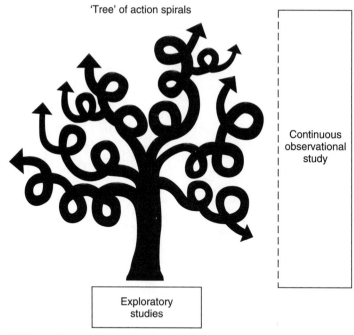

'Tree' of action spirals

Continuous
observational
study

Exploratory
studies

Figure 3.2 *Overall research scheme*

underestimate of the complexity of the project and the common problem, once the scheduled timetable has been overrun, of new professional commitments making competing demands.

Exploratory work

The main purpose of the initial exploratory work was to orientate Angie – a physiotherapist and a newcomer to the Health Authority – to the Oxford nursing scene generally and to nursing in the Medical Unit in particular. In addition, this early work allowed Angie to experiment with her own role as a participant observer in a ward and to test out methods of data collection and analysis.

There were two discrete strands to the exploratory work. The first strand was a series of interviews that Angie conducted with key people in the Health Authority. The data from these interviews helped to establish the context in which the study was taking place and recorded some of the history of Oxfordshire's nursing development work.

The second, more substantial, strand of exploratory work was a case study, carried out in a ward in the Medical Unit which we have called 'Linacre Ward'. This was not Alison's ward, but one for which, as senior sister, she had overall managerial responsibility. Angie conducted the case study over a three month period. As a participant observer, and through a series of interviews, she collected data about ward life at a time when team nursing was first being introduced and developed. The study described the change to team nursing as it was experienced by patients, nurses and other staff. It also captured the nurses' perceptions of the traditional style of practice they were leaving behind and their feelings about how things should be changed.

Findings from the case study have been reported elsewhere (Titchen and Binnie, 1993a; 1993b). Their value at the time was to highlight some of the major issues needing attention in the main study, and they provided tentative principles that we could apply in managing the change process. In other words, the exploratory case study generated some tentative 'theory', which subsequently informed some of the planning and action in the main study. As the action research spirals progressed, this 'theory' was modified and refined.

The observational study

The main study took place mostly in Alison's ward over a two year period. The observational element was designed to capture the perceptions and experiences of people involved in, or affected by, the changes that took place in the ward during that time, thus capturing the 'lived experience' of the change.

This was the element of the study that was approached from a phenomeno-logical perspective. During participant observation and depth interviews, we aimed to ask, with an open mind, what was happening, how were events interpreted and what was it like for people. As an 'outsider', Angie was in the best position to collect most of these data. When she was in the ward, she was free of clinical responsibilities and able to give her full attention to observing the events of ward life, and to listening to and questioning patients, relatives and staff. Furthermore, as an 'outsider' and a non-nurse, it was probably easier for her than for Alison not to take things for granted and to ask naive questions when necessary.

The observational study kept us alert to the unexpected and constantly challenged our assumptions. It revealed how others saw what was happening in the ward and the data helped us to steer the change process in a sensitive, well-informed way. When taken as a whole, at the end of the study, the richly detailed phenomenological data provided material from which we were able to develop a 'theorized' account of the change process and people's experiences of it.

The action spirals

In contrast to the loose, open approach of the observational part of the study, the action spirals provided structure and focus. They also provided a framework for involving others and for moving the change process along. Each action spiral took us through the cycle of planning, action, observation and reflection as many times as was necessary to solve a particular problem, or to establish a particular change. The process began with one obvious, central spiral of work, related to preparing for and establishing primary nursing. As this work progressed, concern arose about Alison's role as a ward sister and a new spiral of work emerged, which focussed on helping her to develop new ways of practising alongside the staff nurses. Yet another spiral was generated when the staff nurses began to struggle with their new primary and associate nurse roles, and so it continued until the 'tree' had developed and included a total of eight spirals. Often, it was data collected in the observational part of the study that alerted us to the need for a new spiral.

Each spiral was managed in a slightly different way depending upon its focus and the participants involved, but broadly speaking there was a common approach. During periods of fieldwork, we met every few weeks, for several hours, for a 'reflective conversation'. We discussed the raw data collected during the preceding fieldwork period. If we identified a major new concern that required attention in order to help the change along, we initiated a new spiral. Having examined the data about a new problem, we considered possible strategies for dealing with it and we proposed an 'action hypothesis' – if strategy X is adopted, change Y may be achieved. We completed the *planning phase* at the beginning of the new spiral by presenting our understanding of the new problem to other people concerned, usually the staff nurses in the ward. Sometimes we presented relevant data to help them appreciate the problem from different perspectives. We then involved them in planning the specific action to be taken.

In this way, planning tended to occur in two phases. The formulation of the action hypothesis and the initial strategic plan concerned the approach Alison should take to the problem, as key change agent and leader of the ward team. The second planning phase focussed on the detail of what participants wanted to do and involved open, critical debate and democratic decision-making.

During the *action phase*, participants initiated changes that had been agreed by consensus and Alison continued to guide the change process, using the strategy deemed to be most effective. Angie also played an active facilitative role in the action phase, occasionally in a structured way, but more often by talking things through informally with staff when she was around in the ward.

Most of the data for the *observation phase* were collected by Angie, but Alison and other participants also sometimes contributed data. Data collection in relation to the action spirals was focussed. We wanted to find out whether the action was actually occurring as planned and whether it was achieving what we had hoped. We also wanted to know how people were responding to the change and to Alison's approach to guiding and supporting them through it. Thus, during participant observation and interviews, Angie looked out for specific events and asked specific questions.

Like the planning phase, *reflection* usually occurred at two levels: within the reflective conversations and during meetings with participants. In reflective conversations, we discussed the new data relating to a particular spiral in order to assess how the change was progressing and to see whether the action hypothesis was supported. We also considered concurrent phenomenological data to see whether they shed any unanticipated light upon the work associated with the action spiral. Depending upon the results, the strategic plan was refined or developed and the action hypothesis modified or changed. And so another turn of the spiral began. Similarly, with participants, we met to hear their views, to discuss progress and to invite suggestions for revising the action plan. Figure 3.3 summarizes the way in which the action spirals progressed.

A brief outline of the eight spirals that formed the skeleton of the project is given below. The first six spirals dealt with the development of patient-centred nursing in Alison's ward, Oriel Ward. The last two spirals ran in parallel to the others and grew out of the work of the Medical Sisters' Group.

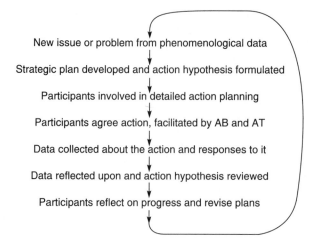

New issue or problem from phenomenological data

Strategic plan developed and action hypothesis formulated

Participants involved in detailed action planning

Participants agree action, facilitated by AB and AT

Data collected about the action and responses to it

Data reflected upon and action hypothesis reviewed

Participants reflect on progress and revise plans

Figure 3.3 *Progression of action research spirals*

Spiral 1: Moving from team nursing to primary nursing

This spiral continued throughout the two years of fieldwork in Oriel Ward. It was conducted in collaboration with all the staff nurses in the ward. When the fieldwork began, the staff nurses had been practising team nursing for nine months, but they were still experiencing many problems working in this way. Primary nursing was an agreed long-term goal, but there was a lot of uncertainty and anxiety about how the system would work in the ward and Alison judged that the nurses were not ready for it. Addressing and studying the transition from one system to another thus emerged as an obvious subject for the first spiral. It was central to the development of patient-centred nursing and a major, very tangible change that all the staff were concerned about.

Much of the work associated with this spiral was to do with the organizational changes described in Chapter 4. But there were also attitudinal and behavioural issues to confront. These are addressed in Chapter 5, along with other changes that occurred in the collective values system, referred to as the ward culture. Alison's overall strategy was to encourage the staff nurses to look critically at the way ward life was organized, to experiment with new ways of working and to take responsibility themselves for developing an effective system to support a patient-centred style of practice. Angie attended staff meetings and 'away days' to collect data, but also to facilitate careful exploration and critical debate of the issues.

Spiral 2: Alison's clinical role in the ward

This spiral was quite unanticipated. It was initiated in response to a strong theme in the phenomenological data showing unhappiness amongst the staff nurses about Alison's clinical involvement in the ward and the way she related to them in practice situations. The nurses found it difficult to adjust to working with a sister whose responsibilities extended beyond the confines of the ward and they found her unpredictable work pattern confusing. As well as showing that Alison needed to renegotiate her clinical role and to rethink the way she balanced her clinical, managerial and research commitments, the data also highlighted serious confusion about the practice development work generally. The strength of feeling and the lack of understanding evident in the data precipitated the first 'away days' (see Chapter 4), which provided the nurses with time and freedom for a level of intense, concentrated work together that was impossible within the ward.

The 'away days' allowed for thorough reflection on the data relating to Alison as the ward sister and for detailed collaborative planning of how her role should develop. This work paved the way for a dramatic improvement in the staff nurses' relationship with Alison, which was reflected in subsequent data. Angie's role as facilitator was particularly crucial in the early part of this spiral of work, because Alison herself was seen as part of the problem and she was also being used as a scapegoat for the general unrest in the ward at the time.

Throughout the rest of the fieldwork period, Angie continued to give specific attention to observing Alison's clinical involvement in the ward and to exploring the nurses' responses to her presence. In addition, Alison's role was inter-mittently reviewed at ward meetings and new ideas were discussed, as she continued to refine and develop ways of practising which supported and enhanced the clinical work of the rest of the team. Most of the data relating to this spiral are presented in Chapter 6, but Alison's strategic use of her clinical role, in relation to many aspects of the development, will also be apparent in other chapters.

Spiral 3: New nursing roles

When the staff nurses began seriously to contemplate taking on the roles of primary and associate nurses, the phenomenological data highlighted their anxiety and uncertainty about what would be expected of them. In addition, they disagreed with Alison about which grades of nurses could be primary nurses and this caused a degree of resentment and some hostility towards the change. It gradually became clear that who should be responsible for what, and what each nurse should expect from her colleagues in the new system, was becoming a big issue, warranting a separate spiral of work. Once the staff nurses actually began to practise as primary and associate nurses, other problems emerged relating to the detail of interpreting the new roles and of managing the boundaries between different roles. The team leader roles were also still relatively new in the ward and developing their function and their relationship with team members became another aspect of this spiral of work.

Planning and reflection in relation to this spiral occurred, as a group activity, at 'away days', ward meetings and team leader meetings and, at an individual level, as part of the personal and professional development work that Alison undertook with each staff nurse. A few staff nurses chose to do some very detailed work on their role development by keeping reflective diaries and they contributed material from them as project data. Most of the data for this spiral, however, were collected by Angie during participant observation and interviews. The work on role development is presented in Chapter 4.

It took a long while for the nurses to feel sufficiently comfortable with their new roles for us to consider this spiral complete. We were then able to move on to Spiral 6, which naturally grew out of this structurally orientated work on roles.

Spiral 4: The Care Plan Project

As team nursing enabled the nurses to become more involved with their patients and encouraged them to think more critically about their care, they became increasingly dissatisfied with the conventional care planning framework and documents that were used in the ward. Alison experienced the same frustration with care plans as the staff nurses and she began to experiment with a new framework that grew out of her own reflections upon the process of clinical decision-making. The staff nurses were enthusiastic about this new approach to care planning and they began to use Alison's framework and to help her to develop and refine it.

Eventually, the level of excitement and activity generated by the care planning initiative prompted a new action spiral to trace and support it. Recognizing its potential, and wanting to harness some of the staff nurses' enthusiasm, Alison bid for local funding to support their involvement in further development of this work. The funding was used to release two staff nurses from clinical work for three months. With supervision and support from us, they were able to become researchers in their own ward, studying the care plan development. They observed and interviewed their colleagues, collecting data on how the nurses had felt about the orthodox care planning system and on how they perceived and were using the new system. Analysis of these data led to further refinements of the new approach. Once the formal part of the staff nurses' project was complete, they both continued, back in practice, to take a special interest in care planning and Angie continued, to the end of the fieldwork period, to collect occasional data relating to the use of the new system.

The substantial amount of work associated with the care planning initiative, and the high profile it had in the ward, gave it a life and identity of its own. It came to be seen more as a small, separate research study than as a spiral of work within the main project. One might say that this spiral spun off into an orbit of its own! (The Care Plan Project is not reported in this book.)

Spiral 5: Ward round behaviour

As the team nursing system developed in Oriel Ward, patterns of communication and decision-making changed. The central co-ordinating role of the 'nurse in charge' diminished and eventually disappeared, as team nurses gradually took over the total management of their own patients' care (see Chapter 4). This decentralization of the daily functioning of ward nursing had major implications for the relationship between nurses and doctors. In addition, as the nurses' focus became more patient-centred, they were conscious of differences in the values and perspectives of the two disciplines, which they had not had to confront in the past. Increasingly, frustration, anxiety and anger were apparent in the nurses' stories about ward rounds collected in the phenomenological data.

Thus, a spiral of work was undertaken with the staff nurses, helping them to negotiate changes in the organization of ward rounds, to explore and understand the interdisciplinary tensions and to try to develop more collaborative relationships with doctors. Alison's strategic role in managing these changes was examined, and she developed her practical role in setting an appropriate example through her own interactions with medical staff. Angie collected data for this spiral of work by observing ward rounds and by interviewing nurses, doctors and patients about their experiences of ward rounds (see Chapter 8).

Spiral 6: Becoming a patient-centred practitioner

This spiral developed at a late stage of the fieldwork, but it was a very important one – in a sense, the crowning glory of the study. For the staff nurses, the work associated with this spiral was a continuation of their role development work. As they became more comfortable with their new responsibilities as primary nurses, they were more concerned with the detail of their actual practice. They found that their greater involvement with patients and families was often very challenging and that their knowledge and creativity were being tested as they increasingly recognized the underlying complexity of many clinical problems.

Alison was very aware of the primary nurses' need for support and guidance from her as an expert practitioner. Trying to help them, she became conscious that much of her own knowledge, about the art of patient-centred practice, had developed intuitively over many years. While both Alison and the staff nurses recognized this style of work when they saw or experienced it, they often found it hard to describe or talk about in any detail.

This spiral was initiated to help the staff nurses to use their new roles, and the whole new system in the ward, to achieve a genuinely patient-centred style of practice. In reflective conversations, Angie helped Alison to analyse and articulate her own practice 'know-how'. Alison, in turn, taught the staff nurses to reflect critically and analytically upon the details of their work with patients and families. This work yielded rich data, mostly in the form of clinical stories recounted to Angie by Alison and the staff nurses, but also sometimes written down by the nurses in reflective diaries or as case studies. Angie watched the nurses at work with their patients, joined their bedside handover rounds and listened to them discussing clinical problems. She also explored the experience of patient-centred practice in interviews with patients, relatives, nurses, health professionals and doctors. These data provided a basis for articulating the elements of the largely hidden art of patient-centred nursing.

Most of the work associated with this spiral is reported in Chapter 7, but the account of the development of clinical supervision in the ward, in Chapter 6, is closely related.

Spiral 7: The changing role of the sister

Soon after her appointment to the Medical Unit, Alison suggested that all the medical ward sisters should meet regularly. At first, Alison acted as facilitator for the Medical Sisters' Group and used its meetings as the main forum for her informal work as practice development adviser. However, her aim was to encourage the group to function as a peer group, sharing experiences and tackling common problems together. Thus, from a strategic point of view, this spiral was concerned with Alison's work within the peer group and facilitating its development. Reflective conversations were used to discuss the group dynamics and, for example, to consider ways of increasing participation or of promoting collaborative work.

From the time the group was formed until the end of the fieldwork period, Angie attended its meetings to collect observational data about Alison's work with the other sisters and, often, to help facilitate group processes. In addition, Angie offered to act as facilitator and data collector for a spiral of work initiated by the sisters, if they wished to use the action research process and to contribute to the study. A major theme emerging in the group's discussions, was the degree to which their roles as ward sisters were changing as a result of the development of a decentralized team or primary nursing system. In particular, the sisters were experiencing difficulties because doctors were still expecting them to behave in the traditional manner. The tasks of clarifying their new roles and of finding ways to reshape their medical colleagues' expectations thus became the focus of an action spiral, which was worked through in collaboration with the medical sisters.

Spiral 8: The staff nurse support group

The Medical Sisters' Group also initiated this spiral, or rather they 'commissioned' it. They felt that the educational opportunities available locally, to help staff nurses as primary nurses, were directed more towards the E and F grade nurses, than towards the junior D grades. They suggested that Angie might help to fill this gap by drawing upon her previous experience with problem-based learning and setting up a professional development group, open to D grade nurses in the medical wards. Angie recognized that this opportunity would not only allow her to make a specific, active contribution to the unit's practice development work, but that it would also give her a chance to study, at close quarters, the problems that junior staff nurses faced in trying to adapt to, and develop for themselves, a more patient-centred style of practice.

During the course of the project, a total of forty enthusiastic D grade staff nurses, from across the Medical Unit, participated in two support groups, but at any one meeting there were usually only around half a dozen nurses. The nurses worked as a group of reflective practitioners, determining the issues they wished to consider and planning exploratory work to get them started. At monthly meetings, they reflected together on their findings and developed or revised their action plans. Angie facilitated the group and also recorded her observations of its progress. The group work was problematic because it was constantly disrupted by participants' irregular attendance, inevitable because of shift work. In reflective conversations, we discussed strategies that Angie might use to maintain focus and momentum in such an unstable group. The emergent findings are reported in Chapter 5.

THE RESEARCH PARTNERSHIP

Our partnership was designed to combine the best of both the 'insider' and the 'outsider' models of action research. There was a division of labour which made the large-scale project manageable but, by each of us contributing to both the action and the research, these two elements of the work remained well integrated.

Alison's role was mainly that of 'actor'. As senior sister in the Medical Unit, she was in a good position to function effectively as the key change agent for the project. She was familiar with the setting and had a legitimate and influential involvement with everyday practice. Less of Alison's time was devoted to the 'researcher' part of her role, but she functioned as project leader, steering every aspect of the study and sharing the detailed tasks of data analysis and final report writing. She also made a minor contribution to data collection.

Complementing Alison's role, Angie worked mainly as 'researcher'. She was responsible for developing the theoretical perspective of the study and for developing data collection, analysis and interpretation strategies. She also actually collected most of the data. With no service responsibilities, Angie was free to take time away from the practice setting to devote to reading the literature and exploring methodological issues in depth. She produced working papers and project reports and wrote the first drafts of papers for joint publication. Angie's 'actor' role was less prominent than Alison's, but she made a significant contribution to the development, mostly through facilitation work. During her fieldwork, she often facilitated spontaneous group discussions or individual nurses' reflections. In addition, she sometimes played a formal role as facilitator in workshops and meetings.

We both experienced the partnership as personally supportive and stimulating. It allowed us to share the excitement of new ideas and challenges, as well as the many problems. We were also able to use it directly to benefit the development work. For example, having two voices, rather than one, to disseminate information and discuss ideas was valuable, as frequent access to all participants was difficult because of shift work. Angie learned to fill gaps in people's knowledge and to reiterate or explain messages that Alison had been trying to convey to staff. Similarly, we both learned to act as 'stooges' for each other in meetings or workshops, particularly when dealing with sensitive matters, with one of us asking a question or raising an issue which was difficult for the other to do.

The partnership was not without its problems and pitfalls. Because of the intensity and immediacy of the 'action' there were difficulties in balancing the partnership fairly and the 'research' clearly lost out at times. Because of the very close working relationship there was the risk of confusing personal confidences with stories that were legitimate data, and confidentiality had to be checked constantly. Furthermore, there was a danger of Angie, in her data collector role, being perceived by staff as 'Alison's spy'. Avoiding this suspicion required absolute integrity from us both in dealing with the data and total consistency in responding constructively to the honesty and openness of the staff. (Discussions of the strengths and weaknesses of the research partnership are presented elsewhere – see Titchen and Binnie, 1993d and e).

DATA COLLECTION METHODS

The research was concerned with the behaviour and the perceptions of people involved in ward life during a period of major change. Data were therefore required about what people did and what they thought and felt, at different stages during the course of the project. The process of managing the change process was also of interest, so we needed a record of the change strategies employed by Alison and the decisions and actions taken by other participants involved in the development work. The three main methods used to capture these data were participant observation, depth interviews and reflective conversations. Documentary evidence provided supplementary data. This data triangulation (i.e. the use of multiple sources and methods to collect data about a particular situation) increased the accuracy and completeness of the data and enhanced the validity of the study (Denzin, 1978).

Most of the data were collected by Angie, but a degree of investigator triangulation was achieved by Alison also providing observational data and by staff nurses contributing diary material. Thus, data relating to some of the same events or issues were collected by different people, again to strengthen validity.

Participant observation

As the project's researcher, Angie participated in ward life, interacting with staff by informally chatting to them, helping them to think through problems or assisting them with simple tasks such as bed-making. However, everyone knew that her main purpose in being there was to observe what was happening and to collect data. Her role was that of 'observer as participant' (Denzin, 1978). She sat in the ward staff-room during breaks and while nurses talked about their work, she joined bedside handover rounds, 'shadowed' individual nurses, or located herself at the nurses' station or in one of the patient bays. Similarly, at meetings, while she sometimes contributed information and ideas, or helped to facilitate debate, her main function was that of observer.

Having observed a particular event, Angie often tried to follow it up with a short, focussed conversation with a key participant. For example, having observed a nurse participating in a ward round, she might take the opportunity at coffee time to ask her what she had been trying to achieve on the round and how she had felt about it. Similarly, when 'shadowing' Alison, she might follow her into the sluice and use the moment's privacy to ask her about an interaction she had just observed, posing questions such as: 'What were you thinking just then?' or 'Why did you decide to do that?'. Thus, the recording of what was happening on the ward was enriched by concurrent accounts of participants' interpretations of events and the thinking behind their actions.

As the nurses got to know and trust Angie, they would often approach her spontaneously and volunteer stories about what was happening in the ward, or about their own practice, because they thought they would be of interest to her. Angie would subsequently write up the stories in her fieldnotes, check them with the nurses concerned and confirm that she had permission to use them as data.

The design of the study required Angie to collect two different types of data. In relation to the action spirals, she was looking for particular events or behaviours and noting participants' responses to initiatives that had been agreed. This kind of observation was guided by specific questions: for example, 'How do nurses react when Alison challenges their clinical decisions?', 'How much do nurses involve their patients during bedside handovers?' and 'What contribution are nurses making to ward rounds?'. On the other hand, in relation to the phenomenological aspect of the study, Angie was required to be alert to the unexpected, to watch and listen with an open mind. This kind of observation was most easily managed when she was simply 'sitting around' in the ward, attending in a very general way to anything and everything, and during informal conversations prompted by open questions such as, 'How are things going in the ward?' and 'How are you getting on with your new patient?' It was common for Angie to have to switch from one observational mode to the other, or sometimes to use both almost simultaneously – posing quite a challenge.

Over the course of two and a quarter years, Angie spent over 400 hours in participant observation. Alison's contribution to the participant observation was less formalized and impossible to measure, because it was subsumed within her role as senior sister. She took the role of 'participant as observer' (Denzin, 1978). In this respect, she often made a mental note of events or conversations that she recognized as relevant data. She reported these observations to Angie who recorded them in the fieldnotes or on tape.

Angie recorded fieldnotes as she observed, or as soon as was convenient after an incident or a conversation. Factual narrative was written on the left-hand pages of a large notebook. If additional material about an incident came to light later, it was added on the right-hand page opposite the initial data. Reflections, interpretations and methodological notes were also recorded on the right-hand page, in brackets. This system maintained a distinction between factual statements of what was observed and Angie's initial interpretations.

After a period of observation, nurses were invited to read fieldnotes referring to them, and any associated reflections. For validation purposes, they were asked to correct the descriptions, if necessary, and to comment upon Angie's interpretations. They were also invited to add further interpretation of their own.

As well as helping to keep track of each action spiral as it progressed, the many volumes of fieldnotes provided, in retrospect, a series of vivid, detailed snapshots of ward life during the peiod of change.

Depth interviews

Angie conducted a total of 141 interviews during the fieldwork period: 54 for the exploratory work and 87 for the main part of the project.

Interview subjects were selected using non-probability judgement sampling, that is, they were chosen, by virtue of their status or experience, as people likely to be able to contribute information or opinions relevant to particular aspects of the study (Burgess, 1984). Apart from seven staff nurses who were interviewed several times, each participant was interviewed only once. The different groups interviewed (with the number of interviews held in brackets) were: key people in the Health Authority to capture the context of the study (12); staff nurses (54); sisters (12); doctors (14); patients (25); relatives (2); health professionals (8); student nurses (6); nursing auxiliaries (2); nurse educators (2); ward clerk (1); liaison sister (1); service manager (1); and visiting sister (1).

Most interviews were initiated because data were being sought in relation to a particular spiral of work and participants were interviewed once to capture their views at that particular time. However, to help gain a longitudinal perspective of the change process, five staff nurses, of different grades, contributed a series of interviews at intervals during the main study. These staff nurses were selected because they were likely to remain in post throughout the project. In fact, one left the ward early in the fieldwork and another left half way through, but two more staff nurses replaced them. These seven staff nurses contributed a total of 25 interviews between them, over a two year period.

Most interviews lasted between 45 minutes and an hour and the majority were audio-taped and transcribed in full by secretarial staff. Interviews were only loosely structured and were designed to allow participants to talk at length about their thoughts and feelings in relation to the changes being made in the ward. As with her observation, Angie's mode of questioning during interviews varied according to the type of data she was seeking. To explore participants' experiences of what was happening in the ward and to allow them to raise issues of concern to them, Angie asked open questions, such as, 'How are you finding things in the ward?' She also encouraged participants to tell stories of their experiences, adapting a technique Benner (1984) found valuable in her phenomenological work. On the other hand, to explore a particular problem, or to follow up responses to a particular change, open questions were still used, but they were focussed on a specific topic; for example, 'Could you tell me about your experiences of taking primary patients for the first time?' In both modes of questioning, Angie used techniques for probing and clarification, and she made a point of reflecting back participants' responses for validation and to give them an opportunity to expand, clarify or interpret what they had said.

If a participant raised an issue during an interview which Angie felt she should respond to, she made a mental note and then, at the end of the interview, she would switch from 'researcher mode' to 'actor mode'. For example, when a doctor demonstrated that he had misunderstood the philosophy underpinning the nursing development work, Angie explained it to him at the end of the interview. Similarly, when a staff nurse reported having difficulty handling a particular situation, Angie returned to the problem at the end of the interview to facilitate some reflection and to help the nurse consider possible solutions.

The interviews yielded enormously rich data. As transcripts became available, they were used to inform the action strategies. Taken together at the end of the project, they made the most substantial contribution of all the data to the theoretical understanding of the development process.

Reflective conversations

A total of 20 reflective conversations were recorded. The reflective conversations were used to maintain the momentum of the action spirals. They were intense, 2–3 hour periods of discussion, in which we reflected upon progress, identified new areas of work and planned strategies for moving things forward. The function of these conversations was therefore not primarily data collection but, as they were audio-taped, a lot of relevant material that Alison added during the reflection phase was recorded. The decisions that we made and our initial tentative theorizing about the change process were also captured as data.

Documentary evidence

Written material relevant to the project work was collected, with permission from appropriate individuals when necessary. The documents included: nursing philosophy statements – for the ward and for the District; formal reports or proposals – submitted by the Medical Sisters' Group or by individual sisters to nursing administration or general management; ward information sheets; noticeboard material; minutes of meetings – from the Medical Sisters' Group meetings, ward meetings and team leader meetings; material from the ward communication book; letters – from senior hospital staff; and 'thank you' letters – from patients and relatives.

Personal accounts of experiences in the ward, during the life of the project, also provided valuable data. These accounts included reports from visiting nurses and a visiting researcher and essays written by staff nurses. Six nurses also kept reflective diaries, for varying periods, and offered them as data. Three of these nurses recorded their transition from team nurse to primary nurse, one wrote about her experiences as a new staff nurse in the ward, another about patient situations she found difficult and another about how Alison helped her to develop patient-centred nursing skills.

PRACTICAL RESEARCH ISSUES

Access

Following ethical approval from the Health Authority's Nursing Research Committee, formal permission for the project to proceed was granted by the Director of Nursing. Access to Alison's ward was straightforward, because she was the local gatekeeper. The project was explained to the staff nurses as something that would help them achieve the changes they wanted to make in the ward. Once the nursing team as a whole had agreed that the development work should proceed, opting out of the project entirely was not an option for individual staff nurses, unless they chose to leave the ward. However, the degree to which they actively participated was negotiable.

The sister of Linacre Ward, the other ward in Alison's unit, was invited to participate. She consented to have the initial case study undertaken in her ward, because she recognized that it could help her to achieve changes she wished to pursue. The staff nurses in Linacre Ward became involved through the sister, in the same way that the staff nurses in Alison's ward became involved through her.

Access to the Medical Sisters' Group was achieved by Alison inviting Angie to the group's second meeting, where the aims of the project and its potential value to the group were explained. The sisters granted permission for Angie to attend their meetings.

Participation

Active participation in the project was variable and in some cases rather confused, probably as a result of the way the project was set up and managed, and the initial methodological uncertainties. Many participants saw the action (the changes within the wards) and the research (the collection, analysis and use of data) as quite separate activities, rather than as parts of the same action research project. They tended to see the research as 'Alison and Angie's project' and to see themselves as willing but passive subjects, rather than as participants in the research. In retrospect, this perception was hardly surprising, given that the project team, which planned the outline of the project and took the major methodological decisions as it proceeded, consisted of only ourselves and the Director of the National Institute for Nursing, who acted as supervisor. Had we had a clearer understanding of the critical social science approach to action research at the beginning of the project, and a full appreciation of the notion of collaborating groups of practitioners engaging in action research (Carr and Kemmis, 1986), we would have started rather differently. For example, the sister of Linacre Ward, another of the medical sisters and one or two of the staff nurses in Alison's ward could have joined the project team. Closer involvement of representatives of participating groups in the overall management of the project might have lessened the perceived split between the action and the research.

As the project progressed, the participants collaborated more actively. The best example of the nurses becoming fully involved in researching, as well as changing, their own practice was in the Care Plan Project (Spiral 4). Here the two staff nurses took key roles in every stage of the action research cycle. The medical sisters initially welcomed Angie to their meetings purely as an observer, but later, when their work on the changing role of the ward sister became established as an action research spiral (Spiral 7), they participated actively in the research as well as the action elements of the work. The setting up of annual ward 'away days' helped the staff nurses to become more actively involved in the main study in Oriel Ward. These days provided a forum in which data could be fed back, reflected upon and debated by the whole nursing team and in which the nurses could use the data as a basis for action planning. The greater familiarity with the project gained at the 'away days' seemed to spill over into everyday ward life and to encourage greater participation thereafter.

Confidentiality

Confidentiality and anonymity were maintained within the project as far as was possible given the nature of the work. The specific limits of confidentiality and anonymity were explained to each participant as they affected her or him.

In reporting the work, we have changed the names of the two wards involved but, as they are known to be the two wards in Alison's unit, their identity will be obvious to local people. All the staff, patients and relatives were given fictitious names, which ensures anonymity for most of them. However, a few staff will be identifiable locally because of their prominent roles. This position was made clear to the individuals concerned when they were interviewed or observed.

When staff nurses were interviewed, or when they told Angie stories during her observation periods, they were assured that their data would remain confidential within the project. Angie specifically asked the nurses for permission to share their data with Alison and, without exception, they gave it. The frankness of the staff nurses' interview data, which at times included strong criticism of Alison, and their relaxed behaviour in Angie's presence suggested that they were not inhibited by Alison's access to the data. When data were fed back to participants, the identity of contributors was obscured, unless prior permission had been gained to share their data.

It was often possible to feed back data of a sensitive nature in a supportive way, helping those concerned to deal constructively with the issues that had been raised. A few times, in the interests of future working relationships, we judged that it was wiser not to feed back the data, or to delay the feedback until a time when it would not be too damaging.

BIAS

The project was undertaken from a value-committed position. Alison had a vision of a patient-centred style of practice, which was supported by senior nurses within the Health Authority and the Institute. She believed that this style of practice could best be developed within a primary nursing system and under a democratic form of leadership. Angie came to the project believing in a style of health care that embraced the values implicit in patient-centred nursing and, from her educational background, she brought a commitment to a learner-centred approach to professional development.

Given our biased starting position, we set out to develop an account of the change process, and people's experiences of it, in as honest a way as possible. We attempted to reduce the effects of our bias in four specific ways. First, during data collection, we tried to maintain an open, non-judgemental attitude to whatever opinions and perceptions were expressed. Second, fieldnotes and interview transcripts were given to participants to read and to correct, interpret or add to. Third, we tried to remain conscious of our own standpoint, so that we could put it on one side and be alert to that of others. Finally, we have made our values public – here and in other publications – so that the trustworthiness and plausibility of our work can be judged in the light of the inevitable bias that must remain, in spite of our attempts to limit it.

DATA ANALYSIS AND THEORY GENERATION

The exploratory case study

Detailed discussion of the phenomenological approach used to analyse the case study data is presented elsewhere (Titchen and McIntyre, 1993). The steps of the analysis process are summarized in Figure 3.4.

The case study highlighted two complex issues that arise when the organization of ward nursing begins to be decentralized. First, there is a major role change for staff nurses, which can be confusing and traumatic (Titchen and Binnie, 1993b). Second, there is a fundamental change in the relationship between the staff nurses and the ward sister, which is again potentially confusing and uncomfortable for both parties (Titchen and Binnie, 1993a). The theoretical insights into these issues, gained from the case study, informed our response to problems that arose early in the main study.

The data analysis procedure developed for the case study provided a model that was adapted for the major, retrospective analysis conducted at the end of the main study.

The main study

Two different approaches were used to analyse data in the main study, each for a different purpose. First, during the fieldwork period, we made a fairly crude, impressionistic analysis of data in order to inform, and subsequently evaluate, our decisions and actions in managing developments in the ward – the *concurrent*

- *Immersion in the data*
  Reading and re-reading the data relating to six nurses; repeated listening to their audio-tapes.

- *Development of first order constructs*
  Identification of issues raised and views presented, capturing them in concise phrases and using the language of participants.

- *Development of second order constructs*
  Conceptualization of first order constructs in broader, more abstract terms, using the language of social science. For example, statements such as 'I'm confused', 'what the hell am I meant to be doing?' (identified as first order constructs) suggested that 'role ambiguity' (the second order construct) was a key issue for participants.

- *Validation of second order constructs*
  Reconstruction of participants' accounts in a concise form, using the second order constructs; presentation of these interpretations of the data to participants to check accuracy.

- *Development of themes and construction of a theoretical framework*
  Identification of second order constructs occurring repeatedly within and across cases as common themes; development of a theoretical framework identifying likely relationships between the eight emergent themes.

- *Testing the theoretical framework*
  Testing the initial theoretical framework against all the remaining data; assessment of the 'fit' of new material within the theoretical framework (does this work here; do boundaries have to be extended or made narrower; are new themes needed?); validation of procedures and interpretations by two research colleagues.

- *Final validation*
  A distillation of the findings written around the refined theoretical framework; presentation of this account to nurses involved; further discussion of issues raised.

Figure 3.4 *Steps of the analysis process*

analysis. Second, at the end of the fieldwork, we undertook a *retrospective analysis*, returning to all the data and analysing it as a whole, in a much more rigorous and systematic way. (Further discussion of our approach to data analysis, and the literature that influenced it, are included in Titchen and McIntyre, 1993; and Titchen and Binnie, 1994.)

The concurrent analysis formed an integral part of each action spiral. It occurred during reflective conversations. We read the raw data from the preceding period of fieldwork before meeting. Then we discussed our initial impressions of the data, noting how people were responding to changes that had already been made and identifying new issues and concerns. We refined our initial impressions by comparing our individual responses to the data, returning to the data to check things out when necessary and exploring specific issues further. From this detailed discussion, we could draw conclusions about which aspects of the development work were progressing successfully, which were problematic and where attention was needed.

This process of concurrent analysis allowed us to formulate and test *action hypotheses*. These were proposals for action which we anticipated would initiate, support or guide a desired change. We planned data collection to record the effects of the action. Subsequent analysis of these data enabled us to judge whether a hypothesis had been falsified, whether it needed refining, or whether it stood up as a valid proposition. The formulation and testing of action hypotheses was the first stage of generating theory about effective strategies for managing the development of a patient-centred nursing service.

The retrospective analysis was a mammoth task. It began with detailed work which involved analysing the interview transcripts of the seven nurses who had been studied longitudinally and selecting out and analysing any fieldnote data that related to them. We worked independently on this material, in order to cross-check the analyses and ensure a consistent approach. We followed the first three steps of the case study analysis process (see Figure 3.4).

From this intimate contact with a sample of the data spanning the whole period of fieldwork, we were able to identify and label 144 themes which occurred in 72 pairs, each pair representing opposite poles of a continuum. Recollection of one theme, such as 'work perceived as a slog' or 'deep relationships with patients', prompted us to recall a strand of data representing the opposite, such as 'work perceived as a challenge' and 'superficial relationships with patients'. One set of themes characterized the perceptions and experiences of participants during the early days of the fieldwork, while the opposite set of themes characterized some movement towards, or achievement of, quite different perceptions and experiences later in the development.

Eventually, the 72 pairs of themes were grouped as six grand themes. The first grand theme embraced everything associated with the organizational aspects of ward life and the second, everything associated with the ward culture, its norms and values. The third grouped all the themes related to Alison's leadership in the ward and the fourth combined the themes associated with doctor–nurse relationships. The fifth drew together everything concerned with the nurses' actual practice, involving their work with patients and families. Finally, the sixth grand theme included themes relating to the development of the Medical Sisters' Group and the work the group undertook. As these grand themes emerged, we conceptualized them as representing different aspects of the nurses' complex transition or 'journey', from traditional practice to patient-centred practice. It seemed that this broad, central journey was made up of several specific journeys, which all had to be negotiated at the same time. They became:

- The organizational journey
- The cultural journey
- The leadership journey
- The doctor–nurse journey
- The practice journey
- The medical sisters' journey.

The six journeys, each with a series of paired themes, provided the initial theoretical framework for developing an account of the change process. We tested and refined this initial framework by applying it to all the data. This was a long and painstaking process, the theoretical framework being either supported or modified as it was challenged by each piece of data. After two months of working together at this task, the framework was fairly robust and standing up well to the data. The six journeys remained as the core structure of the framework, but our refinement of the themes had reduced them to 47 pairs.

We prepared an outline of each 'journey' in chart form. Then we identified the strategies we had used to stimulate and guide the transition from each 'starting point' to each 'end-point'. This was relatively easy because we were so steeped in the data and we had lived through the development work ourselves. We shared the initial writing of the 'journey' chapters between us and then exchanged drafts for critical comment. In a further attempt to validate our theorization of the 'journeys', we sent drafts to some of the nurses who had been involved in the project and asked them to comment on the faithfulness of our account.

Finally, we considered the journeys together and identified three strong, overarching themes running across them. We were able to draw out a number of *theoretical principles* which may guide others engaged in similar work. These principles are general statements about the approach to change that we found effective. As Brown and McIntyre (1981) emphasize, principles developed from action research in this way cannot be assumed to be necessarily valid. However, the principles can be said to be hypothetically valid and useful for further work.

GENERALIZING FROM THIS STUDY

Action research is a qualitative research strategy. It involves the study of particular individuals in a particular situation; they are not claimed to be representative of any broader population. Findings cannot therefore be generalized on the basis of probability theory, as they can from experimental research. However, opportunities for generalizing to other settings may arise in two different ways and both are relevant to this study.

First, where the findings and the emergent theoretical ideas are supported by similar findings in other empirical work or by social science theory, then some generalization elsewhere is likely. It is worth emphasizing though, that it is the abstract account that will be generalizable, and not the *specific* data in which it is grounded.

Second, by providing a detailed picture of the project setting and a rich description of the change process studied, it should be possible for readers to make comparisons with their own settings, problems and experiences. Readers may then judge for themselves the degree to which the findings and the 'theorization' fit their own situations. Presenting this study in seminars and workshops, we have found that many nurses readily recognize situations that we describe and identify with the experiences of participants. This provides some confidence that our project findings will be of relevance to a wide audience of nurses.

Part Two

Chapter 4

The organizational journey

'The ultimate solution must be a restructuring of the system of work organization and nurse training ... For example, one might try systems of ward organization which give nurses more continuous and intensive contact with patients; this would require new techniques for dealing with the stress that would arise initially.'

Menzies (1960, p. 16)

INTRODUCTION

Work organization methods can either help or hinder the achievement of a particular style of nursing. By providing the boundaries within which individual nurses operate, they create or limit the opportunities each nurse has to function in particular ways. In this chapter, we trace the introduction and development of an organizational system designed to give nurses both the freedom and the support they need to practise in a patient-centred way.

The two central themes of the organizational journey are 'decentralization' and 'role development'. Manthey (1980) argued that *'decentralized decision making seems . . . to be the organizational framework within which humane treatment of the sick can most effectively be provided and maintained'* (p. xvii). If work is predictable, repetitive and fairly simple, then it seems reasonable for a central authority to design standard procedures for relatively unskilled workers to perform. When applied to nursing, it follows that if the nurse's work is perceived as no more than a series of practical tasks (such as washing, toileting, bed-making, temperature-taking) then it is reasonable for a central administration to establish rules and procedures for patient care, to be carried out by a nursing workforce of junior and unqualified grades. If, on the other hand, nursing is recognized as a complex activity, addressing an infinitely variable array of human problems and experiences and demanding intelligent, sensitive, creative responses, then each practitioner must have the authority and the skill to make a fresh decision in each clinical situation. It follows from this argument that a decentralized organizational system in the hospital ward is a prerequisite for the achievement of a patient-centred style of nursing.

Devolving authority for decision-making from the centre to individual nurses immediately changes the roles of both practitioners and managers. Each group has a new contribution to make within the organization, new skills are required and new relationships need to be negotiated with colleagues at every level. While the primary nursing literature gives an outline of what the new nursing roles are in a decentralized system, it says little about how nurses with a traditional background can be helped to develop these new roles, or about the difficulties that they are likely to encounter in the process. Our project data show that taking on new roles in a decentralized system can, at first, be confusing and difficult and that it takes time and careful facilitation to help nurses become comfortable with the scope and the boundaries of their new authority. This chapter focusses upon the development of primary and associate nurse roles.

Resource implications

The potential of any method of work organization is limited by the resources available. The main resource required to provide a twenty-four hour nursing service is obviously nurses, but exactly how many nurses are needed to run any particular service, and what grade they should be, are difficult questions. Certain principles guided the structuring of nursing teams in our study wards:

- Only *registered* nurses are legally recognized as qualified to manage the total nursing care of patients.
- In an acute hospital ward, where patients may be in an unstable condition and new nursing decisions have to be made every shift, direct patient care should be provided by qualified nurses.
- Nursing auxiliaries should only be employed to *assist* qualified staff with direct patient care, and to relieve them of housekeeping and clerical work.

Starting with these principles, Alison's earlier work (Binnie, 1987) had made a case for employing a high proportion of registered nurses in acute hospital wards. While the case was argued primarily on professional grounds, the rich skill-mix was also shown to be cost-effective. Given the small pay differential at that time between qualified and unqualified staff, replacing auxiliaries with staff nurses, within a fixed budget, resulted in a very small reduction in numbers being exchanged for a considerable increase in skill. Now that qualified nurses are significantly more expensive than auxiliaries or health care assistants, the economic case is, at first sight, harder to sustain. However, experience has shown that the direct involvement of a qualified nurse in each patient's care, on every shift, seems to speed up decision-making and consequently increases the throughput of patients. This view was supported by an audit report from external consultants (Wilton, 1994), which stated that the hospital's nursing skill-mix appeared to be justified by a relatively low cost per patient episode. Further evidence of the value of a rich skill-mix came from a comprehensive study, carried out across a number of hospitals, by the Centre for Health Economics, University of York (Carr-Hill *et al.*, 1992).

Following Alison's early skill-mix project carried out in the Surgical Unit, other wards in the hospital used opportunities afforded by natural wastage and the transfer of students to supernumerary status gradually to increase the proportion of registered nurses in their nursing teams. Thus, the skill-mix we inherited in the medical wards at the beginning of the project was robust enough to handle a decentralized system. Indeed, the qualified staff were bored and frustrated within the existing system and were eager for more responsibility (Binnie, 1988).

Decentralization cannot occur unless there exists at least a substantial core of registered nurses in the ward team. Just how big that core needs to be can be calculated using the concept of 'caseload size'. Nurses in any ward are likely to be able to state the number of patients one nurse can reasonably be expected to care for on a late shift. They will probably be able to say how many patients they would comfortably like to look after in an ideal world and how many they can actually cope with in the high-pressured, cost-conscious real world. In the study ward – a busy acute medical ward – nurses considered five patients to be their ideal caseload, but up to seven to be realistically possible. In the twenty bed ward, taking six to seven patients as the 'caseload size', in order to devolve authority from the central nurse in charge to the practitioners at the bedside, a minimum of three staff nurses each shift was needed. From this starting point, a rota of three teams of nurses could be built up, each capable of taking total responsibility for its own caseload of patients. In most wards, the core of registered nurses is likely to need supplementing with additional staff to cope with the total workload on the busier shifts (such as weekday mornings and operation or ward round days). Whether these additional staff are qualified nurses, students or auxiliaries/health care assistants, will depend upon the nature of the ward's nursing work. How many additional staff are needed, and when, can be estimated fairly accurately by nurses in the ward. In addition, dependency studies are useful for validating these judgements and for fine-tuning the match between workload and numbers of staff available.

It was not our intention to provide a blueprint for the staffing levels required to run a patient-centred nursing service. Every ward is different and staffing needs should be assessed locally. However, it is important to start such an exercise with a picture of the kind of nursing service that is to be delivered and with clear principles outlining how qualified staff should be used within the service. Manthey (1980, p. xv) points out very firmly that primary nursing will not solve staffing or skill-mix problems and argues that the system should not be used to justify increased expenditure. However, it is quite likely that attempts to devolve decision-making in a ward – to small nursing teams or to primary nurses – will highlight existing funding or skill-mix problems and these need to be resolved before development work can proceed.

DECENTRALIZING THE SYSTEM

Establishing a decentralized nursing system is the key organizational development required to facilitate the delivery of patient-centred nursing. If nursing decisions are to be tailored to the specific needs of individual patients and made, whenever possible, with their involvement, then the authority for making those decisions must rest with the individual nurse caring for each patient. If decisions about nursing care are to be truly patient-centred, nurses with authority to make decisions must have the opportunity to form a relationship with each of their patients and to observe them closely. In other words, the size of each nurse's caseload must not be too big to allow her close personal contact with each of her patients and at least some direct involvement in their care. Furthermore, if nurses are to address more than just their patients' immediate needs each shift – if they are to plan and manage their nursing in a comprehensive way – then they must be assured continuity of contact and involvement throughout each patient's stay in hospital.

Thus, three essential features of a decentralized nursing system at ward level are:

● Authority for decision-making devolved to nurses at the bedside.
● Predictable continuity of care.
● A manageable caseload size.

The 'ends' system

At the beginning of the project, Alison had already started to develop a team nursing system in the study ward, but it was in its early stages and the nurses could readily recall the previous system and, indeed, were still much influenced by it. The nurses described the earlier method of work organization as patient allocation, but in fact it was an impure form that fell somewhere between patient allocation and team nursing without continuity. On each shift, the sister, or in her absence one of the more senior staff nurses, had been 'in charge'. Dividing the ward geographically in half, the rest of the nurses had then been allocated to work at either one 'end' or the other. For morning shifts, there had usually been two nurses at each 'end' and in the evenings, only one. An attempt had generally been made to allow nurses to work at the same 'end' for several consecutive shifts, but because the duty rota had not been arranged with continuity in mind, this could not be guaranteed and was not predictable. Consequently, nurses could never plan their work with a particular patient beyond the present shift and relationships were always at risk of being interrupted.

'Doing the baths'

Lack of any predictable continuity of care had inevitably limited the focus of the nurses at the bedside. Their main concern had been the completion of practical tasks which were structured informally by a ward routine determining roughly when things should be done: first baths, then 'obs', drugs, lunches, and so on. Looking back, the nurses recognized how restricting the system had been.

In the old system, when a nurse didn't have ultimate responsibility for a patient, you didn't get so involved. (Sophie)

In patient allocation, you never looked after the patient long enough to get the whole picture. (Carol)

Nurses also appreciated that the lack of continuity had sometimes been inefficient.

If you don't look after the same patients every day, there's a longer period of time before you actually realize a lot of things that need to be done. (Carol)

The constraints on the nurse at the bedside had been further compounded by the division of labour built into the old system. While the nurses at the 'ends' had been responsible for providing all the direct 'hands on' care for patients, they had been expected to leave all the planning and co-ordinating of their patients' care, and all communication with relatives and other disciplines involved with their patients, to the nurse in charge. Because information from doctors or from other departments could take some time to filter down to nurses at the bedside, they had often felt they '*didn't really know what was going on*' with their patients. As the people most directly in contact with patients, nurses at the bedside are the people patients are most likely to turn to for information and advice, yet, in the old 'ends' system, these nurses had been particularly ill-equipped to respond to their patients' questions.

The staff nurses reported that, as students, they had been encouraged to think of their patients as a whole. They had been taught that nurses should address their patients' psychological and social needs, as well as providing physical care, and they believed that this was how things should be. Once qualified, however, they had found that the system denied them the opportunity to practise in the way they thought they should and gave them little chance to use much of the knowledge and skill they had acquired. Like the new graduates in Kramer's (1968) study, these staff nurses had experienced 'role deprivation'; they had not been fulfilling the roles they had been prepared for and this had frustrated them. As one nurse grumbled, '*Nobody's willing to give you any responsibility.*' In addition, many of the staff nurses working in the old system had almost lost sight of their patients as people and had become bored with the endless rounds of routine tasks.

The frustration and boredom experienced by the nurses while they worked in the 'ends' system, and the sense they had gained from their training that things, at least in theory, could be different, made them open, indeed cautiously eager, for the changes that Alison's arrival in the ward heralded.

Being 'in charge'

Being in charge had been the role reserved for the most senior nurse on duty each shift. The sister had always been in charge when she was on duty, with the more senior staff nurses usually filling the gap when she was not. Junior staff nurses had much less frequently had a chance to be in charge and this was usually at weekends or in the evenings, when nobody more senior was available. Being in charge had carried a lot of responsibility and had not been regarded as boring. It had been a demanding role, but, like the traditional bedside role, it was still not the kind of nursing work the staff nurses believed they had trained for.

The nurse in charge had been responsible for any important clinical decisions that needed to be made during her shift. Much of the patients' care had been determined by ward routine and standard procedures. However, when circum-stances demanded deviation from usual practice, it was the nurse in charge who had generally decided what should be done. This nurse had been expected to keep a supervisory eye on the other nurses, particularly students and auxiliaries, and nurses had reported back to her on how they were progressing with their work and any significant changes in the condition of their patients. Opportunities for 'hands on' patient care had been relatively rare for the nurse in charge. She had been expected to carry out certain technical tasks that juniors were not permitted to perform, such as administering intravenous drugs, but otherwise most of her work had kept her away from the bedside. Being in charge had involved a lot of 'desk work', arranging admissions and discharges, communicating with other departments, dealing with telephone enquiries and so on. It had also meant being the focus for communication with doctors and with other professional staff visiting the ward. Here, though, the nurse in charge had often found herself on unsure ground, for her own lack of clinical involvement meant she was frequently relying on second-hand information when she was discussing a patient's condition. The difficulty in obtaining enough accurate information about patients to do her job really well could be frustrating for the nurse in charge and sometimes embarrassing (Binnie, 1988).

Aspects of being in charge of the ward had been challenging and interesting, but the role contained inherent contradictions which had often made it unsatisfying. It had meant that the most experienced nurse on duty had least contact with patients, and was least accessible to them, and it had meant that the nurse most relied upon to contribute to multidisciplinary decisions could be the least well equipped to do so.

Being in charge had often provided a stimulating change for staff nurses who were tired of the heavier routine work, but when they were frequently in charge, they had missed the patient contact. Changing from one role to the other, as many of them did, meant adjusting constantly to a somewhat disconcerting change of status. As in any classically bureaucratic system, status had been invested in roles rather than in individuals. When in charge, the nurse was important and had authority to make decisions. When she was not in charge, the same nurse slipped a notch down the hierarchy and had to tolerate being less visible and having to ask permission. In this way, the bureaucratically structured 'ends' system had both depersonalized and disempowered the staff nurses. They had not been free to practise as adult professional nurses.

Strategies for creating effective teams

'It is understandable that the nursing service, whose tasks stimulate such primitive and intense anxiety, should anticipate change with unusually severe anxiety. In order to avoid this anxiety, the service tries to avoid change whenever possible, almost, one might say, at all cost, and tends to cling to the familiar even when the familiar has obviously ceased to be appropriate or relevant.' (Menzies, 1970, p. 22)

The climate in the Medical Unit, when Alison took up her post there, was not as rigid or formal as the climate Menzies had experienced in traditional wards in the late 1950s. But the legacy of the carefully ordered bureaucracy, in which each nurse was expected to know her place and to accept it obediently, was still palpable. There was a degree of openness to change and a readiness to accept that it was necessary, but the nurses had no experience of change in their professional world and did not see themselves as having the power to initiate or influence it. As one nurse put it,

I don't think I ever thought about how I could change things . . . because I didn't feel that I was in a situation to do anything about it. (Terry)

Alison began the organizational changes in the ward with a top-down approach. There was an expectation that she would lead the changes and she felt a certain urgency about getting the development started – the ward was unsettled and the staff turnover had been high. The staff nurses' passivity and inexperience in handling change, as well as the absence of any mechanism in the ward for involving them formally in decision-making, also weighed against the more democratic approach that Alison would have preferred. The staff nurses were not particularly enthusiastic about the way the early changes were introduced either, but they went along with them and most were prepared to acknowledge the benefits.

> *It was imposed, we were told exactly what to do . . . it was a case of having to really, but it was alright when it happened. I think it is natural people would be a bit dubious, a bit sceptical . . . but once it was underway and we understood a bit more, it wasn't so bad. But . . . we didn't have much choice over the matter.* (Carol)

Alison's first step was to introduce the organizational framework for the beginning of a team nursing system. Once it was in place, she anticipated that there would be time enough, as the ward team matured, for negotiation about improving and developing it. Another very early top-down initiative was the setting up of a structure in the ward that would allow all the nurses to participate in decision-making, in relation to both patient care and ward management. The purpose of imposing these initial organizational changes was to create the framework for a decentralized system which, as nurses learned to use it, would facilitate the emergence of bottom-up initiatives. Thus, after a couple of years, when the primary nursing system was being formalized, as the final phase of decentralization, the nurses themselves were very actively able to direct the shape and pace of change, using Alison as a sounding-board and consultant – she was no longer simply an authority figure to follow.

Establishing predictable continuity

Dividing the whole ward nursing team into several, smaller, permanently established teams provides the organizational basis for predictable continuity of care. Each team can be given responsibility for the continuous nursing of a group of patients. In this way, the number of patients with whom each nurse works closely is limited to something manageable and, by the same token, each patient is likely to be cared for by only four or five nurses throughout his or her stay in the ward, instead of a potentially much larger number.

Establishing a team nursing system sounds quite easy in theory but, in practice, a whole new set of ground rules may have to be negotiated for managing the duty rota if continuity of care is to be achieved with any degree of consistency. In Oriel Ward, three teams were created. Each team carried a caseload of around six or seven patients – the actual caseload size was managed by calculating a crude total dependency score for each team and allocating each new patient to the team with the lowest score. Each team was made up of five or six full-time nurses, of comparable grade-mix, and one or two part-time nurses. To ensure continuity, the duty rota had to be organized so that there was a minimum of one nurse from each team on duty for every shift, including night duty. In addition, to ensure that appropriate expertise was always available and to provide supervision for junior staff, the grade-mix for each shift had to be balanced across teams (i.e. the team rotas could not be planned in isolation from each other).

Providing continuity within teams placed additional demands on the duty rota and, consequently, the amount of flexibility for staff was less than when the rota was planned for the ward as a whole. Nurses' concerns about reduced flexibility caused some initial resistance to a team rota and prompted some frank discussion in the ward about values and priorities. Alison made a point of responding to grumbles about the rota by bringing the issues behind them into the open for debate. The question of whether the rota should be planned primarily with the patients' or the nurses' interests in mind had to be confronted. The nurses' right to expect a socially acceptable rota was acknowledged, but the notion that it should be infinitely adaptable to every nurse's social calendar was questioned. Compromise had to be agreed. With Alison acting as prompt and facilitator, the following ground rules were negotiated:

- *Holidays:* Only one nurse from each team should be away on holiday at a time; holidays should be planned well in advance.
- *Night duty:* Only one nurse from each team should rotate to night duty at a time; night duty should be planned well in advance. (A few of the nurses worked permanent night duty – some full-time, some part-time. This arrangement reduced the need for other staff to rotate to night duty and so improved continuity on day duty. It also accommodated nurses who preferred night duty and took some pressure off those who did not.)
- *Swapping:* Swapping of individual shifts, or of planned night duty or holiday, should only be negotiated within teams.
- *Sickness:* This should be covered, whenever possible, by adjusting the rota of the team affected; gaps should be filled by staff from other teams, if available, or by bank nurses if not.

In some ward settings, agreeing a fixed core rota may help nurses to plan ahead and may reduce the time spent producing the rota each month. Some wards may be able to improve either continuity or flexibility by adjusting nurses' shift times. In the study ward, neither of these options was attractive to the nurses and, as there were no strong organizational or financial reasons to pursue them, we did not push the nurses to explore these options further. We mention these additional strategies to emphasize the importance of flexibility and an open mind when it comes to duty rotas – anything is worth trying if it promises to improve continuity, looks attractive to staff and is not prohibitively costly. One cannot expect to get all the right answers first time and it is necessary to keep on experimenting until the best possible solution emerges.

Getting the team rota system right is crucial for the development of a patient-centred style of practice. Attempts to establish a team or primary nursing system are easily thwarted by frequently disrupted continuity if nurses do not adequately address the sometimes sensitive issues associated with rota planning.

Devolving decision-making

There are essentially two strands of decision-making in ward nursing: clinical decision-making, associated with the care of individual patients, and managerial decision-making, associated with the running of the ward and the supervision and support of staff. It was always Alison's intention, as the sister ultimately responsible for the ward's nursing service, to retain overall control of the style of clinical and managerial practice developed in the ward, but, within that broad remit, there was considerable scope for involving staff nurses in decision-making of both kinds and for delegating specific responsibilities to them.

Creating team leader roles was an important early step in the process of decentralizing both clinical and managerial decision-making. These roles were designed for experienced senior staff nurses who were familiar with the nursing specialty, committed to the development of patient-centred nursing and ready to begin to make a significant contribution to the ward's management. The first appointments were made from within the ward team, but subsequent vacancies were open to internal and external candidates. Unlike the responsibilities of the traditional nurse-in-charge, which were assumed purely for the duration of a shift, by whichever staff nurse happened to be the most senior present, the responsibilities of the new team leaders were permanent and continuous. They were expected, on a continuing basis, to organize their teams effectively, to guide and oversee the clinical work of their team members and to support their professional development.

Devolving clinical decision-making

The presence of the team leaders facilitated the decentralization of clinical decision-making, which was a gradual process achieved in two distinct phases. Initially, decisions about how individual patients were to be nursed were devolved to teams. Each patient was allocated to a team on admission to the ward and continued to be cared for by that same small group of nurses throughout his or her stay. Plans for the patient's care were proposed or reviewed by individual team members when they looked after him and were discussed with team colleagues at handovers. Key nursing decisions were thus made by consensus within the team. The team leaders, and Alison as sister, monitored the team decisions and intervened to guide and advise, whenever their expertise was needed. This team nursing system provided a comfortable half way stage in the process of decentralization. Nurses at the bedside were no longer simply following routines or obeying directives from the central figure in charge. They were expected to think for themselves about individual patients, whom they now knew much better and with whom they were working on a continuous basis. However, at this stage, individual staff nurses were not expected to carry the full burden of clinical responsibility. They were, as always, accountable for their own contribution and for their individual actions, but the team leaders, by retaining authority for overseeing their teams' clinical work, held the major responsibility for clinical decision-making.

Team nursing provided a structure within which nurses could experience continuity, learn to manage closer relationships with patients and families, and develop creative ideas for more patient-centred care, but all within the protective constraints of shared decision-making and supervision by a team leader. Team nursing was eventually found to have its limitations as a system for promoting patient-centred care. But, at the beginning of the project, it gave nurses the opportunity to develop skills that they would need for more independent practice, without overloading them with responsibility that they were not ready to carry and without exposing patients to unreasonable risk.

The second phase of decentralizing clinical decision-making was the introduction of a primary nursing system. This system was superimposed, as it were, upon the team system. The team structure remained intact but, within it, overall responsibility for managing the nursing care of individual patients was devolved to individual team members. Responsibility for decision-making became no longer a shared team affair, but rather the *personal* responsibility of the primary nurse. The team continued to work together, sharing the daily care of their caseload of patients, but where one nurse took on the role of primary nurse for a patient, her team colleagues acted as her associates. Team leaders, like other team members, took their own primary patients and acted as associates for others. They remained available, as experienced practitioners, to advise and support others and, as associate nurses, they could make suggestions and challenge decisions made by primary nurses, but it was no longer their particular task to oversee all the clinical decision-making within their team. The onus to seek out and use the expertise of more experienced staff was transferred to the primary nurses. As responsible practitioners, primary nurses were not expected to need someone to 'check up' on them, but they were expected to take the initiative to seek out and use the advice of experts in the ward when it was likely to be of benefit to their patients.

A key feature of the strategy to decentralize clinical decision-making was not rushing the process. Having set up the framework of the team system fairly quickly, we waited until the nurses themselves were confident that they were ready for more independent roles. Evidence that they were recognizing the limitations of team nursing and were frustrated by shared responsibility seemed to be a good sign that they were maturing as practitioners and were ready for more individual responsibility. In spite of our very active support of the nurses' development, it took 2 years from the start of team nursing to reach a point where everyone was ready to consider changing to primary nursing. It was nearly another year before the transition was made.

Devolving managerial decision-making

A primary nursing system demands individual staff nurses capable and confident of managing their own practice and making their own clinical decisions. The traditional bureaucratic style of nursing management did not encourage the development of these skills. Indeed, it tended to stifle the intelligent, alert questioning and creativity that this level of autonomy requires (Menzies, 1970; Fretwell, 1980). Our aim was to reverse this process and to create a ward management system which offered opportunities for nurses to think independently. Our strategies for decentralizing clinical decision-making were therefore paralleled by strategies for decentralizing managerial decision-making.

Our first task was to establish forums in which nurses were specifically asked to raise issues of concern to them, to challenge ward practices, to discuss proposed changes, to present new ideas, to exchange views and, finally, to reach responsible decisions about nursing practices and about ward life generally. At an organizational level, our strategy was simply to set up regular meetings and, until they became well established, to make sure they actually occurred in spite of the many competing activities in a busy ward.

Meetings were set up at three levels: ward, team leader and team. Ward meetings were held monthly and were open to all ward nurses. A file was kept in the staff-room in which nurses could write down problems or suggestions they wished to have discussed at the meeting and Alison added her own agenda items. The ward secretary took notes of the meetings and typed them up so that decisions were recorded and could be reviewed and so that absent staff could read them. Ward meetings provided an important opportunity for all staff nurses to contribute to shaping ward life and to influence the pace and course of our development work. Throughout the project, Angie attended ward meetings, not only to collect data about what occurred in the meetings, but also to participate by feeding back her observations on the ward's progress.

Team leader meetings were established for two purposes: to create a senior staff policy group and to provide a support group for the team leaders. They were not set up until the second year of the project, when the team leaders were maturing in their roles and beginning to make a distinct contribution to steering the ward's development. A team leader had complained to Alison that she found it difficult to support her in ward meetings when she did not fully understand her strategy or what she was trying to achieve. Alison then realized that she needed to take the team leaders more into her confidence, sharing her ideas and involving them in plans for moving the development forward. They often had a more intimate feel for the mood of the ward and the concerns of the staff and could give good advice on timing and strategy for change. In turn, team leaders had their own problems with managing their teams and appreciated the opportunity, in a private meeting, to share with each other and with Alison any difficulties they were having. They were able to seek advice, for example, on how to improve team morale, how to deal with tensions between individuals and how to sustain the momentum of change. Providing a formal support mechanism for the team leaders proved to be an effective strategy for promoting decentralized management, for well-supported team leaders were able to resolve many problems within their own teams at an early stage and without ever having to bring them to Alison. Furthermore, encouraging staff to resolve difficulties at team level, rather than always 'turning to Sister', was a way of promoting independence, maturity and confidence in problem-solving.

Individual team meetings were less formal affairs, sometimes planned and sometimes snatched when the ward was not too busy and the moment seemed right. They were organized by the team leaders and Alison was only present on rare occasions when she was invited to help resolve a particularly difficult problem. Team meetings were an opportunity for team members to sit down together and discuss anything of mutual concern. For example, they might review how they were working together, or discuss a particularly distressing case they were all involved with. Again, at a different level, the meetings were an opportunity for peer support, as well as for problem-solving and for planning and reviewing change.

Restructuring communication channels

In the team system, nurses' information needs changed. Their close, continuous involvement with their own patients, and their increased responsibility for clinical decision-making, meant that they needed to be kept well informed of every detail of their own patients' progress and care. Their contact with other patients in the ward, however, was now more limited. Nurses in one team might be called upon briefly to help colleagues in another with their patients, they may need to answer bells for colleagues in another team who were busy, and they could possibly be required to deal with the sudden collapse of a patient who was not in their team. For these reasons, it was still important for all the nurses in the team system to have *some* information about all the patients in the ward, though not at the level of detail required for their own patients. Clarifying the precise nature of these two levels of nursing information helped us to design a shift handover system that met the nurses' needs in the team system.

Essentially, the handover was divided into two phases – one in the office and one at the bedside. The office part of the handover was attended by all the nurses on the oncoming shift and it provided them with general information about all the patients, which would include name, age, diagnosis, resuscitation status, an indication of dependency level and any other crucial information. The nurses were encouraged to be concise and factual when giving this report and to avoid lapsing back into old habits of reporting everything that had happened that day. They prompted and teased each other when the report began to ramble. When managed well, the office part of the handover could be completed in about 15 minutes.

The bedside part of the handover was designed as an opportunity not only for team nurses to pass detailed information about their patients on to each other, but also for them to review and discuss together their patients' care. Its purpose was twofold. First, at a technical level, it was an effective way of passing on a lot of detailed information. The impact of actually meeting the patient at the handover was much greater than a verbal description. In addition, the visual cues in the bedside scene were easier to recall than a list of instructions and seeing the patient, equipment, charts, and so on, prompted more questions and elicited a more precise communication. Second, and most important, the bedside handover was intended to involve the patient. If the patient had not met the oncoming nurse before, a proper introduction could be made. Hearing the handover meant the patient could be confident that the oncoming nurse was properly informed about his or her care and could prompt, correct or add information if necessary. The patient could also join in the discussion about his or her progress and plans.

The introduction of a two-phase handover at the lunchtime shift change was readily accepted and it soon became a highly valued part of daily ward life. However, the idea of using the system early in the morning and at the evening handover to night staff was not popular. Indeed, it was resisted by the nurses until near the end of the project. They defended their position on the grounds that a bedside handover would take too long at these busy times and would result in nurses getting off duty late. They also admitted that they liked their cup of tea and chat together, which was part of the morning and evening handover ritual. Eventually, after encouraging the nurses to talk informally to staff in another ward who had already changed all their handovers, Alison persuaded them to try the two-phase system in the mornings and evenings. She encouraged the nurses to acknowledge the frustrations they experienced with the old handover system and helped them to explore honestly their motives for clinging to it. The trial that followed was an immediate success – the nurses recognized that the quality of their communication was vastly improved and inevitably more patient-centred. Furthermore, even with a quick cup of tea during the office phase, the new handovers proved more efficient and allowed nurses to be off duty more promptly than before. This story illustrates well how change in a ward can take time and how the change agent needs to be patient, not deterred by initial resistance and prepared to wait for an opportune moment to try again.

Redesigning handovers addressed the issue of communication between nurses on different shifts in a team system. Communication channels between nurses and other health professionals visiting the ward during a shift also needed to change to accommodate decentralization, but the nurses themselves tackled this problem by introducing, and then gradually diminishing, the role of a co-ordinator for each shift. Other than supporting and reinforcing this transition, no special strategies were required from us.

The flattened hierarchy

The idea of decentralizing the organization of nursing was generally welcomed by nurses in Oriel Ward, but, when they began to experience it in reality, many of them were hesitant, some even hostile, at first. There were also organizational difficulties as a result of the nurses' inexperience and uncertainty in handling the new system. But gradually the system began to work well, with the staff nurses enjoying their new freedom and additional responsibilities.

Responses to organizational change

For all its faults, and the staff nurses were quick to recognize them (Binnie, 1988), the old 'ends' system was comfortable, secure and unthreatening. Decentralization challenged the nurses and many of them found themselves ill-prepared for life without the protective shield of routine and bureaucracy.

I used to be quite laid back. Now I'm permanently twitched and worked up. I'm sure it's the job, the changes . . . I think the changes are good, but its the stress of the changes, the stress . . . it's just such a big upheaval. (Carol)

We found it a strain at first. It was a lot to cope with. (Sophie)

The nurses were used to turning to an authority figure when they were in difficulty and, as Alison was their new leader and the initiator of the changes, they relied heavily on her guidance in the early days. Although she spent a considerable amount of her time working alongside the nurses in the ward, she also had other responsibilities and they found her absences difficult to deal with.

We struggled a lot to start with . . . she would explain the principles, but then we would run into trouble . . . we would have to wait for days before we could see her and ask her things. (Carol)

At the beginning of the development, the nurses also questioned Alison's priorities.

At that time we didn't feel she was supporting us very much in our nursing. We felt that all she was interested in was the organization of the ward and not the nursing care and the patients. (Sophie)

Alison considered that establishing a team nursing system was an essential prerequisite for patient-centred nursing and a crucial first step in the process of practice development. She gave a lot of attention, in the early days, to getting this structural base right and, not wishing to overload the staff with too much change at once, she was inclined to allow patient care to continue much as it was at that time. Although Alison did talk about her plans at ward meetings, it would seem that she did not make enough effort to explain this specific change strategy to the nurses. However, before too long, beneficial effects of the changes became apparent.

As we found team nursing working, we realized the good things Alison was doing for the ward. (Ursula)

Two years later, staff nurses were totally committed to the decentralized system and quite clear about the benefits of the changes they had experienced.

I never wanted to stay on the medical floor . . . I had hated it before, but here I am two years later, so there obviously was a difference. (Janice)

Nurses talked about the constant challenge they experienced in the system and how it kept their interest in nursing alive and made them feel they wanted to stay on in the ward. Many said that now they could not imagine working in any other system.

I asked myself, 'Am I ever going to find anywhere else where I am treated as a professional nurse, where I am trusted to use my professional judgement?' (Mike)

This nurse went on to explain what was so rare and so valuable about working in a decentralized system.

In my previous experience of general nursing . . . I was always being checked up upon. I could never understand why I spent three years learning to be a professional nurse. It's been really great, the abolition of all these controls and checking up. (Mike)

Those nurses who lived through the early days of the ward's development and who eventually went on to become confident primary nurses had no doubt, on reflection, that the organizational changes were ultimately worthwhile, providing them with opportunities to practise in much more satisfying ways. However, building a stable and efficient decentralized system was a gradual process and many obstacles had to be faced and overcome as the original team system was refined and developed into a mature primary nursing system. The development and eventual demise of a co-ordinator role was one of the factors that helped to ease the organizational transition.

The rise and fall of the co-ordinator

The nurse in charge (in the 'ends' system) automatically disappeared with the introduction of team nursing – team nurses were 'in charge' of their own patients' care and were no longer expected to look to a central figure to tell them what to do. However, during the early days of team nursing in Oriel Ward, this 'being in charge of one's own patients' was experienced as a new and heavy responsibility. Nurses at the bedside felt they needed to have uninterrupted time with their patients to get to know them well and to manage all their care effectively. They did not feel able to take on their new responsibilities at the bedside and, in addition, cope with frequent interruptions from doctors and other health professionals visiting the ward. For this reason, the nurses wanted to retain a central figure on each shift, not as a supervisor with authority to dictate how they should care for their patients but, instead, merely as a co-ordinator who could communicate with others on their behalf.

There was a tendency, initially, for staff nurses used to being in charge to fall back into their old role when acting as co-ordinator. Other nurses experienced this behaviour as 'interfering' with their team nursing work. To help to clarify the distinction between the old and new central roles, and to guide those acting as co-ordinator, Alison produced a written 'role description' summarizing what the nurses said they wanted from the co-ordinator. Essentially, at first, it was to collect information or queries which needed to be passed on to other health professionals from nurses at the bedside and, then, to return to them with information, responses and new instructions concerning their patients. The co-ordinator was also expected to be available to advise student nurses and had a few additional administrative responsibilities, such as organizing meal breaks and dealing with bed management and telephone enquiries. In this way, the co-ordinator was expected to protect the other nurses from being distracted from what they then saw as their primary task of caring for their patients at the bedside.

Initially, the co-ordinator role was perceived to be effective.

Most of the time the system of co-ordinator works really well on the ward . . . If they know what they're to do, and the team know that they have to go to the co-ordinator to tell her what to say to the dietician and the physio, then they'll see to all that and generally make sure things are running smoothly. Then I think it takes a lot of pressure off you. (Moira)

But satisfaction with the role was short-lived and its limitations soon became apparent to the nurses. The main problem was that communication through an intermediary was not as effective as direct communication between the key parties involved. The problem was similar to that inherent in the 'in charge' role, namely that the nurse liaising with other health professionals or relatives was not the nurse who was actually caring for the patients.

Being co-ordinator is like the old 'being in charge'. You don't know half the patients. (Sophie)

With team nursing, however, the frustrations of an indirect communication system were greater because, as the team nurses became more involved with their own patients, they found they had a great deal more to say about them. Increasingly, the team nurses found themselves asking the co-ordinator to direct people to them, so they could talk face to face, and they asked to be interrupted to take phone calls about their own patients. It seemed that as the team nurses became more confident in their new role, they progressed from seeing their work exclusively in terms of providing highly individualized bedside care, to recognizing that their more intimate knowledge of their patients also gave them a legitimate role as participants in clinical decision-making and as advocates for their patients. Being interrupted to make an active contribution to their own patients' management became gradually more acceptable to the nurses and the need for the co-ordinator diminished accordingly.

You know the patient a lot better than the co-ordinator might know the patient. There are only certain things the co-ordinator can do. (Moira)

As the liaison function of the co-ordinator was reduced, it became possible for the person filling that role for the shift to take a clinical caseload as well. The later version of the co-ordinator was thus merely a team nurse nominated to take on a few extra administrative tasks, such as sorting out admissions and discharges, and to keep her or his eyes open to direct doctors and others visiting the ward to an appropriate nurse at the bedside. As the team nurses grew in their roles and began to experience some of the challenges and satisfactions of continuity and involvement that came with decentralization, the profile and status of the central figure were lowered. Whereas being in charge in the 'ends' system had been seen as important, being co-ordinator in the team system came to be regarded as a rather tedious distraction from work with patients. After six months of team nursing, the possibility of scrapping the co-ordinator role altogether was already being raised by the nurses at ward meetings.

Finally abandoning the co-ordinator role was a relatively painless step for the nurses, but it initially caused some difficulty for other staff who visited the ward. As the nurses gained confidence in managing their own caseloads within the team system, they also became comfortable negotiating with each other for assistance, over when to have meal breaks and about which team should accept the next admission. The need for a central figure to orchestrate these internal workings of ward nursing simply disappeared. But the need for some mechanism to oil the wheels of communication between nurses and other people arriving in the ward did not disappear, and it was not until satisfactory new arrangements for facilitating communication had become well established that absence of a co-ordinator ceased to be problematic for doctors and other health professionals.

Complaints from doctors that, without a co-ordinator, they could never find the right nurse were initially commonplace and there was evidence of physio-therapists and dieticians wasting time looking for nurses or waiting for them. These problems were raised on a number of occasions at ward meetings and were a major issue for discussion at the 'away days' (see below). Alison took the position that it was only reasonable to remove one communication system (i.e. having a co-ordinator available) if an alternative one, that acknowledged the needs of other disciplines as well as nurses, could be put in place. Thus, she challenged the nurses to develop new mechanisms for communicating efficiently and effectively with other staff. Gradually, through trial and error and with persistence and persuasion, a new, workable system evolved.

There were a number of simple strategies that were effective. The nurses redesigned the large white board at the nurses' station which indicated where patients were located in the ward. Team colour-coding was used and space was made for indicating the name of the nurse on duty caring for each patient, and for indicating when referral to another health professional was required. Most importantly, the nurses became disciplined about keeping the board up to date – an inaccurate board giving misleading information had inevitably infuriated other staff and brought forth cries for the return of the co-ordinator. A message pad for junior doctors was also introduced to alert doctors to minor tasks that needed doing. This helped to avoid unnecessary bleeping of doctors and meant that, when they came to the ward, doctors did not have to spend time tracking down every individual nurse to check that all was well.

The development of the ward clerk role was a key factor in the eventual success of decentralization. The ward clerk spent most of her time at the nurses' station and was present every weekday morning, which was when the greatest number of health professionals visited the ward and nurses were hidden behind curtains or in the bathroom. The ward clerk was keen to expand her role and responded readily to the suggestion that she might act as receptionist, taking responsibility for greeting staff visiting the ward and making sure that they were promptly directed to an appropriate nurse. The ward clerk also learned to take over much of the bed management work formerly carried out by the co-ordinator. The nurses kept her informed of their patients' discharge plans and she was then able to liaise with the Admissions Office over booking beds.

Teething troubles

Achieving a decentralized ward nursing system was a gradual process which the nurses did not find easy. The nature of the nurses' difficulties changed over time as the system developed and as they grew professionally. Very broadly, their experiences can be categorized as occurring in three phases. Initially, there was ambivalence about taking new responsibility; it was both wanted and feared. Then, within the team system, there was the enjoyable participative freedom of shared responsibility, but, at the same time, a frustrating degree of confusion about who was to do what. Finally, anticipating primary nursing as a helpful means of clarifying individual responsibility, there was then anxiety that the comfortable egalitarianism of team nursing would be lost in favour of a new hierarchical order in which primary nurse was boss and associate nurse was underling. As the difficulties associated with each of these phases were confronted, and as solutions were negotiated, there was the additional frustrating experience of the time lag between deciding what to do and actually making it happen. The timing of change in such a complex environment was crucial and interference from external factors not uncommonly thwarted the nurses' plans and produced a series of false starts and restarts which could make morale and momentum difficult to maintain.

'I was used to having someone in charge'

Facing up to the realities of devolved responsibility took some considerable adjustment in both the managerial and clinical areas of practice. As one nurse put it,

> *I was used to having someone in charge to make decisions . . . I just gradually got used to the fact that you do make decisions at the time.* (Carol)

The habit of relying upon an authority figure was quite hard for the nurses to break and, in the early days, Alison frequently found nurses, who said that they wanted to be more independent, still referring relatively trivial managerial problems back to her. It took time too for the nurses to feel confident about sustaining the smooth, efficient running of a shift without the presence of Sister, or an 'in charge' figure in her place.

> *I used always to think, if Alison was here she would know how to deal with it, but I think people are more and more becoming able to deal with things.* (Rosemary)

Clear, effective delegation of specific managerial responsibilities also took time to negotiate and manage successfully. Sometimes nurses accepting managerial responsibility found it difficult to be firm enough with their colleagues, as often happened when the management of the duty rota was first devolved.

> *This is one job that I delegate that always comes back to me. They are not following the rules which they have all negotiated and agreed to.* (AB)

The nurses' lack of confidence sometimes made Alison reluctant to delegate and, from time to time, she needed prompting by the nurses and by Angie. Later in the development, when Alison complained about an excessive burden of administrative work, a ward sister colleague suggested that she was not using her team leaders enough. As a result, Alison reviewed the team leaders' workload with them and they agreed they could share some administrative tasks. Letter baskets were provided for each of them in the ward office and then, when Alison screened her post, she was able to pass things on for them to deal with, as the following fieldnote illustrates. Sharon (a team leader) has a memo on 'work experience students'.

Alison has asked me to find out what people think about this and I'd like your opinion. (Sharon)
She's been delegating things to me too. I've got a few things in my pigeon-hole. (Sophie, a team leader)

In clinical matters, the nurses' tentative reaction to new responsibility was most evident in their tendency to refer important decisions to the team leaders or to leave difficult problems for them to sort out, rather than using their expert advice and retaining responsibility themselves for seeing issues through. Thus, in the early days of team nursing, nurses noticed that, in managing patients, *'nothing seemed to move along until the team leader picked it up'* and that *'the team falls apart when the team leader is not here'*. From the team leaders' point of view, they felt that they were *'dumped with all the work'*, especially being *'left to sort out all the social problems'*.

Increasingly, as problems like these were debated in team meetings, nurses began to take more initiative and generally to thrive on the new challenges, but a vague fear of independent professional action remained for some time, discernible often in small, subtle ways. A story told by one of the other medical sisters illustrated this phenomenon well.

Passing the Buck

There was this whole notion of professional nursing and trying to get them to make decisions themselves, but allowing them to do that gradually. I remember a staff nurse popped her head around the corner and said, 'I'm going to give Mrs Jones two Distalgesic. That's alright isn't it?' and she swept off, not even waiting for my reply. I called her back and said, 'You just asked me to make a decision.' She said, 'Well, yes, because you are on duty.' I said, 'What would you do if I wasn't here?' and she said, 'Oh well, I would give them.' So I said, 'Can you give your rationale for giving them?' Eventually, I said, 'I am not making this decision for you. I want you to make this decision.' And she actually went off and phoned the house officer and asked him if she could have a prescription for the Distalgesic.

She and the others fairly soon realized that I wasn't there to make decisions for them. I didn't mind talking their decisions through with them, but I wasn't going to make them. In fact, it was just wanting to pass the buck, so that if they made the wrong decision they could say, 'Well Sister knew.' (Medical Sister)

Everyone responsible for everything
Team nursing provided space for the nurses to flex their decision-making 'muscles' within the unthreatening context of shared responsibility. They could propose changes in a patient's care and discuss their ideas with team colleagues and, in that way, directly influence what happened to a patient, without experiencing the full burden of being personally responsible for total management of the nursing. However, once into the second year of team nursing, the

down side of this initially comfortable arrangement became evident and ultimately produced the impetus to move on.

As the nurses became more confident in the close, continuous relationships that team nursing allowed, the potential for creative and highly personalized nursing became increasingly apparent to them. Within their teams, they were becoming much more involved with patients and their families and were more proactive in managing care and discharge planning. Working in this way was more demanding than before and, because every nurse was more or less equally involved with every patient in the team, there was a significant increase in each nurse's workload. As individual nurses came on duty, each felt responsible for chasing progress and reviewing every problem with every patient, and this was exhausting. Alison had a taste of this problem herself when she worked for a month as a full team member.

I find it frustrating because everybody is responsible for everything and I am not sure exactly what I am responsible for. The problem is the forward planning and the discharge planning and the health education, who is actually responsible for it? . . . It's not that they're not taking responsibility, it's just you've all got to do it for everybody all the time. (AB)

When later, with primary nursing, there was a much clearer division of labour in the teams, one nurse recalled the extra effort associated with shared responsibility.

If you go back to team nursing, you felt you were trying to be involved with all six or seven patients. That was hard work. (Ruth)

On the other hand, if at times the pressure of a clinical caseload felt overwhelming, it was easier, when responsibility was shared, to opt out.

Before, when I was only a team member, I sort of had an excuse not to know the answer. I could send them to someone else. (Janice)

When, as was usually the case, nurses did make an effort to get involved with a patient's management, they often found themselves 'bumping up against each other' and sometimes the patient seemed to get lost in the process.

Quite often I think that there can be too many staff nurses making too many decisions . . . there's too many chiefs . . . If you have a lot of staff nurses who are very strong minded and they think that their decision is right for the patient and they disagree, they have to sort it out, but often I think the patient gets forgotten. (Moira)

Angie reported a specific example of a nurse, who was ready to make a commitment and to take personal responsibility, being held back and frustrated by the limitations of the team system.

She was raring to move on and she talked about some of the other nurses who were really longing to move on and take on full responsibility. She described the difficulty she had had with a patient who she had been working with for three consecutive days and they had developed a very deep relationship. They had really discussed his care and developed plans together. Then, on the fourth day, on the late shift, another nurse came on and started to interfere – this is the word she used, 'interfere' – and she felt really upset about it. She said,

'I was the key nurse, but because it hadn't been made explicit, my authority wasn't being accepted.' (AT)

As the nurses' practice matured and as they gained confidence in handling clinical decisions, the frustrations of 'everyone being responsible for everything' began to outweigh the benefits of the cosy camaraderie they had valued so highly in the early days of team nursing. Alison judged that this was the time to promote the idea of primary nursing, for it offered a potential solution to the confusion of the situation. Alison's intention was to build upon the co-operation, support and sharing which were the strengths of the team system, and to add in primary nursing in order to clarify individual roles and responsibilities within the teams. While the nurses appreciated the rationale for introducing primary nursing, they were hesitant, because they feared it would bring with it a new hierarchy.

Fear of a new hierarchy

We had initially anticipated that only the team leaders would take on the role of primary nurse. The literature emphasizes the considerable responsibility carried by a primary nurse and indicates, as a consequence, that the role should only be taken on by experienced qualified staff (Ersser and Tutton, 1991). In early primary nursing developments in the UK, such as the Burford and Beeson Ward projects (Pearson, 1988; 1992), and in Alison's previous surgical ward development, this pattern of having a small number of senior staff acting as primary nurses to fairly large caseloads (six to eight patients) was the one that had been adopted. In the relatively stable environments of the community hospital and the elderly care rehabilitation ward (Pearson, 1988; 1992), the size of the primary caseload seems to have been manageable. In the acute surgical ward, Alison had found that the intensity of the relationships, the speed of change in patients' conditions, the frequent demand for new nursing decisions and the short length of stay of many patients, were all factors that made it virtually impossible for nurses, however experienced, to remain closely involved with every patient passing through their care. In practice, primary nurses inevitably found themselves supervising at a distance, whilst associate nurses filled the key nursing role for some patients. At times, it seemed as if the primary nurse were more like a 'mini sister', directing a small team, than a true primary nurse who was both key decision-maker and main care giver.

In Oriel Ward, when the possibility of primary nursing was first being considered and the model described above was still the likely one to emerge, the prospect of being *only* an associate nurse was not very attractive to the experienced staff nurses who were not team leaders. Used to a system in which status was closely associated with grade, title and notches on a precisely marked career ladder, the nurses automatically judged the new roles in strictly hierarchical terms.

I qualified just over two years ago and . . . I couldn't possibly stay in primary nursing at this moment in my career, because I couldn't be an associate nurse. I just couldn't be a minion, because I'm afraid that's what it is in a way. You are being dominated by a primary nurse. (Carol)

While this nurse was making her case on the grounds of status, it could also be argued that she was indirectly making a point about her skill and expertise being wasted. It seemed that the original distribution of primary and associate roles needed reconsidering. Having the few primary nurses overburdened with responsibility, while other well-established members of staff felt their talents were underused, was not a sensible situation.

When another senior sister began her development of primary nursing on the medical floor, a year earlier, she addressed the problem of primary caseload size in an acute setting and agreed with her team that it was reasonable to expect E grade nurses to carry a *small* primary caseload. This arrangement meant that team leaders and E grade staff nurses were the primary nurse for some of the patients in their team and associate nurse for others. It meant that when any one of these nurses was on duty, caring for all the team's patients, she or he could focus special attention on the broader management issues and closer involvement with her or his own few patients, knowing that someone else would be doing the same for other patients on the next shift. Alison had been impressed with this solution to the caseload size problem in the acute ward setting. She anticipated having E and F grade primary nurses in the study ward, but still felt that D grade nurses were too inexperienced for the role.

As moving on to primary nursing became a real option in the study ward, the issue of D grade nurses not being primary nurses became the major barrier to progress. The D grades unanimously opposed being excluded from the role and won wide support from their colleagues. It was argued that, with team nursing, the D grades were already making decisions and participating actively in the management of patients. They saw becoming an associate nurse as having this responsibility removed from them, as being 'demoted' to someone who would merely carry out the orders of the primary nurse. No real enthusiasm for introducing primary nursing was sustainable while this problem remained unresolved.

The nurses formally challenged Alison on the D grade issue. Alison explained that the 'bottom line' in this matter must be that patients were not denied access to expertise because the nurse in charge of their care was a junior member of staff. The agreement that emerged was as follows:

- A D grade nurse could act as a primary nurse, once she or he was established in the ward and when both the nurse and the sister felt the nurse was ready for the responsibility.
- A D grade nurse could only take on *one* primary patient at a time. She or he would continue to act as associate nurse for other patients cared for by the team.
- Part of a D grade primary nurse's responsibility towards her or his patient must be to seek out and use supervision from a senior colleague.

This agreement represented a significant shift in Alison's position. As she said, '*I have stood up on conference platforms all over the country and argued that the primary nurse must be an experienced nurse.*' That she was prepared to accept this kind of challenge from the ward nurses and negotiate with them in this way was an important lesson for them. It helped them to realize that they were not dealing with an immutable authority; they were part of a new development, which they had power to influence. Indeed, their active contribution to shaping the development was welcome and perceived as crucial for its success.

On the other hand, this episode also illustrated that underlying the development were certain core principles, about commitment to patients' well-being, which were not negotiable. In this example, there was room for flexibility and experiment over who exactly might take on the primary nurse role and in what circumstances, but making sure that every patient had access to the professional opinion of an experienced nurse was essential. Insisting upon the use of supervision, as a condition of being a D grade primary nurse, was Alison's way of protecting this principle.

In practice, the agreement about the D grades stood the test of time and proved to be a good solution from several points of view. The concern about hierarchy vanished without trace, because there was a separation of role from grade. Any qualified nurse, from sister to newly registered staff nurse, might be a primary nurse, but experience and expertise determined the size of the primary caseload and the degree of clinical autonomy exercised in decision-making. Once the D grade nurses were allowed to take one primary patient, their complaints about feeling underused and undervalued quickly disappeared. Once they experienced being a primary nurse, they recognized the responsibility and the emotional demands of the role and there was no clamour for a bigger caseload. It seemed that the experience of being a primary nurse stretched the D grades in a healthy and stimulating way, while limiting their caseload protected them from being overwhelmed by demands they were not ready for.

I found it quite strange, sitting there with his care plan in front of me. Normally, I find it easy to write the care plan, but, in this case, I found it really very difficult. I felt that I had to do a really deep assessment, a really full assessment ... because I felt more responsible. This was my first primary patient and I knew that this was the only patient for whom I had to write a care plan. I felt I had to do it really well and I found it very difficult to assess the patient. (Janice)

Supervision was often negotiated less formally than Alison would have liked, but an appreciation that it was in the patient's interests, as well as ones own, to check out key decisions with a senior colleague was readily established. Furthermore, on occasions when a D grade found herself primary nurse to a patient with particularly complex or demanding problems, a close supervisory relationship with Alison or a team leader was always established.

False starts

Resolution of the D grade issue brought a surge of enthusiasm for moving on to primary nursing. It was agreed that individual teams should begin allocating primary nurses to patients as soon as they felt ready. Teams recognized that they were at slightly different states of 'readiness' (for example, one team had relatively new members of staff), so it seemed right to leave the final decision to start primary nursing to the individual teams. However, even with this control, they found the change difficult to sustain. Having started primary nursing, they often found themselves 'lapsing back into team nursing'. Perhaps a key member of the team left, or the ward went through a particularly busy phase leaving nurses little energy for the extra effort required to take on a primary caseload. Sometimes they found themselves prevaricating over taking on primary patients, particularly if they were anticipating days off, and then patients did not get a primary nurse for several days or sometimes not at all. At times, the nurses got disheartened by their 'false starts' and Alison needed to encourage and reassure them and to remind them that taking a primary caseload was demanding and difficult because it was new.

The ward runs itself

At the end of the project, a decentralized nursing system was running smoothly. Routines no longer dominated the nurses' daily clinical work. Instead, they were actively managing and prioritizing their own workloads and discussing their plans with their patients.

> *They come and say, 'I've got somebody who is rather ill, OK? I won't see you for an hour or so. Is that alright?'. I was perfectly happy with that because I knew where I was.* (Patient)

The nurses were no longer automatically passing things up to someone more senior, but, whenever possible, they dealt with problems themselves. They were also observed taking personal responsibility for making referrals to other disciplines, for communicating with relatives and for co-ordinating their own patients' discharge arrangements.

A sister visiting from another hospital was impressed with how smoothly the ward ran without a co-ordinator.

> *I was surprised how well the ward functioned without a co-ordinator. I wasn't sure how it would work, but it works really well. Things like doing their own drugs and their own doctors' rounds . . . it was surprising how it wasn't chaotic . . . I think the ward clerk with her extended role, that helps a lot. . . . I've spoken to the physiotherapist and the speech therapist and the OT and they all find it helps their work.*

Individual nurses were observed taking responsibility for issues as they arose and they consulted and negotiated with colleagues when a consensus was necessary. In this way, without recourse to a central figure, new admissions were booked into the ward and allocated to a team, meal breaks were negotiated, help was arranged for a busy team, and the rota was reorganized or bank nurses were booked to cover sickness. Similarly, nurses began to demonstrate that they recognized that they all had a responsibility to make the decentralized communication system work and this was appreciated by others.

> *It doesn't work well where people dismiss you saying, 'He's not my patient' and don't stop . . . On this ward, they don't have that problem now. They are actually very helpful . . . they will go out of their way to find someone . . . I think that's a crucial part of it. People actually respecting the system and trying to get it to work, because if they don't, you get stuck. It needs that co-operation between the disciplines, as well as in one team.* (Senior Registrar)

At a policy level too, decentralized decision-making became evident. Nurses gradually got used to participating in discussion about how the ward should be managed and ultimately took it for granted that it was their prerogative to suggest changes or to be consulted about any proposals. For example, a staff nurse confidently reported that at the second 'away days', '*We decided to make some ground rules*' – a far cry from the early days of waiting to be told what to do.

Alison reviewed these 'away days' and compared them with the same event the previous year.

They were much more ready to come up with suggestions and decisions. They didn't particularly look to me for solutions. If we discussed a problem, they were working at coming up with the solution themselves . . . whereas last year they were looking to me – 'the expert'. (AB)

By the final year of the project, managerial responsibilities were widely shared across the nursing team. Team leaders played an active role in every aspect of managing the staff in their teams and they contributed to short-listing, interviewing and orientation of new team members. With Alison's support, they conducted performance review interviews and, at team leader meetings, they regularly reviewed how their team members were functioning, both individually and as a group. Other managerial responsibilities were shared out, with more emphasis being placed upon an individual's particular interests and aptitudes than their seniority. One nurse took responsibility for meeting regularly with the domestic supervisor to liaise over catering and cleaning matters and another became the ward's health and safety representative. There were link nurses for infection control, wound care and diabetes who attended local specialist meetings and fed updating information back into the ward. Organizing and monitoring training in back care, blood glucose monitoring and resuscitation were each the responsibilities of yet other nurses.

Being able to devolve so much of the ward management work previously handled by the sister, left Alison free to contribute to the ward in new ways. In particular, she was able to give time and attention to helping the nurses develop their roles as primary and associate nurses. The smooth running of the decentralized system depended to a great extent upon the nurses clarifying and becoming comfortable with their new roles. Developing these new nursing roles proved to be a much more complex and difficult business than we had anticipated.

DEVELOPING NEW ROLES

Roles define the behaviours and responses that others expect from us in a particular context. Taking on an established role for the first time can be a daunting experience. Novices can feel uncertain about what is expected of them and underconfident about their skill to perform in the role. Gradually, through trial and error, and by observing accomplished role models, novices come to terms with the new role. It becomes a comfortable part of a social repertoire that the actor can take on or leave off with little conscious effort.

Taking on a brand new role, one that is only loosely defined and that the individual has not seen played before, is even more challenging. When new roles emerge, or are created in response to a particular social change, as was the case in this study, then interpreting these roles in specific situations can be confusing initially. The precise scope of new roles is often unclear and their boundaries with other roles may be blurred. When the nurses in the study first adopted the roles of primary and associate nurses, they experienced this kind of role ambiguity.

Role ambiguity

Establishing a primary nursing system was recognized as a key organizational goal for Oriel Ward for nearly two years before staff nurses actually began to take on the roles of primary and associate nurses. During this long preparatory phase, there was a great deal of discussion in the ward about what the new roles would involve. In addition, primary nursing literature was made available in the staff-room and many nurses were able to attend local study days designed for potential primary nurses. Thus, by the time primary nursing was being formalized in the ward, most of the nurses had a reasonably good *theoretical* grasp of what their new roles would involve.

During the first 'away days', the nurses wrote down what they considered to be the components of the primary and associate nurse roles. They produced comprehensive and well-informed lists.

The following list was produced for the primary nurse role:

- To take overall responsibility for the patient's nursing.
- To work with the patient and associates to prescribe, implement and evaluate care.
- To provide individualized care for patient and family.
- To negotiate a plan of care with other disciplines.
- To communicate effectively.
- To teach, advise and support.
- To be accountable for the patient's nursing.

And the following list was produced for the associate nurse role:

- To assist in planning care.
- To implement the plan of care in the primary nurse's absence.
- To reassess the plan if care needs altering.
- To provide feedback to the primary nurse.
- To offer ideas and experience.
- To support the primary nurse.
- To be accountable to the primary nurse.

It seemed that they had grasped the essence of the special primary relationship, were clear about personal responsibilities associated with each role and comfortable with the prospect of being called to account for their individual decisions and actions. However, experience was soon to show that there is a great difference between knowing in theory and knowing in practice. What seemed relatively clear and simple, when discussed in abstract terms, became surprisingly complex and difficult in the real world of ward life. Several nurses articulated this experience.

> *I knew the principles, but I didn't appreciate the involvement and the responsibility ... You've just got to do it.* (Sophie)

> *I was quite clear in theory about primary nursing, but I had no idea what it would be like in practice.* (Moira)

The practical difficulties with interpreting the new roles were most evident in tensions that occurred between primary and associate nurses. Individuals found themselves unclear about just how much was expected of them and how much they could expect from colleagues. Sometimes lack of confidence lay behind this tentativeness.

I'm still not feeling completely confident about taking primary patients. I'm still not very clear about what the role actually involves. I don't always make the decisions that the primary nurse should make, but I think that's because we're not used enough to primary nursing. We're in the transition phase. (Ruth)

While primary nurses were underconfident or uncertain about the scope of their responsibilities, associates felt they could not safely assume that primary nurses had everything under control. This was particularly a problem for the more experienced nurses when acting in an associate role. They found themselves still checking up on everything that was happening, for all the patients in their team, and getting involved in problems that they should be leaving the primary nurse to deal with. Rachel recognized this behaviour in herself.

I certainly have a feeling that I should be trying to do everything for everybody, even though they are not my primary patients. And yet that means you can't do anything well for anybody really. Rosemary calls it 'letting go' ... I think that is where the problem comes. If an associate doesn't have confidence in what somebody else is doing ... That is something that has just come to me, that you can only let go when you have confidence that the primary nurses are doing what you think they should do. (Rachel)

Associate nurses who, while only trying to be helpful, unintentionally stepped into a primary nurse's territory were regarded as interfering. It was a delicate position to be in. As one nurse put it, *'I'm finding treading on other people's toes a problem at the moment.'* Sometimes, though, primary nurses could be found to have brought the 'interference' upon themselves by not thinking sufficiently far ahead or by not communicating their intentions clearly: *'I suppose it comes down to you not having actually laid down the plans for what you want.'*

Ambiguity about the boundaries of the new roles was experienced as particularly uncomfortable because the nurses were reluctant to confront or challenge each other about their work. For example, a care plan might have been changed without, in the primary nurse's view, good reason, but rarely would she challenge the associate concerned to justify the change. Similarly, in the associate role, nurses often wanted to make suggestions about the management of a colleague's patient, but, although they knew this was legitimate, they found it difficult to do.

You think there might be something that could be done slightly differently or slightly better. I wonder whether we ought to discuss people's care more. I know we're supposed to do that, but I don't know that we really do. We need to make it OK to air those views ... I mention things and then afterwards I sometimes think, 'I hope they didn't think I was being snotty, trying to take over their role, or being bossy.' (Janice)

Alison described her own experience of role boundary tension. Her story shows the kind of feelings that can be generated when people are new to their roles and not quite sure what to expect from each other. Alison had been Paul's primary nurse for several weeks.

Overstepping the mark: Part 1

Because I have been nursing him very closely every day, I am very attuned to his symptoms. And I know him. I know his personality. I know his reactions to his illness . . . He had been doing well, after recovering from his confused state and being so ill, but on Thursday he wasn't quite so well. He started getting tired, he wouldn't eat and he wasn't making so much effort. On the Friday, he was a little bit worse again. Nothing terribly obvious. I couldn't put my finger on it. I said to the registrar, I don't know what it is, but he's not quite so well . . .

I then went off for the weekend and Clare and Mike looked after him. Obviously they didn't know him as well as I did, but they decided over the weekend that he wasn't making enough effort and that he was regressing psychologically and that he needed to be pushed. They discussed it and when the consultant came in they talked to him about it. They all agreed that he was to be encouraged to get up more and perhaps go home with his wife for a few hours and generally to be pushed.

I came in on Monday late shift and they were very good. They took me aside and explained all this . . . I appreciated that. But I could feel myself reacting in quite a negative way. I felt a bit that they had taken over and they had changed the direction of my patient's care. They had taken the initiative to discuss it with the consultant and they had made plans for Paul to go out with his wife. I could feel myself reacting to it. But at the time I didn't tell them how I was feeling, because I thought I was being possessive and feeling put out. They had just picked up things over the weekend and they were giving their account and doing it nicely.

I thought I should recognize that they were making a valuable contribution as associate nurses. So I was very gracious about it and thanked them, but I felt unhappy and uncomfortable about it. I had this underlying feeling during the day, as I worked with Paul, that they were wrong. It wasn't like Paul to give up. I watched him during the day and it was true that he was unusually irritable and was withdrawing. As I listened to him, I realized that he was suffering from sensory overload. He was very irritable about the television being on and about not being able to get any sleep. I thought, 'This man is not regressing, he's been so ill, but in the middle of the ward, with so much going on, he just can't get any rest – what he needs is a good night's sleep and some peace and quiet, some space of his own'. When I suggested that, he said, 'Oh yes'. I arranged a single room and moved him in straight away and his wife was so pleased. And I cancelled him going out anywhere, because he clearly wasn't well enough.

That night, at home, I was thinking about my reactions to Clare and Mike and I decided that in fact I was right, that they had overstepped the mark. They were right as associates to present their observations of my patient and to give their interpretation and make suggestions, but it wasn't urgent that anything was done and they knew I would be back on Monday. They shouldn't have talked to the consultant and changed the plan and negotiated it with his wife. They should have said to me, 'We've been watching Paul over the weekend and we think he's been regressing and we think it might do him good to go out. Perhaps you should talk to the consultant'. Then I thought, 'Now, dare I tell them that? Will they feel I am undermining them? Will I set them back?' I decided that it was important that we should all learn from these situations and that I needed to discuss it all with them. (AB)

However sound one's intentions, it is all too easy, when playing a new role, to fall back into old patterns of behaviour. Here, Clare and Mike, trying hard to be effective associates and succeeding in some ways, made the mistake of falling back into the old staff nurse pattern of dealing with whatever problems arose during their shift. They had not yet learned, in practice, to discriminate between decisions that an associate nurse should make and those it was more appropriate to leave to the primary nurse. Alison had more experience of working in a primary nursing system, but she too was at first not sure of her ground and had to take time to examine her feelings and to consider the principles at issue, before she was confident enough to confront her colleagues.

Strategies for clarifying roles

For new roles to be effective in an organization, they have to be understood and accepted, not only by the role holder, but also by others who need to relate to the role holder. Facilitating both the development and the negotiation of new nursing roles required careful, sustained work, some of which was best achieved away from the ward setting.

Time out

Away days
The demands of a twenty-four hour nursing service make it extremely difficult for all the nurses belonging to any one ward to meet together. Ward meetings in Oriel Ward came to have an important place in ward life, but it was unusual for more than half the ward's nurses to be able to attend any one meeting. Those present felt pressured to get back to their patients and some had to keep one eye on the ward, and so the kind of work that could be accomplished was limited. Ward meetings could not give nurses space for deep, detailed exploration of an issue and, because of the inevitable attendance problem, it was not possible for the whole group to participate in the process of negotiating, planning and taking responsibility for change.

The scale of the change we were promoting was more than the nurses could handle whilst at the same time continuing to meet the demands of a busy ward. Towards the end of the first year of the project, evidence began to emerge of serious confusion, uncertainty and unhappiness about the new system generally and about the new nursing roles in particular. Strong criticism was being directed at Alison, as leader of the development, and there was considerable tension in the ward. Something had to be done to help the nurses resolve the muddle and conflict. Ignoring the practicalities, Alison said,

> *The ideal setting for this would be 'away days', because there is an awful lot here that needs mulling around and it would be very helpful to do it in a big group.* (AB)

We considered the idea of staff from each of the two wards in Alison's unit covering each other, to allow each ward team to have time out all together. This was not beyond the realms of possibility, but it would have been very difficult to organize and it would have put pressure on the staff, requiring them probably to forego their days off one week and take days in lieu at a later date. Angie then asked an obvious question, knowing that a positive response was unlikely, '*Is it possible to close half the beds for a short period?*' She pointed out that beds did get closed when a ward needed decorating, so why not also to accommodate important staff development?

Alison laughed at the reactions she could imagine from doctors and managers to a suggestion that, in such a busy service, beds might be closed for nurses to have 'away days'. But then it occurred to her that there was, at that time, a ward closed for refurbishment on another floor. The nurses from that ward had had some study time together and they were now being used around the hospital to fill staffing gaps. The ward was due to reopen in three weeks time. Would it make any real difference to anyone if that reopening was delayed by just a few days? Alison went to see the sister of the ward that was closed and she felt that, as her staff had benefited from the time the ward closure had given them, they could be persuaded to cover two other wards for just an extra few days. Alison put her case to the consultants concerned and then, via the hospital's general manager, to the Hospital Board. The proposal was accepted.

We planned the first 'away days' not merely as study days for the staff to learn more about primary nursing; the message we wanted to convey was that 'this is time for you'. The days were to be as much about listening to each other's experiences and ideas, as about imparting knowledge and interpreting theory. Going somewhere pleasant, having nice food and structuring the days in a relaxed, informal way were thus important guiding principles in the design of the 'away days'. (Ward fund money was used to cover expenses.)

The two day programme was structured as a workshop, focussing upon roles and relationships within the ward, its key aims being:

- To develop a clear, shared understanding of the roles of the team leader, team member, primary nurse, associate nurse and ward sister.
- To develop action plans for individuals and groups to help them establish their new roles more comfortably.
- To achieve a clear, shared vision of the way forward.

Much of the work was done in small groups to make sure that everyone had a chance to be heard and to participate, but introductory sessions and feedback sessions involved the whole group, so that the cohesion of the ward team was maintained and developed. Presenting project data to the nurses at the beginning of sessions was a powerful way of helping them to confront the tensions that had existed in the ward. The individual sources of the data remained anonymous, but everyone knew that everything they heard belonged to someone in the group who had been sharing their recent experiences of ward life. Sometimes individuals were able to identify closely with the data and confirmed that it represented what they too had felt. Sometimes they were surprised by the data, occasionally even shocked that they had been so unaware of what their colleagues had been experiencing. The data helped to bring issues into focus very quickly and, because the interview material recorded nurses speaking very frankly, responses to it were correspondingly open and honest.

The material we presented in these first 'away days' was very sensitive. Both the data and the nurses' responses to them exposed strong feelings about the new roles. There were feelings of uncertainty, inadequacy, frustration and resentment. With such emotionally charged material, the workshops required careful facilitation to make them productive. Had we not been experienced facilitators ourselves, we would probably have invited an outsider with the necessary skills to join the workshops.

An exercise we found especially useful was 'role analysis'. In small groups, nurses were asked to imagine themselves in a particular role and, using simple brainstorming, to answer the following questions:

- What am I here for? (i.e. What is my purpose within the organization?)
- What is expected of me? (i.e. What do other people expect me to do?)
- What should I offer? (i.e. What qualities and skills should I bring to this role?)

Having produced long lists in answer to each of these questions, the groups were asked to analyse them as role descriptions, considering whether they were reasonable and realistic. They were also asked to examine the paired roles of team leader and team member, and primary nurse and associate nurse, to ensure that the pairs were compatible and complementary in function. These role analyses provided a firm basis for clarifying misconceptions, for negotiating roles that were both acceptable and achievable, and for comparing actual experiences with expectations. Gaps in skill and confidence were acknowledged and appropriate development work was planned.

The first 'away days' gave dramatic new impetus to the development work. Written evaluations indicated that participants had found the two days very enlightening.

I learnt a great deal about people's feelings.

I've learnt so much about myself and feel very critical of things I've done and thought about the changes.

I've discovered that I am not alone. Many people are in the same boat with similar hopes, fears and aspirations.

I realize that people are willing for us to be perfectly open with one another, without taking offence.

I've learnt more about the people I work with, how they think and what makes them tick.

The experience of listening and sharing had greatly strengthened the cohesion of the ward team

Having a chance to debate issues with colleagues helps our understanding and I feel has strengthened a sense of belonging to a team.

I feel that people are not going to be judgemental about your honest opinion now when you're back at work.

I felt we became closer as a group – both as a team and as a ward.

The specific goal, of clarifying the new nursing roles, was perceived as having been achieved and much of the conflict that had arisen out of the confusion was felt to have been resolved.

I found that things I had thought were quite clear actually weren't so. The roles have now been defined and I know (hopefully) what is expected of me.

Most strikingly, the evaluations suggested that the workshops had energized the nurses and enabled them to go back to their wards with new enthusiasm and a clearer sense of direction.

It spurred me into action. I feel I'm going somewhere.

I feel set up with a whole new round of ammunition with which I intend to go forward and improve my practice and working relationships . . . I feel more motivated by those two days . . . and see my direction as a lot more clearly defined.

We are all keen to get on with it!

I'm bursting to put it all into practice. On the whole, I've found it more enjoyable and stimulating than I would have thought possible.

The first 'away days' undoubtedly marked a turning point in the development of both wards. Morale improved enormously, the tension and unhappiness disappeared completely and the nurses found the confidence to formalize primary nursing and to begin exploring their new roles more creatively and more openly. Inevitably, however, as the development progressed, new issues emerged and new difficulties arose and, as time went by, new staff who had not experienced the workshops joined the wards. We felt it was crucial to build into ward life permanent mechanisms that would maintain the healthy openness we had created, maintain the enthusiasm and commitment now so much in evidence and enable the ward to remain constructively responsive to change which, regardless of the project, was increasingly a feature of hospital life.

The possibility of making 'away days' a regular annual event had to be explored. Alison shared her experience with the other medical sisters and they considered the feasibility of all the medical wards having the same opportunity the following summer. The sisters recognized that, by taking advantage of the regular summer ward closure and redeploying staff in a carefully planned way, each of the six medical wards in turn would be able to release all their nurses, from day and night duty, to have one or two 'away days', without creating any additional disruption to the service. 'Away days' every summer have since become an established feature of life in the medical wards, and other departments in the hospital have also begun to make similar arrangements.

The surge of energy and enthusiasm that always followed 'away days' helped greatly to maintain the momentum of development work and generally kept staff feeling that they were coping with the impact of other changes that were occurring in the hospital. Although new topics appeared on the programmes, interestingly, primary and associate nurse roles were revisited, by popular request, every year. This was partly for the benefit of new staff who, confronted with the roles for the first time, experienced difficulty negotiating their delicate boundaries. But, in addition, more experienced staff found that new concerns emerged which, once shared and examined, could lead to helpful refinements of their roles.

Team days

At least once during the year, between the annual 'away days', each team had a day away from the hospital, with all the team members present. Each team negotiated with the other teams to cover their shifts for the day, knowing that they would be asked to return the favour in due course. Usually one of the team members offered to host the day at her home, others contributed food and often there was some kind of social activity planned for the end of the day. The team days were essentially modelled on the annual ward 'away days', but as they involved only six or seven nurses they were more intimate and better suited to addressing the personal, detailed aspects of working together. Alison did not attend the team days and left the team leaders and their group to draw up their own agendas, unless, as was sometimes the case, a team leader asked advice on how to handle a specific issue. Again, roles were a recurrent theme in the team days. The teams were trusted to use their time out constructively and the investment paid back handsomely, both in terms of the fund of good ideas brought back to contribute to the ward's development, and in terms of the strong team cohesion that emerged.

Variety and refreshment

Traditionally, time out from clinical work for staff nurses had been relatively rare and confined to study days or courses. Inevitably, the demands of workload and the limitations of staffing levels and funds made substantial increases in time out for individual nurses impossible. But, with a little imagination, flexibility and give and take between colleagues, we found that it was possible to create new opportunities for them outside the ward. The need for nurses occasionally to have time out for themselves was highlighted early in the project. Nurses compared themselves with Alison, noting that, although she worked long hours, her work was varied, whereas for them, every day was much the same.

> *(Alison) can be involved with practice . . . in research, (and) in lots of other things. That's a very enviable position. She can recharge her batteries. She seems to gallop along . . . She can put so much into her work because, even though she is putting a great deal into it this month, it is not what she was doing last month and that is a rest as much as anything else. It would be really nice to withdraw and enter into something else with just as much enthusiasm, because it was different enough for it to be a change . . . The only sort of rest I get is a two week holiday.* (Mike)

Recognizing the value of variety in one's working life, as well as the importance of space and time to think, Alison consciously began to seek out opportunities for individual nurses to be involved in a range of activities that would enrich their professional lives. For example, nurses were given time out for self-directed project work that was likely to be of value to the ward. One nurse noted that her team leader, who was '*depressed about the way the team was developing a few weeks ago,*' seemed quite different after a short period of study leave.

> *She came back looking really positive and full of ideas and looking forward to putting them into action.* (Janice)

When Alison ran workshops or study days for other nurses, she sometimes asked one or two of her own staff to help her and to make a contribution. As nurses developed their own special interests and responsibilities, opportunities arose for them to attend meetings on behalf of the ward. When visiting nurses and even occasional VIPs came to the ward, as they did increasingly as the development work attracted publicity, Alison asked nurses to talk about their work and to act as host to visitors. Talking to outsiders about what they had achieved, and finding that these people were interested and perhaps impressed, made the nurses feel good about themselves and their work and it helped to build their confidence as individuals and as professionals.

Ensuring that individual nurses had time out was more a general professional development strategy than specifically a role development strategy, but it complemented the group 'away day' work, which grew out of the striking need for role development. Furthermore, the insights and increased confidence that nurses acquired from their various time out activities helped them to grow into the primary and associate nurse roles, which demanded greater professional independence and maturity.

Facilitating learning from experience

Developing new roles involves a continuous dynamic between experience and thinking. Nurses are first presented with the *idea* of a new role, which they may grasp intellectually, but that is very different from translating it into everyday behaviour and relationships. During the project, the time out strategies provided opportunities for nurses to explore the components of their new roles, to negotiate ground rules and boundaries and then, subsequently, to share problems and to consider modifications and refinements of the original ideas. Through this process a clear conceptualization of the new roles evolved. It left the nurses fairly certain about *what* they should be doing, but gaining confidence in *how* to perform in the new roles was something that had to grow from experience.

Relating theory to practice

Working alongside the nurses in practice, Alison was alert to specific examples of confusion or tension that occurred because a nurse was not entirely fulfilling the obligations of her new role, or because she was trespassing on someone else's 'territory'. Using the immediate situation and explaining what was happening in terms of the theory that the nurses all knew, helped them to modify their behaviour at the time and to work through difficulties in a constructive way. The immediacy of this kind of learning gave the nurses a real 'feel' for their new roles. As one nurse put it, '*It was actually doing it that helped it become clearer.*'

Alison gave an example of the way she actively tried to raise an awareness of role boundary issues and to steer things in the right direction.

There was a stroke lady who was Rosemary's patient. She had been unconscious and her prognosis had seemed very poor. A couple of days before, I had talked with Rosemary, Sophie and Dave about role boundaries. I helped Dave to wash this lady and to sit her up, as she was much better. Afterwards we both commented on how her condition was changing and we talked about the implications for her treatment. It was a real opportunity for him to talk through with me what we should do and what we should leave for Rosemary. We talked about how it would be different if Rosemary were off for three days, but, as she was back that afternoon, we should leave certain things for her. (AB)

Sophie, also acting as an associate nurse in this case, picked up the story and explained how the team respected the primary nurse's special relationship with the patient's husband and how they waited for the primary nurse to take the lead in making an important decision.

The primary nurse was off duty and the team were posing the question, 'Should the patient be fed naso-gastrically?' There was some uncertainty about this decision because all other treatment had been withdrawn, but the woman was really beginning to improve. The primary nurse had established a strong bond with the husband who was getting confused about the conflicting reports of what was going to happen to his wife. We decided to wait until Rosemary came back so that she could discuss the issue of feeding with the patient's husband. Rosemary had given me a good handover, so I knew all about the husband . . . and how to handle him. I understood his feelings. This was a good example of the associate nurse and primary nurse working well together. It enabled me to spend useful time talking with the husband, clearing things up and helping to prepare him. Then when Rosemary came back, she talked with the doctor and the husband and we made a joint decision. (Sophie)

Situations like this one, where associate nurses had to consider whether to make a decision or whether to wait for the primary nurse, were common. The associates were, on the one hand, anxious not to 'step on the primary nurse's toes', but were also, on the other hand, concerned not to ignore a problem that needed attention. In thinking through these dilemmas, Alison asked the associate nurses to consider four factors:

- Any contingency plan indicated by the primary nurse.
- The urgency of the patient's problem.
- When the primary nurse would be available.
- The significance of the decision.

A skilled primary nurse could be expected to think ahead, to anticipate likely changes in her patient's needs and to indicate in the care plan how colleagues should respond to these changes in her absence. Naturally, however, the primary nurse could not plan for every eventuality. If there were an unexpected turn of events in the primary nurse's absence, then the associate must take over, particularly if the new situation was an urgent one. If the new problem did not require immediate attention, then the associate must weigh up the pros and cons of postponing a decision, taking into account how long it would be before the primary nurse returned. In particular, decisions that would significantly change *the direction of the patient's care* should involve the primary nurse whenever possible.

Examining the role boundary question in this way with the nurses emphasized the fact that the associate role is not a passive one. Some of the literature gives the impression that the role of the associate is little more than carrying out the primary nurse's instructions. Particularly in an acute hospital setting where patients' needs can change very quickly, the contrary appears to be the case – the associate needs to be an alert, active partner in the patient's care, capable of making responsible clinical decisions, but also sensitive to occasions when it is in the interests of the special primary relationship and the overall management of care not to intervene. However she or he handles these decisions, the associate nurse should be ready to give an account of her or his work to the primary nurse who is in charge of the patient's care.

Demonstrating new roles

In an established system, such as traditional nursing, a novice can observe and copy the behaviour of experienced role models. This happens at both conscious and unconscious levels and is an extremely valuable way of learning. When new roles are developed, however, good role models may be in short supply. In the early days of the project, several nurses pointed out the disadvantage of not having role models.

I can't really conceptualize how primary nursing will be, because it is outside my experience. (Rosemary)

Alison was the only person in the ward who had previous experience of the new roles and she adopted a conscious strategy of making her own practice, as a primary or associate nurse, as visible as possible. She tried to make her decisions in each role explicit, so that the nurses could see not only what she had done, but also why she had done it. She talked openly about her feelings and concerns in each role and about her responses to others and her expectations of them, thus bringing the detail and the fine-tuning of the roles to life.

Rachel learned from observing Alison and from comparing her behaviour with her own.

Alison said that because she was the associate nurse, and you had been doing all the work with (the patient), she didn't feel it was really appropriate for her to try and do some detailed, in-depth work with the patient . . . because she was a bit confused and having more than one person try to work closely with her would be too much. So she said that she was quite low key . . . (AT)

Yes, I think that is something Alison has learned to do that maybe more of us should learn to do. I'm sure I'm guilty of doing the opposite. I tend to feel I have to do everything for everyone, even when I'm an associate. (Rachel)

As well as providing the nurses with a model of the primary and associate roles, Alison was also able to demonstrate the skills of confrontation and negotiation that were necessary to deal with role boundary problems. When primary nurses complained about associates doing either too much or too little for their patients, or when associate nurses complained about primaries not communicating their plans or not valuing the associate contribution, then Alison would facilitate discussion between the two parties. She would show how it was helpful to confront these tensions openly, because individuals could then account for themselves, apologize if necessary and always learn from the experience. The spirit of the confrontation was usually warm, sympathetic and constructive, and humour and light-hearted exaggeration were often used.

By taking on the roles of primary and associate nurse, Alison also experienced role boundary problems first-hand so that, as an actor in the situation herself rather than a detached facilitator, she was able to show the value of being open and honest when colleagues got things wrong. The continuation of the story of Claire and Mike 'overstepping the mark', reported above, provides an example of this kind of role modelling.

Overstepping the mark: Part 2

I thought about it and decided that it was important to tell them. . . . I really thought about how to present it to them. In the end, I explained exactly how I had been feeling and that first of all I had thought I was wrong and that's why I didn't say anything to begin with. I said that I had gone away and thought about it and decided that they were right up to a certain point, but wrong beyond that . . . I wanted them to realize that it isn't easy to get these things right and that I had had to think about it before I was sure; that we are all learning together . . . They were fine, not at all defensive. I think I handled it OK, though I'm glad I had given myself twenty-four hours to think about it. (AB)

Knowing what is expected

Developing a clear, shared understanding of the scope and the precise function of each new role involved thorough debate and careful negotiation. But even once the ground rules were clear, it took time and practice, led by Alison's example and considerable nudging along, before the nurses really felt that they knew what was expected of them and before they were able to practise in their new roles with confidence.

Primary nurse in name only

Telling signs of the nurses' early tentativeness as primary nurses were their hesitation over taking new patients on to their caseloads and their frequent reluctance to tell their patients when they did finally decide to assume the responsibilities of primary nurse. Being assertive about instructing colleagues acting as associates and having the confidence to prioritize their workload in favour of their primary patients were other new behaviours that emerged quite slowly. Indeed, when primary nursing was formalized, it was initially hard to tell that very much had changed, other than that there was an individual nurse's name beside a patient's name on the white board at the nurses' station.

At first, the decision to take on a primary patient was left to individual nurses. If nurses felt that they could cope with another patient, or if they established a good rapport with a patient and the patient's family on admission and wanted to see through the care they had initiated, then they would volunteer to be the primary nurse. In this way, nurses did not feel pressurized to take on bigger caseloads than they could manage, but equally it left room for prevarication. They soon recognized that taking on a primary patient involved a significant commitment and demanded extra effort and energy. Furthermore, the personal responsibilities of primary nurses were very visible within the teams and there was a sense that, if nurses were going to be primary nurses, they wanted to be seen to do the job well. Consequently, if circumstances were not quite perfect – perhaps the nurse was going to be off duty the next day, or was feeling tired from the demands of caring for another patient – then it was all too easy not to take the next patient who was admitted and to hope that someone else in the team would volunteer the next shift. The result of this system was that many patients were not allocated a primary nurse for several days and some patients never got a primary nurse at all and so were effectively 'team nursed'. The nurses were disappointed that things often turned out this way.

> *I don't feel completely happy with it. I thought it would be easier than it actually is. I thought that every patient would have a primary nurse when they came in, but in reality it's not worked out like that . . . We fluctuate between team nursing and primary nursing.* (Ruth)

> *When we started it wasn't that well planned. It tended to be somebody who you looked after for a long time that maybe became your primary patient . . . I like this patient, or I have worked with this patient a lot so I know a lot about them, so I will take them on . . . Until very recently, only patients who were in for a long time got primary nurses . . . I remember a few people . . . who I looked after who stand out in my mind and that was because I called myself their primary nurse.* (Rachel)

The problem of patients continuing to fall through the primary nursing net became a major concern. Interestingly, by this stage of the project, the staff had 'matured' and they 'owned' the problem and set about designing a better system, without automatically turning to Alison as 'the expert'.

We decided we'd make some ground rules, like every patient should have a primary nurse and we should try and decide who the primary nurse was when the patient came in. So now we actually say to someone, 'Do you want to have such and such as your primary patient?' (Ruth)

The nurses recognized the importance of team-work in making the system run well. Simply thinking about their own workloads was not enough. They had to look ahead to see which team members were going to be on duty, then consider each caseload and weigh up who would be the most appropriate person to accept the new patient. They also had to trust each other to be considerate and fair. But the decision got made early and there was no more prevarication – in Rosemary's words, '*You have to take the plunge.*'

Initially, patients were often unaware of having a primary nurse, even when a nurse had been allocated to them. They recognized the team system and could name two or three of the team members who had been especially involved in their care, but they were not always aware that one of these nurses had special responsibilities as their primary nurse. Some of the nurses admitted that they did not always tell their patients that they were the primary nurse.

I think the patients think of it as team nursing. I don't tell people that I am their primary nurse. I don't know what others do ... I suppose it's really an unnatural sort of reticence on my part. I hadn't really thought about it. (Moira)

It seemed that taking the first tentative steps towards being a primary nurse involved, for many of the nurses, simply putting their name up against the patient's on the white board and making sure that the care plan was written and up to date. Being more explicit about the role and, in particular, making it clear to their patients that they were in charge of their care, involved a commitment that, initially, some lacked the confidence to make.

When they first experienced the new system, nurses found that there was less distinction in practice between their roles as primary and associate nurses than they knew there should be.

The other day Alison asked me to think about the difference between my role as a primary nurse and my role as an associate nurse. I went home and thought about it. 'Well, I hand over the basics ... but with patients with complex and numerous problems, I find it very difficult to set the direction of care for them'. I think that that's wrong. I think that there should be a difference between the way I'm acting as a primary and associate nurse. (Moira)

The nurses' failure to assert themselves confidently as primary nurses fuelled the role boundary tension. If primary nurses were not explicit about being in charge of their patients' care, and did not provide a clear sense of direction and specific instructions for their team members, then associates felt obliged, to a certain extent, to take over and to get on with things. When some primary nurses were underconfident in their roles, it was hard, especially for the more senior nurses, to feel they could concentrate fully on their own primary patients. They still felt they had to 'check up' in detail about all their team's patients, instead of feeling comfortable that the other primary nurses would do all that was necessary when they came on duty. Trying to be an effective primary nurse oneself, while still carrying this feeling of being responsible for everything in the team, was experienced as exhausting. Thus, for some nurses, primary nursing was initially more of a burden than it should have been, while for others, functioning as primary nurse in name only, there was little significant difference.

Practising confidently

As the project progressed, there was a sense that nurses were much more relaxed about the new system. They had plenty to say about enjoying being a primary nurse and they had far fewer problems to report. Sophie's confidence and enthusiasm typified this new mood.

> *I feel I'm on the final bit now. We are now getting the feel and experience of becoming quite good with primary patients ... In relation to receiving new patients, my attitude has really changed. We are really in there now from the word go. ... Rather than thinking of leaving the assessment until tomorrow, I can see the advantages of doing it straight away ... Over the last three months I've really enjoyed my patients. I'm feeling successful as a primary nurse.* (Sophie)

The nurses were clearly beginning to feel more at home in their new roles and were able to appreciate, in more detail, what was expected from them in each.

> *We all know our responsibilities as a primary nurse ... You know damn well what you're supposed to do.* (Janice)

> *I suppose I've come to understand what primary nursing is. I've found actually taking on primary patients is getting easier and I'm finding out what my role is ... When it started, if you took on a primary patient, you didn't get any more involved than anybody else, but now you definitely feel there's a difference in your involvement in different aspects of their care ... you take a major part in the decision-making ... but I wouldn't say that it is perfect yet.* (Ruth)

There were reports of being able to switch much more comfortably between the primary and associate roles and of nurses being able to weight their workload on a shift in favour of primary patients, confident that team colleagues would be giving special time to other patients who were their primaries.

Sharon commented upon the value of the new division of labour within the team.

> *(Primary nursing) organizes things better ... It is more efficient because there is a named person responsible for everything. It works well, whereas with team nursing you had to check up on everything.* (Sharon)

Once the more senior nurses became established in their new roles, they were able to act as role models and guides for junior staff and for newcomers to the ward. Sophie recognized this teaching function as an important element of her role as team leader.

> *I am now able to explain more easily to other team members about primary nursing. For example, I can quiz them about their care plans, because I know what we are looking for.* (Sophie)

This development took pressure off Alison as the only 'expert' and it helped make the new system stable and self-perpetuating.

As the nurses became confident in the primary nurse role, they described feeling different about their work. The personal involvement with primary patients seemed to draw greater commitment from them and the challenge of personally taking charge of a patient's nursing was highly motivating. Many nurses talked about their increased sense of professional responsibility.

Before I had a primary patient I could see the difference between having a patient as a team member and as a primary nurse, but I didn't expect it to feel very different. To my surprise, I found I did feel different. I felt more responsible. (Janice)

Becoming established as a primary nurse, and meeting the challenge of the responsibilities invested in the role, was described as a very positive experience and as associated with a general increase in job satisfaction.

It's been much more satisfying and fulfilling – a complete package. There's more responsibility and it's more rewarding than just being part of a patient's care . . . you feel more in control. Before, each nurse was doing part of the care, so it seemed more fragmented. (Sophie)

Once primary nurses felt able to take their new responsibilities seriously, they were no longer hesitant about telling patients and families that they were their 'special nurse'. Indeed, as the nurses' confidence grew, they were not simply mentioning the fact that they were to be the primary nurse, but also explaining in some detail what could be expected of them in this role. Patients were able to single out their own primary nurses and were clearly developing special relationships with them. Alison noticed that if a primary relationship was working well, when she acted as an associate nurse, even though patients recognized her as the ward sister, it was the primary nurse who seemed most important to them.

There was also this very subtle thing that amused me with Mark's patient. When the lady was discharged, Mark and I were both on the ward. The daughter came up and she went to Mark first. She had a big cake with 'thank you' iced all over the top and she gave it to him and really thanked him very warmly for all he had done. Then, in that order, she came and sought me out and thanked me for what I had done. I thought, 'Yes, this family have got it exactly right.' I had been a key associate, but Mark had been the primary nurse . . . The fact that I was the sister didn't come into it really. (AB)

Reflecting on the experience of growing into a competent primary nurse and of working in a decentralized system, Janice weighed up some of the costs and the benefits.

It might seem like hard work and a lot of extra work, but it is definitely worth it for the rewards, once you get there. It's what the two visiting nurses picked up on. They noticed how dedicated everyone is and how little moaning there is, even though it's so busy. (Janice)

Establishing a primary nursing system was not an end-point, but rather a foundation or a starting point, providing an organizational framework and specific roles that gave nurses the freedom to practise in a new way. A crucial step in helping them to make the most of the opportunities offered by the new structure was creating a ward culture that challenged them to work creatively and that supported them in closer, more intense, professional relationships. This aspect of the development work is described in the next chapter.

Chapter 5

The cultural journey

'The first requirement for the successful application of the primary nursing concept is an atmosphere in which individuals feel free to learn, to risk, to make mistakes and to grow. The philosophy of the nursing department and its leaders must demonstrate this trust and give support to nurses whose attempts at comprehensive care lead to unorthodox activities.'

Manthey (1980)

INTRODUCTION

An organizational culture is the unique configuration of norms, values, attitudes, beliefs and behaviours which characterize the interactions of groups and individuals as they attempt to achieve organizational goals (Eldridge and Crombie, 1974). Language, rituals, myths and ideologies are the symbolic forms in which this organizational culture, or ethos, is enshrined (Pondy *et al.*, 1983). In the study ward, commitment to achieving a patient-centred style of practice represented a change of organizational goal for the nursing service. In the previous chapter, the structural changes introduced to support this new goal were described, but, as Clarke (1978) pointed out, structural changes alone do not alter the way people think about and experience their work.

We found that the cultural legacy of traditional nursing inhibited the kind of independent thinking and behaviour required for patient-centred practice and limited the development of nurses as professionals. We had to develop strategies for helping the nurses to confront and challenge institutionalized attitudes and behaviours. Outmoded rituals and myths had to be exposed and new customs and new language, reflecting the new ethos, had to be allowed to emerge.

Socialization – the process by which a culture is learned or absorbed – occurs because human beings need approval and reward (Bredemeier and Stephenson, 1962). The individual conforms because to do so is instrumentally useful or pleasurable. But when the purpose or value of accepted forms is forgotten, or is no longer relevant in an organization, then adherence to prescribed conduct becomes pointless, ritualistic behaviour (Merton, 1968). In the early days of the project, there was evidence of this kind of dysfunctional ritual and much of our work took the form of consciousness-raising, enabling nurses to question established norms. We proposed, modelled and reinforced new ways of thinking and behaving which were constructive and meaningful in the context of patient-centred nursing. Eventually, a new culture emerged which was experienced by the nurses as supportive of their new ways of working.

Four main themes characterize the ward's 'cultural journey'. The first concerns the nurses' gradual transition from passive to active participants in shaping the style and quality of life in their ward. The next two themes are associated with their move away from a 'worker' mentality and the development of a professional approach, first, to their practice and, second, to their own continuing education. The final theme is about changes in the way nurses related to each other – rather than being merely sociable work companions, they became concerned, supportive colleagues.

SHAPING WARD LIFE

This theme parallels the organizational process of decentralization described in the previous chapter. The structures that were created to promote decentralization provided the nurses with forums for contributing to debate and decision-making about how the ward should run, but then the nurses had to learn how to operate within them. We had to develop strategies to support this learning process.

Doing what you are told

Before the introduction of team nursing, the centralized system of ward management, with its well-defined routines and procedures, left little scope for individual nurses to use their initiative and creativity. Furthermore, the formal hierarchy in the ward, with its clear pecking order, left most nurses feeling that they had no power to influence or challenge the way the ward was run.

> *I don't think I ever thought about how I could change things . . . because I didn't feel I was in a position to do anything about it.* (Terry)

The absence of ward meetings, or of any other formal opportunity to express an opinion or to participate in decision-making, is likely to have reinforced this perception. As the nurses had not experienced ward life any differently, they tended to accept the status quo.

> *That's how I'd worked where I came from before. So to me, it was normal.* (Pat)

There were clear examples of the old culture still at work when the new structures were first introduced. During eraly ward meetings in Linacre Ward, the sister found that, '*Everyone just sat around and looked at me and waited for me to instigate everything.*' However, the sister herself was stuck in old behaviour patterns, which undermined her intentions to encourage participation from the nurses.

> *Lorraine's (the sister's) style of leadership appears essentially autocratic. She made all the final decisions, without asking the others what they thought. Discussion in the group tended to be between her and the individual nurses and not between nurse and nurse. No one was asked to be responsible for carrying out the decisions made.* (AT – Fieldnote)

We observed team leaders in both wards adopting similar behaviour, which suggested that they had little experience of a more facilitative style upon which to model their own behaviour. In addition, when individual staff nurses were asked to carry forward initiatives proposed at a meeting, progress was often slow. They were unaccustomed to this kind of responsibility and seemed to expect new developments to be managed by a senior figure.

Lukes (1986) argued that '*the sheer weight of institutions*' influences people's thinking and perceptions. Consequently, '*they accept their role in the existing order of things, either because they see it as natural and unchangeable, or because they value it as divinely ordained and beneficial.*' The nurses did not believe that the organization and culture of ward life was entirely beneficial for either themselves or patients, but they saw things as unchangeable and ordained by authorities that were invisible and inaccessible. Historically, the religious and military origins of the nursing hierarchy, and the weighty influences of gender, class and low status, have all contributed to the socialization of ward nurses into passive, limited roles. The ward culture reflected in our early data suggested that these factors were still influential in modern hospital wards.

A powerful force in maintaining the traditional non-participative, non-challenging culture was fear of the ward sister. Early studies by MacGuire (1961) and Revans (1964) found the legacy of the 'dragon' ward sister much in evidence, and Manthey (1980) saw nursing as still influenced by its '*punishment-oriented heritage*'. In our project, staff nurses appeared to be afraid that they would be punished or reprimanded if they challenged the established order, even though there seemed to be little justification for this fear. For example, in the case study, nurses often reported not agreeing with the sister or with practices she had established in the ward, but they did not challenge her. However, Mary, an experienced staff nurse, told a story which illustrates how the nurses' perceptions were determined as much by the traditional culture as by their experiences of an individual sister. The account below is summarized from an interview.

Expecting her to be Fierce

Mary decided to apply a particular dressing to a patient's pressure sore. Her colleague was not happy about this decision. When Mary pressed her for an explanation, the nurse responded, 'Sister doesn't like it'. Mary concluded that her colleagues were frightened to approach Sister to suggest new things. She felt their fears were unfounded because when she had presented her rationale for using the dressing, Lorraine (the sister) had accepted her argument. Mary thought that students and junior nurses expected a traditional sister to be 'a bit of an ogre' and, as Lorraine was 'a bit of the old school', they expected her to be fierce too. (AT)

When team nursing was introduced, the nurses were, in theory, free to manage the care of their own patients in an individualized way and there was no longer any need for the traditional routines. However, some of them lingered for a while, showing again how people's behaviour can lag behind structural change, because the principles behind the change have not become embedded in the culture and have not been properly internalized by the individuals involved. For example:

A lot of people come on to the ward . . . talking loudly and Sister would say, 'Be quiet' or 'It's rest time.' I mean, gosh, that went out with the Ark, but still, you know, we have our rest periods and they haven't changed and I don't think things like that will without a lot of special encouragement. (Amanda)

Nurses were often aware that they were conforming to cultural patterns which they did not believe in and which they recognized no longer served what they considered to be the best interests of their patients.

Strategies for increasing participation and democracy

We needed to show the nurses that their unwilling conformity was no longer necessary and to help them use the power that the new structure gave them to change things. They needed convincing that the invitation to use the new meetings as forums for questioning outmoded practices, and for contributing their own ideas, was genuine. They also needed to develop the confidence and skill to participate effectively in debate and decision-making within the meetings.

Facilitating participation

Our strategy, initially, was to include items on ward meeting agendas that were of immediate concern to the staff nurses. We anticipated that this approach would motivate them to participate in decision-making, because the issues were especially relevant to them. We aimed to demonstrate how change in ward practice could be achieved democratically. In the following excerpt from a reflective conversation, Alison articulates the detail of this strategy and illustrates its use.

Three Sets of Keys

I try to sense the things that irritate the nurses and which make their life difficult . . . I analyse the problem and then usually share this at a ward meeting, feeding back to staff what I have observed. Sometimes I might propose a solution or an alternative, but that will be for them to discuss, modify or whatever. Equally, they will be invited to suggest their solutions. At the ward meetings, I would hope to come up with some idea to try out that was felt to be a joint proposal.

A concrete example is the business of the drug keys. I had observed bad practice, in that the drug trolley was being left open. When it was locked, I had observed nurses wasting time chasing the nurse with the drug keys. Nobody was ever sure who had the keys and, from working in the ward myself, I had experienced the frustration that this caused. The nurses themselves hadn't particularly voiced this problem, but it was clearly an underlying niggle every day. The way we organized the storage of drugs was more appropriate for the old drug round procedure and did not help the nurses follow the new practice of each nurse giving the drugs to her own patients. I raised the problem at a ward meeting and tossed out the idea of perhaps having three sets of drug keys, one for each team. And then, together, we worked out a protocol for how this might work. (AB)

By her own example, Alison conveyed that it was acceptable to voice frustrations and to point out anomalies in ward life and so, quite overtly, she gave nurses permission to challenge the traditional way of doing things. We both encouraged the nurses to put forward their own concerns and ideas at meetings and, when they did, we took what they had to say seriously. When nurses presented a problem or raised a question, we often turned it back to them, to encourage them to share responsibility for planning and decision-making. Proposals for change were discussed and modified until everyone was in agreement. Developing a consensus in this way reinforced the message that everyone had a right to contribute to decision-making and that everyone had some responsibility for determining how the ward should run.

Alison was not present at all the nurses' meetings, so it was important that team leaders, particularly, learned to manage meetings effectively, as well as to participate in them. Alison helped nurses to learn these skills by encouraging them to observe her when she chaired a meeting and then discussing it afterwards. She also created opportunities for the nurses to chair meetings when she was present and gave constructive feedback on their performance. Developing the chairing and facilitation skills of other nurses helped to establish democratic practices as the norm in ward life.

Encouraging experimentation

The growth of a participative culture encouraged nurses to question the status quo and to put forward ideas for changing things. Responding positively to these ideas and using them in the development of ward life meant giving nurses freedom to try them out in practice. Thus, an important strategy complementing that of facilitating participation was encouraging nurses to experiment with new ideas in a responsible and thorough way. Our intention was to shift their view that things were either unchangeable or that change could only be initiated by a senior figure. We created opportunities for nurses to experience the whole process of coming up with a new idea, negotiating a plan for change, testing out the idea, refining it and, finally, seeing it established as a new norm. In this way, nurses gradually began to recognize that they genuinely had power to influence the style of life and practice in their ward.

The 'Three Sets of Keys' story demonstrates how this process of experimentation could work. Very importantly, Alison initiated a discussion of the possible consequences and risks of the experiment and involved the nurses in developing a protocol, which laid down rules for the proposed system, to make it as safe as possible. She showed how the freedom to experiment needed to be coupled with responsible caution. Experimentation inevitably involves some risk, not least that change might make things worse rather than better. People often learn from their mistakes and failures, and helping nurses to take responsibility for things going wrong was another aspect of building a democratic culture. To this end, experimentation was not discouraged even when it was felt the chances of success were low. The strategy of standing back and letting things run their course sometimes had a place. For example, each team experimented with a model of its choice as a framework for care planning and then fed back their experiences to the rest of the ward. Alison could see, at an early stage, that some of the experimental care plans were far too cumbersome to be workable, but she kept her reservations to herself, judging that it would be better for the nurses to come to their own conclusions and, also, that out of their struggle might come valuable new ideas.

Ward meetings were the main forum for discussing and agreeing possible experiments. As they were minuted, there was a mechanism for ensuring that experiments were reviewed, with those involved being asked to report on progress and to make recommendations for retaining, modifying or abandoning the scheme being tested. Ensuring that there was a review process and encouraging review of progress to be seen as an integral part of experimentation were other strategies for developing a responsible approach to innovation. Without these strategies there would have been the risk of flawed changes being introduced on a trial basis, but then lingering on and eventually becoming established as the norm.

The creative team

Change in any aspect of the ward culture was always a gradual process. The transformation of the passive, disempowered nursing team into a lively, confident group of creative individuals was no exception.

As already mentioned, the nurses were initially tentative and cautious about participating in meetings and needed a lot of prompting and encouragement to take on specific responsibility for carrying forward anything that was agreed. They tended to follow Alison's lead, responding to her suggestions for change and waiting to be asked, rather than volunteering, to become involved with project work. But gradually, new ideas began to emerge from all grades of staff and their confidence about personally making a contribution to ward life increased.

> *Every team is bubbling up with excitement at the moment. The Ash Team decided to colour code their documentation and have been out and spent a lot of money on new files and they have just done it. They didn't ask me – which is great!* (AB)

The ward communication book began to fill with problems and suggestions for discussion at ward meetings and the meetings themselves became increasingly lively, with nurses readily exchanging views and putting forward their ideas. Alison's role became less directive and less dominant. She commented, after the second 'away days', upon the nurses' growing independence as a group.

> *At the 'away days', if we discussed a problem, they were working at coming up with the solution themselves and often the idea would come from them, rather than from me. Whereas at last year's 'away days', there was more looking to me as 'the expert'. That wasn't the case this time.* (AB)

By the second 'away days', the nurses were also demonstrating that they had learned how to explore problematic issues together, how to negotiate rules for new behaviour and how to plan the implementation of change.

A democratic way of working became established as a valued new norm and nurses came to accept responsibility, individually and collectively, for shaping the life of their ward. For example, they discussed the part of the midday handover that took place in the ward office and were critical of themselves, admitting that they wasted time with 'messing about and chit-chat'. They felt that this was selfish behaviour because it meant that people were delayed in getting on with their afternoon work. They negotiated new guidelines for the handover and agreed to caution each other if there was any tendency to slip back into old habits.

By the second year of the project, the nurses no longer waited to be told what would happen or what they should do. They were alert to new problems arising and to changing circumstances and took the initiative to put forward proposals for how things should be managed. For example, at the end of the project, when it was planned that Alison should have some sabbatical leave for writing, the nurses discussed possible ward management arrangements for her absence and proposed that one of the team leaders should act as sister, rather than having an outside senior nurse 'borrowed' to fill the gap. They put forward sound reasons for their proposal and so it was accepted.

The opportunity for every nurse, regardless of grade, to participate fully in shaping ward life was greatly appreciated. The nurses enjoyed the sense of active involvement in the ward, of feeling able to contribute and being *more able to voice an opinion*, and they liked the comfortable sense of belonging that came from feeling *part of the team*.

LEARNING TO WORK PROFESSIONALLY

The transition from traditional nursing to a patient-centred style of practice required a shift in the nurses' focus, from the completion of a series of tasks, to the development of therapeutic relationships and the prescription of carefully individualized practical strategies. This shift of focus required a change in the whole ethos surrounding the nurses' work. The existing 'worker' ethos, which implied that nursing, like industrial labour, consisted of well-defined jobs to be completed to a predictable timetable, became untenable. It had to be replaced by a 'professional' ethos, which emphasized nurses' commitment to provide a personal service for their own patients and acknowledged the wide discretion each nurse must be able to use in fulfilling this commitment. We had to create a climate that accommodated and supported a professional way of working and we had to help individual nurses to adapt to the greater responsibility, independence and flexibility it involved.

Getting through the work

The old culture, in which 'work' was seen as practical tasks structured within a rigid routine, was hard for the nurses to leave behind, even though they recognized its limitations. One nurse, recalling her student days in Oriel Ward, described the almost frenetic rounds of ward activity that characterized the old system.

> It was horribly busy, rushing around all the time doing obs and temps . . . I absolutely hated it and I never wanted to work here. (Janice)

Unpopular though the system had been, its values lingered long after team nursing had been introduced. For example, some nurses felt guilty if they stopped to talk with patients. Still nagging at them and contradicting their modern, conscious belief that talking to patients is important, was the old attitude that talking with patients is not real work. Similarly, although the nurses wanted to work flexibly, prioritizing what they did according to the particular needs and wishes of their patients, they seemed almost haunted by the traditional imperative that baths and bed-making must be finished '*by the time the lates came on*'. The habits of needing to be seen to be busy, of rushing to get through 'the work' and of clock-watching, both in relation to the traditional ward routine and in relation to getting off duty on time, all seemed to be deeply embedded in the nursing culture, making the worker ethos difficult to shake off. These findings recall Clarke's (1978) account of nurses who saw properly constituted 'work' as '*expending physical energy doing something, during the time they were paid for*' (p. 77), and they are similar to Johns' (1989) observations of nurses who wanted to attend to their patients' psychological needs, but found themselves too locked in to the culture of 'mucking in together' to get through the work.

Another aspect of the worker ethos was the tendency to accept orders from people in authority without question. While nurses would say they had a role as 'the patient's advocate' and believed they had their own professional contribution to make to their patients' care, it seemed all too easy for them to slip back, unaware, into the old pattern of taking orders from others, particularly from doctors.

Removing the Charts

It was quite an interesting problem of a man with a phaeochromocytoma, which is a tumour that causes blood pressure to go out of control. It is operable, but because the blood pressure is all over the place, patients have to have some rest and drug control before they go to theatre. This patient was very anxious about his blood pressure . . . and the more he knew it was all over the place, the more he worried about it. And that upset his blood pressure even more. The doctors had said, 'Just take his charts away from his room and don't let him see them.' The staff nurse's care plan said that he was anxious and one of her aims was 'to relieve anxiety'. The strategy she prescribed was to take his charts away, so he couldn't see them. Now it wasn't clear to me whether that had been negotiated with the patient. So I asked her and she said that the doctor said that's what you must do – so that's what you must do . . . She just hadn't questioned that. (AB)

This story illustrates the contradiction found in much of the data, particularly in the early part of the project and, as in this case, still appearing occasionally in the final year. The nurses believed strongly that they should be working in a mature, professional way, but the reality was that, in their practice, they had learned to function more like obedient workers. Shedding the habits and the implicit values of the culture they no longer believed in, and embracing the professional ethos they aspired to, involved a considerable struggle.

Strategies for developing a professional work ethos

Many aspects of the development work contributed to the creation of a professional work ethos. Some have already been described in Chapter 4, including the creation of more independent roles and of opportunities for nurses to extend their responsibilities beyond the confines of their daily practice. In Chapter 7, the ways in which nurses were helped to use their relationships with patients more effectively and to manage complex clinical decision-making are highlighted. All these strategies played a part in drawing nurses away from the limited and tightly controlled working practices associated with traditional nursing and in enabling them to work in the more open, professional manner that patient-centred nursing requires.

In addition, we developed specific strategies to promote greater awareness of what it means to work professionally and to encourage attitudes and behaviours within the nursing team which supported professional ways of working. We used opportunities at meetings and 'away days' to talk explicitly about the nature and value of a professional approach to work, in relation to the kind of service the nurses wanted to provide for their patients. By practising alongside the nurses, Alison was able to identify when they were still operating in 'worker mode'. She used these situations to help them examine their own behaviour and to recognize the implications of clinging, albeit unintentionally, to old habits. Reflecting on real situations in this way was a powerful consciousness-raising strategy. It brought nurses face to face with the reality of the professional responsibilities that individuals had to carry if they were seriously committed to patient-centred practice.

Alison encouraged nurses to take responsibility for managing their own work. For example, she did not tell nurses when to take meal breaks, but made it clear that they were expected to organize breaks themselves, negotiating cover for their absence with colleagues. Similarly, she did not tell nurses when they should go home – *'It's up to you. If you feel you have finished your work and your colleagues are happy that you have handed over to them properly, then, by all means, go home.'* She made it clear that commitment to patient-centred practice was not compatible with rigid shift working, but required nurses to support each other in accommodating their varying personal workloads.

Alison used 'permission-giving' and facilitation strategies to help nurses let go of the old ward routines and to encourage them to let the special needs of their patients determine how they spent their time. In particular, when working alongside the nurses, she tried to make it both permissible and possible for them to give priority to spending time with distressed or anxious patients, so that this work was no longer seen as a luxury, subordinated to the routines of practical tasks. Sometimes Alison would free nurses of other work so that they could concentrate on the patients who needed them most. She might take on some of the extra work herself, or suggest how it could be postponed or shared out to colleagues. By showing how work could be organized in this way, Alison gave a clear message that making focussed time for patients in particular need was important. She also demonstrated that, by working flexibly and by using colleagues appropriately, the more time-consuming psychological aspect of nursing care could often be given the priority that nurses felt it deserved, even during a busy shift.

Finally, to complement this practical, visible effort to release nurses from the influence of the old routine-orientated culture, every opportunity was taken to help nurses reflect upon how they used their time and the degree to which they felt their work mirrored their beliefs and values about patient-centred practice. Supervisory discussions, informal conversations and staff development reviews were used to promote this kind of reflection and the use of reflective diaries was encouraged.

Professional commitment

The emergence of a professional work culture in the ward happened gradually, with nurses initially asserting themselves independently and responsibly in some areas of their work, while remaining passive and unthinking in others. However, over time, there was increasing flexibility in their work and greater conscious, personal commitment, both to patients and to colleagues.

Eventually the nurses were managing their time in a confident and independent way. The duty rota was organized competently by an E grade staff nurse, within guidelines agreed at a ward meeting. Around the basic shift structure, nurses were observed negotiating with their team colleagues exactly when they started or finished work. Many nurses came in early or stayed late to do something particular with a patient or to finish important work for which they felt personally responsible. Nurses were often seen in the ward outside shift times, and out of uniform, when they chose to attend meetings or when they made time for project work. Substantial chunks of non-clinical time (half a day or more) were usually scheduled within the duty rota. When nurses were in the ward for shorter periods of unscheduled time, they might negotiate with their team colleagues to take time in lieu, but sometimes they did not bother. Far from abusing the freedom they were given to manage their time, the nurses tended to give more time to the ward than they had done previously and than was 'officially' required. Indeed, at times, Alison became anxious that some nurses were giving too much of their own time to the ward and she would talk to them about getting a healthy balance between their commitment to work and their need for personal time. However, in general, being in control of their own time changed the way nurses felt about putting in extra effort for their patients and for the ward.

> *You are always staying late and putting in extra time ... but you readjust the way you look at it. Because I want to do it and I take the decision to do it, it doesn't seem stressful.* (Sharon)

In relation to managing their clinical work, the nurses also gradually became more flexible, structuring their time each day around the particular needs of their own patients. They took note of the way Alison worked when she carried a caseload and they learned from her role modelling.

> *Alison spends a lot of time with the patients and that is correct, but sometimes the more mundane things, the tasks like making the beds, aren't done ... But she does stay behind to do the work she hasn't done.* (Janice)

A year later, the same nurse commented upon how differently this way of working felt compared with the constant 'rushing around' she had experienced earlier.

> *Everything is much slower for some reason, though the workload is hard ... a slower, more relaxed pace and the ward is for patients and you have time ... You have to have time and patience with the patients and to see their problems – not the medical problems necessarily, but how they see things.* (Janice)

Another staff nurse captured her own letting go of task-focussed time management in her reflective diary. This excerpt from the diary shows the gulf that can exist between what nurses believe they should do and what they actually do in practice.

Camouflaged Task-Oriented Nursing

On Saturday . . . I was on a late. . . . At about 5 p.m. I suddenly realized that I was working the shift in a way I'd not done before. Instead of rushing around doing all the outstanding things which needed doing, such as taking out a venflon, organizing transport, etc. I was actually going around my patients giving them all the nursing care I could.

I suppose I'd moved on from organizing my work around tasks that needed doing and was actually organizing my time around the patients and therefore doing those tasks which I had to do, but also nursing the person at the same time – incorporating the tasks into my care. And so I . . . walked Elizabeth down the ward and back instead of just giving her tablets etc.

I don't know why I suddenly started working in this way – perhaps because I've found the confidence to stop rushing around trying to do the things I have to do and found that I could slow down and give the care I should be giving . . . Despite being saturated with the patient-centred approach to nursing care and . . . finding task-oriented nursing an anathema, I hadn't realized that I was actually working in a task-oriented style! I'm incredibly surprised, not to say somewhat horrified, that I have been working from such a bad basis of practice! In theory, I totally reject task-centred care and yet I suddenly realize that my practice has been task-centred, although so well camouflaged that I hadn't even realized. (Barbara)

The emergence of new cultural norms in the ward helped to pave the way for patient-centred practice. Gradually shedding the rigidity and the task-focussed thinking and behaviour inherited from the traditional culture seemed to free the nurses to be more open, attentive and responsive to their patients. Becoming more responsible for planning and directing their own work challenged and motivated them. Supported by the new professional ethos in the ward, the nurses were able to begin exploring the therapeutic potential of a more patient-focussed approach to their work.

LEARNING AT WORK

In the traditional system, initial training was generally considered to be a sufficient educational basis for a life-long professional career. After qualification, nurses were expected to develop their skills and confidence through experience, but there was little or no expectation that continuing education should be part of their working lives. Furthermore, the emphasis upon accepting the established order and working to standardized procedures did little to encourage the intellectual curiosity of nurses. As Fretwell (1980) found, the traditional ward routines *'stifled the spirit of inquiry'*.

The notion that professional education should end at qualification has now become untenable. New knowledge, ideas and techniques so frequently confront the practitioner, in every profession, that regular educational refreshment and updating has become essential to maintain an appropriate level of competence and to retain public confidence. In nursing, the UKCC's (1994) requirement that evidence of continuous learning should be a condition of periodic re-registration shows that the profession is seriously embracing this principle. At the level of everyday ward practice, new incentives for qualified nurses to continue learning are provided by the explicit personal accountability accompanying primary nursing and by the challenge to be creative that comes with a patient-centred approach to care.

At the beginning of the project, the nurses were aware of the pressures to keep themselves up to date and they generally believed that continuous learning was a good thing. However, the existing ward culture was antithetical to learning. Creating a new climate, in which work was experienced as intellectually stimulating and as providing rich learning opportunities, was a way of releasing the energy and creativity that the nurses needed to develop and sustain a patient-centred style of practice.

Missed learning opportunities

Nurses initially construed work and learning as separate activities and, as they often experienced work as 'exhausting', they had no energy left for learning. They were, indeed, observed to be working extremely hard in the ward and looking tired when they went home. Their practice drained them and they sought recreation, stimulation and relief from stress outside of work. When the nurses' workload relaxed a little, they saw this as an opportunity for a well-deserved escape from work, rather than as an opportunity for educational refreshment.

> I'm not prepared to stay behind after my working hours on the ward. I have to go. I need to go home to have a break . . . When Alison asks if nurses would like to go to the library, surely she must know that people are not likely to go, that they are more likely to go home? You need to get away from the stress to have a break. (Janice)

The nurses talked a lot about wanting to develop professionally, but they conveyed no sense of knowing how to take responsibility for their own continuous learning. When Alison joined the ward, they looked to her to motivate them and to provide educational opportunities. In the early days, Alison's efforts to support nurses in this respect often failed, because they could not sustain their initial interest and enthusiasm alongside their negative feelings about their work: 'I'm just too tired to sit in the library and study'.

During the course of each shift, coffee breaks and meal breaks were seen as opportunities to escape from 'what was going on out there' and conversation about life outside the ward was favoured as a pleasant distraction from work. Often, during breaks, the nurses also shared experiences of frustration in their work or related amusing incidents from their practice. These exchanges seemed to function as opportunities for 'letting off steam', an emotional release to counter the pressures of work.

There was little evidence of nurses actively seeking to learn from talking about their practice. On a day to day basis, there was limited criticism of the standard approaches to patient care and a lack of curiosity about alternative ways of working with patients. Nurses were rarely observed challenging each other's decisions or offering different perspectives on a clinical problem.

> I wonder how I would feel if I'd worked hard over a care plan and someone said, 'What do you think about such and such?' No one's ever said that to me. So I wonder whether people aren't saying it, but whether they actually feel it? (Janice)

The nurses said that they wanted to be stimulated and challenged at work and that they would value honest feedback about their practice, but when Alison responded by commenting critically upon their work, and by asking probing questions about their care of patients, the nurses reacted in a negative way.

> *When Alison said, 'Have you tried this? Have you done that?', I immediately got my defences up, because I had tried really hard with this patient. It has been a real slog lately and . . . I am not very good at taking criticism, but maybe because nobody has ever questioned what I do . . . When Alison is trying to be constructive, you think she is criticizing you.* (Rachel)

The nurses were unable, at first, to recognize that Alison was trying to help them to learn. Her observations and questions made them feel anxious, inadequate or defensive, because they assumed she was making unfavourable judgements about their performance.

In her study of a traditional nursing service, Menzies (1970) reported senior nurses complaining that junior nurses *'are irresponsible, behave carelessly and impulsively, and in consequence must be ceaselessly supervised and disciplined.'* The nurses' early responses to Alison's attempts to stimulate critical thinking showed that the traditional expectation that criticism from a senior figure implied a reprimand, was still firmly embedded in the ward culture. The nurses could sometimes catch themselves being influenced by this traditional legacy, even when they knew that Alison's intentions were educational rather than punitive.

> *Mark described how he and Rachel were getting into a panic because a patient didn't have a care plan and Alison was coming on to the team on the late shift. In retrospect, he realized that this was 'ridiculous' and 'not at all in line with what Alison was hoping to be able to offer the team.'* (AT – Fieldnote)

In addition, Angie's role was initially viewed with suspicion. The arrival of a researcher, collecting and feeding back data about the nurses' practice, was inevitably the cause of some anxiety. Nurses tended to feel that Angie's questioning was rather stressful. It took them time to appreciate that her observations and questions were designed, like Alison's, to stimulate growth and learning, as well as to seek data.

Strategies for promoting curiosity, openness and debate

Repeatedly asking open questions and encouraging informal discussion of practice issues were two simple, but effective, strategies used to develop a more critical and enquiring culture in the ward. During bedside handovers, Alison would interrupt the exchange of information about patients, saying, for example, 'That's an interesting problem. I wonder what is behind all that?' Sometimes, she would initiate discussions in the ward corridor, as nurses walked from one patient bay to another. Alternatively, when it seemed appropriate and always careful not to undermine nurses in front of their patients, she would open up the discussion at the bedside, involving the patient concerned and, perhaps, a relative. Although at first, as mentioned above, the nurses were inclined to misconstrue Alison's questions and sometimes felt threatened by these exploratory discussions, they gradually became used to them and recognized the value of Alison's approach.

Alison opens our eyes to new ideas, new ways of looking at things ... When she takes an interest in our patients, she says 'Have you thought of this or that?' She helps me to think about a much wider area than I have been used to. During handover, she will ask questions about the patient, about things that I hadn't really thought about. (Sophie)

Similarly, over coffee in the staff-room, Alison took every opportunity to stimulate lively, informal discussion about practice issues. She would present something that was puzzling or worrying her about one of her own patients and would ask the nurses to give their opinion. She would also prompt discussion about general issues that had some relevance in the ward at the time, such as the difficulties of caring for confused patients, for example.

Alison's aim was to show the nurses that she was interested in them as professional people, not just as workers who had to get through the chores in the ward. By sharing her own questions and doubts, by seeking their opinions and by respecting (if not always agreeing with) what they had to say, Alison tried to nurture the nurses' self-confidence, so that they could engage in debate without defensiveness. She aimed 'to give permission' for greater openness in the ward and to demonstrate how challenging the status quo or questioning a colleague's practice could be handled constructively. Gradually, the nurses became more relaxed about Alison's questions and, slowly, their own critical faculties were aroused.

Alison took an interest in us and our development, which we had never felt before ... By helping us to be more aware of why we were doing things, we started to question our own practice. (Ursula)

In time, as the habit of exploring and discussing clinical problems together became established in the ward, Alison often took a less prominent role in facilitating the debates that occurred. She would sit back and listen and only intervene occasionally, to nudge things along or to suggest a new avenue of enquiry.

In the staff-room, four staff nurses try to help Henrietta to identify her patient's problems and aims of care. They help her to see what she, as a nurse, can do ... Later Alison told me that she had deliberately allowed silences and had been consciously not leaping in and taking over, so as to allow some peer group teaching and learning. (AT – Fieldnote)

Angie supported and complemented Alison's work in this area during her fieldwork. Her data collection task gave a legitimate reason to talk informally with nurses about their work and her questions often prompted them to look afresh at taken for granted aspects of ward life. It was thus not difficult for her to use her fieldwork to make a contribution to the development of a more open and critical culture in the ward. However, she had to remain aware of the dual function she was fulfilling and to maintain a clear distinction in her own mind between the two different activities in which she was engaged.

It was crucial for us both to remain sensitive to the nurses' readiness to learn and to cope with a more challenging culture. At first, for example, we were cautious about raising difficult issues, or pushing nurses to explore a problem, when the ward was exceptionally busy. We did not want them to experience a more enquiring approach to work as simply adding to their pressures. On the other hand, sometimes helping nurses to stand back for a moment, to consider how they were responding to an apparently overwhelming workload, could be constructive and could release tension.

Gradually, nurses began to take a more critical and curious approach to their own work, but they continued to find it difficult to challenge each other's practice and to give critical feedback. They felt that they should be able to be honest with each other and to discuss their practice openly, but they were inhibited by fear of causing offence and of straining close working relationships. In response to this problem, we encouraged them to explore the issue of openness within their individual teams of only six or seven team members. This work began at the ward's second 'away days'. A 'trust and honesty session' was included in the programme which allowed each team space, time and privacy to talk about their concerns, to explore 'undercurrents' in team relationships and to plan strategies for working more openly together.

The trust and honesty session wa3 a very popular one. Each team handled it differently . . . I moved around the teams to help a little bit. For the Ash Team, it was quite painful and it was just opening up . . . What was clarified was that they had a lot of work to do . . . The Elm team talked about giving criticism and feedback and they negotiated ground rules about how they would talk to each other. (AB)

A further strategy for helping nurses to learn from their work was to suggest that they might establish 'critical friendships'. A 'friendship' could be developed between two nurses who already felt comfortable working together. The idea was that they should identify an area of their practice that they both wanted to develop, and then they should meet regularly to give each other constructive, critical feedback on their progress. In these 'friendships', the nurses needed to be honest with each other, while also being sensitive and supportive. 'Critical friends' were also advised to exchange feedback on the effectiveness of each other's helping strategies. In this way, we hoped that the nurses would develop the skills of facilitating learning from practice, as well as developing in particular substantive areas.

Only a few nurses chose to establish 'critical friendships' in a formal way, but those who did seemed to find them both valuable and enjoyable. One pair of nurses, for example, decided to work together on developing their care planning skills and they met, whenever they could, to read and discuss each other's care plans. One of the problems of maintaining a 'critical friendship' in a hospital ward is the shift system. The nurses who experimented with these relationships often found the momentum and enthusiasm of working together difficult to sustain when frequently interrupted by one of the pair disappearing for a few weeks for night duty or holiday. Possibly for this reason, rather than many strong 'critical friendships' growing up between pairs of nurses, what actually emerged were less formal 'critical groups' within individual teams.

The groups that Angie established for D grade nurses across the Medical Unit provided learning opportunities away from the wards, but learning was focussed upon everyday practice issues confronting the nurses who attended. Angie facilitated two confidential, supportive groups in which nurses shared their interests, experiences and difficulties. Angie's aim, within this safe, comfortable context, was to encourage nurses to adopt a more critical and creative approach to their work and to take responsibility for their own learning. Drawing upon her earlier experience in physiotherapy education (Titchen, 1987a; 1987b), she offered the nurses a cyclical problem-solving framework to structure their work together. Participants were invited to determine their own agendas. Then Angie helped them to explore and clarify the problems they had identified and to develop action plans for addressing issues back in their own wards. Nurses subsequently reported upon and evaluated their actions and their plans were elaborated or redrawn as necessary. Angie developed a record sheet, based on the steps of the problem-solving cycle, which facilitated a systematic approach to the group sessions and ensured that agreed actions were regularly reviewed.

Angie adopted a facilitation style and used processes and skills drawn from the work of Rogers (1983), Boud *et al.* (1985) and Heron (1989). To get some feedback on her facilitation work, and on the group processes that developed, she invited a colleague within the hospital to observe two group sessions as her 'critical friend'. As well as being helpful for Angie, this initiative provided an opportunity for her to introduce the idea of 'critical friendship' to some of the nurses.

The lively, critical community

From quite early on in the project, nurses began to recognize that, under Alison's leadership, it was acceptable to be critical about the ward generally and to express an opinion about how things might be changed.

> *There is quite a lot of thinking going on and debate about what is right and wrong and helpful. There is a growing amount of freedom to do that, and it comes down to having the skills and knowledge to make use of the freedom when you've got it.* (AB)

By the final year of the project, not only were informal critical debates very much part of ward life, but they also had greater depth and substance. Nurses were observed exploring a general issue, or a particular clinical problem, in a lively but careful and thorough way.

> *Yesterday we were having coffee and Rachel bounced into the staff-room and sat down and said, 'I've got an ethical problem I want to discuss with you all'. They really discussed this problem properly and discovered that there were no easy answers. They were using each other and me and taking it very seriously.* (AB)

The more stimulating climate in the ward may have been one factor contributing to the nurses' gradually increasing motivation in relation to individual and group project work. Another influence here was the nurses' growing recognition that their learning and development could be directly relevant to their everyday practice. The number of projects initiated by nurses certainly increased and, by the latter part of the study, all the nurses in the ward were committed to pursuing some particular interest, often with responsibility for bringing back new ideas and information for their colleagues. Nurses commented that they had never worked anywhere where there were so many people involved in projects, and visiting nurses were struck by the industry and enthusiasm that all this project work represented.

The value of project work, as an opportunity for learning and professional growth, was illustrated vividly by 'The Care Plan Project', the most substantial of the projects to emerge.

(The Care Plan Project) gave me time out to focus on one issue. To do it in partnership has definitely been brilliant . . . and to be doing something which is ongoing in the ward, to have been able to spark off some of the care plan discussion. It has given me confidence in myself when speaking in groups or publicly. It has improved my interpersonal skills in dealing with people that, as an ordinary staff nurse, I wouldn't even have dreamed of speaking to, like (the Director of Nursing). I've learned to think on my feet a lot through the workshops . . . and it helped my patient-centredness, having the opportunity to observe Alison closely and ask her all those things. (Rosemary)

Learning from criticism of one's own decisions and behaviour was much harder, but the following story indicates how important it was for the nurses' professional development.

Ruth's Story

Ruth described herself as being afraid of looking inadequate in Alison's eyes. Alison had observed an interaction between Ruth and a doctor in which Ruth appeared disinterested and ill-informed about her primary patient. Alison fed back her observations to Ruth, explaining why she thought the interaction was poor and how it suggested a lack of involvement with her primary patient. Later, Ruth told Angie, 'I felt angry because it wasn't positive and because I don't get much feedback. When I did get it, it was negative and demoralizing.'

Angie explained to Ruth that Alison was trying to create an open learning environment in the ward, where people could be honest, and that she was asking people for feedback on how she was helping them to learn. Ruth said she would tell Alison that she had reflected on the feedback and was now trying to change her behaviour as a result. Angie suggested that Ruth should tell Alison that she had initially felt angry, but had later thought the criticism was justified.

Two weeks later, Angie asked Alison if Ruth had spoken to her. Alison replied, 'Yes. I was so shocked, I don't think I dealt with it very well. I'm quite cross with myself. It was on a late shift and I was staying to write a care plan. I was going off for the weekend and I'd spent half an hour talking with a patient and I thought I must write this into an assessment. This was Friday night and it was very late. Ruth was on night duty and I was sitting in the staff room, exhausted, trying to write my care plan. She had obviously summoned up her courage and just walked round the door. She didn't sit down and just blurted out, straight at me, "I want to tell you that when you criticized me the other day, I was very upset, but since then, I've really been thinking about what you told me and I've been trying to use it." She did it really well, but she was standing only just in the room, just round the door. I was so taken aback. We talked about it then a bit, but I should have asked her to sit down and I wish I'd asked her more about how she was using what I had said. I asked her what had prompted her to say this to me suddenly, after all that time, and she said that talking with you made her think about it.'

Circumstances in the busy ward were often far from perfect for giving and receiving critical feedback sensitively and openly, and a colleague's frankness might be experienced as painful, even when well intentioned. Nonetheless, nurses continued to work hard at being honest with each other and, in this way, at helping each other to learn from practice. The team leaders, in particular, became increasingly confident and skilled at confronting tensions between team members.

> *Alison reported that she had observed Sharon and Kate in a supervision session. There had been a history of tension between the two and Kate had been defensive when Sharon had tried to give her feedback before. In this session, Kate had looked slightly defensive (arms folded) at first, but then suddenly she got some sense of why she was stuck and what the problem was that Sharon was trying to get across to her. Sharon reported that the session went quite well and that Kate had accepted her criticisms.* (AT – Fieldnote)

In the D grade support groups, Angie was able to help nurses take a fresh, critical look at some common practice problems. The problems nurses brought to the groups included low motivation and high stress levels, role ambiguity and role boundary tensions, dissatisfaction with written care plans and communication difficulties between nurses and doctors. Being helped to explore problems like these in a logical and thorough way was a new experience for the nurses and, like newly qualified nurses in the study reported by Lathlean *et al.* (1986), some had difficulty analysing and theorizing their practice and identifying salient issues.

Given time, however, the group process enabled nurses to see their problems in a different light. For example, nurses from one ward initially felt that the main problem with their care plans was that they were being written in different ways by each team, whereas nurses from another ward were concerned that their care plans were written by rote and were therefore not useful in practice. After a lively, free-ranging debate, nurses from both wards agreed that the major problem with their care plans was that they were 'nurse-centred' rather than 'patient-centred'. This new conceptualization of the problems led to specific action plans aimed at finding ways to identify their patients' perspectives and concerns and writing the care plans with their patients.

CARING FOR EACH OTHER

Just as we had to develop the intellectual climate in the ward, we also had to pay attention to its emotional climate. We had to build greater tolerance and sensitivity into the ward culture, in order to support nurses who were beginning to carry more personal responsibility and who were becoming more directly exposed to the distress and suffering of their patients.

The sociable team

In the traditional nursing system, relationships between staff, and between staff and patients, were formal and distant. Nurses were advised 'not to get involved' with patients and they were expected to keep their emotions hidden behind a professional mask (Jourard, 1971). Menzies (1970) showed how this denial of emotion and avoidance of real human relationship in ward life served to shield nurses from the reality of their patients' pain. She also showed how nurses' traditional dependence upon rules and procedures functioned to protect them from the stresses of personal responsibility.

During the case study, nurses talked about being unable to express emotions at work and about feeling unsupported in distressing situations.

Anna and I talked about the death of a patient yesterday. She said, 'I wanted to talk about this with someone, but (peers) are on nights or annual leave. I thought about talking to Sister, but decided not to. I talked to my husband – he's very good. He listens, but he can't really fully understand, not knowing the ward.' (AT – Fieldnote)

The nurses in Linacre Ward saw the sister, in particular, as maintaining the traditional emotional reserve that was part of the ward culture.

Sister is lovely. She has helped me to do my job, but she's not a person you can go to and have a little chat over something that has upset you . . . so I just go home and there is no one to share it with . . . She's a bit of the old school – although I think she is changing now – with an attitude that they should sort of get on with it . . . She does care, but she gives out that attitude of being closed in and unapproachable. (Tina, nursing auxiliary)

In contrast, the early data from Oriel Ward showed no evidence of the distance and formality inherited from the traditional system. Indeed, a striking feature of the ward, which had been present well before Alison's appointment, was its relaxed, friendly atmosphere. The nurses valued informality – the previous sister and the staff nurses had always called each other by their first names and they had often gone out together socially. The ward was welcoming and was a popular place for doctors and other hospital staff to meet for a chat and coffee with the nurses. The nurses described themselves as '*a close-knit brood*'. In their daily practice, they supported each other by '*mucking in to help each other get through the work*', and they shared their feelings about distressing situations.

However, this apparently comfortable ward atmosphere and the friendly sociable relationships between the nurses had limitations which began to show under the pressures of change. For example, when team nursing was introduced and nurses started to work more independently with their own caseloads, they often complained of feeling isolated and of finding that their colleagues did not offer to help when they were exceptionally busy. Under the old 'ends system', when nursing work was still structured in terms of tasks, 'getting through the work' was essentially a communal effort. Nurses could easily assess how their colleagues were coping with their workload by how near they were to completing the routine tasks. If one nurse was behind with her work, another could easily step in to help. Once team nursing was established, individual nurses structured their own work differently each day, according to the needs of their patients, and so they could not automatically judge how their colleagues in other teams were getting along. There was no ready common currency for measuring their progress. Supporting each other in the team system required nurses to take an active interest in each other's workload, purposefully enquiring whether, and in what way, help was required. This kind of intentional concern for each other was not part of the culture of the 'sociable ward team', and nurses who were unwilling to admit that they were struggling were often left unsupported.

The 'sociable team' had difficulty coping with the arrival of new staff nurses recruited by Alison because they were keen to be involved in the development of primary nursing. The newcomers, with their bright ideas and different practices, were ostracized by the existing staff.

Initially, the nurses were very friendly and quite welcoming, but once the novelty wore off, I found them quite defensive and they left me to work on my own when I had heavy patients and needed two people. You would have difficulty getting someone to come and help and you'd find that everyone had gone off to coffee without mentioning it to you. (Kathryn)

Kathryn reported that three other new staff nurses had told her separately and spontaneously that they felt undervalued and had not been made to feel part of the team. It seemed that the prospect of change in their familiar world made the existing 'sociable team' feel threatened. The apparently cosy atmosphere in the ward seemed to mask an underlying insecurity and intolerance of different ways of working, which the beginning of the development exposed.

The 'sociable team' was also not good at dealing with conflict or uncomfortable problems. Nurses talked and complained together about someone who had upset them or someone who they disapproved of in some way, but they were reluctant to confront people openly about their concerns, preferring to maintain a facade of all being well.

There were a couple of occasions when apparently I'd upset the other team members by things that I had done . . . (but) they didn't actually come to tell me. One particular incident was after a period of nights that I was on. We had been deciding who should write care plans at night and we'd felt that if somebody was admitted, the nurse on night duty could write the care plan and it could be reviewed the next day by the day staff. So I carried on and wrote the care plans for patients that we admitted, even though they weren't in my team. People misconstrued this as me interfering in their team . . . and they got really upset about that. I felt I was just doing what we agreed. (Kathryn)

The 'sociable team' was essentially friendly and well meaning, but it lacked the tolerance and maturity required to provide genuine care and support for its members in difficult circumstances. It had much in common with Johns' (1992) 'harmonious team' which maintained a facade of togetherness, in a traditional ward setting, by brushing conflict under the carpet.

Strategies for creating a climate of concern and support

If nurses are to develop a patient-centred style of practice, they have to become involved in emotionally demanding relationships with patients and they are challenged to take risks and to make difficult decisions. How well nurses cope with these personal demands must depend considerably on the degree to which they feel they can rely on respect, understanding and support from their colleagues. Thus a crucial element of the project was the development of a culture in which nurses actively supported each other and in which stresses and tensions were quickly brought to the surface and dealt with in constructive ways.

Our strategies mirrored some of those already described, except that they had a different focus. Role modelling and 'permission giving' were again particularly important. In her everyday work, Alison tried to give high priority to looking after staff, on the basis that if she did not care for them, they would not be able to care for their patients. She also hoped that by showing genuine concern for the nurses, they would learn to show similar concern for each other. She particularly tried to support team leaders, so that they in turn would be able to respond helpfully to their team members. The following fieldnote gives a glimpse of this approach in action.

> Sharon begins to pour out all the difficulties the team is facing with their patients. Alison listened supportively and offered help . . . Later, Sharon told me that she was 'off-loading' and that 'It helps to have a moan – I didn't expect her to be able to do anything.' (AT – Fieldnote)

Giving nurses support when they needed it sometimes meant making difficult choices. For example, Alison saw a nurse about to go home from her night shift looking extremely miserable, so she stopped her and took her in the office to see what was the matter. Listening to the nurse and helping her to work through her feelings took half an hour, at the beginning of a busy morning. Alison knew there were dozens of things that needed doing in the ward, but she chose to stay and talk with the nurse. By making time for nurses when they needed support, even in difficult circumstances, Alison hoped to make them feel that they were valued and that they could rely on her. Similarly, when Angie was in the ward, she also looked out for cues indicating that nurses were stressed or anxious and would offer to listen and talk things through.

Role modelling was a valuable strategy for helping nurses to deal with tensions and conflicts. Uncomfortable subjects were brought into the open, at ward meetings, with members of an individual team, or in one to one discussions, and Alison showed how these issues could be explored honestly and constructively. For example, a nurse in the Oak Team began to talk vaguely about leaving the ward only a few months after her appointment. Although she said that she liked the ward, she was clearly unsettled. When Alison explored the problem with her, it emerged that the nurse's regular rotation on to night duty was causing problems in her marriage, so she felt that she would have to leave. When Alison presented this situation to the Oak Team, they decided that they would share the nurse's night duty between them, because they valued her presence in the team and did not want her to leave. There were individuals in the team who liked working at night and they negotiated a fair way to share the extra burden of night duty between them. The nurse concerned was delighted and surprised at the solution that emerged and she stayed on in the ward for several years, making a strong and valuable contribution.

Using project data was another way of helping nurses to express openly what they really felt and to confront difficult problems. Angie would summarize what nurses had told her about an issue, maintaining their anonymity, but showing the strength of their feelings by using their language as much as possible. Once this material was out in the open, and seen to be acceptable, nurses felt able to own the problems that previously nobody had had the courage to raise.

By encouraging open discussion and demonstrating the value of listening to different perspectives we brought greater tolerance into the ward culture. 'Trust and honesty' sessions, as well as serving their original function to promote critical debate, were also helpful in stimulating the nurses to consider the degree to which they were generally sensitive and tolerant towards each other in their teams. They helped to raise awareness of the value of consciously caring for each other on a personal level, as well as on a professional level.

As nurses increasingly took responsibility themselves for maintaining the climate of openness and support, those who contributed particularly well in this area were given positive feedback to reinforce the sense that this was a valuable aspect of the ward culture.

The caring team

Some of the nurses who had been in the ward before Alison's arrival expressed concern that the development of a more professional approach to work would spoil the relaxed, friendly atmosphere. In time, however, they discovered that their fears were unfounded. Indeed, to cope with the demands of patient-centred practice, the nurses learned that they had to make a greater effort to care for each other and that this increased the cohesion of the ward team and created a culture that was more supportive, rather than the reverse. The 'caring team' that emerged was more tolerant and more actively concerned for the well-being of its members than was the original 'sociable team'.

Over the course of the project, there was a major change in the way nurses supported each other's clinical work. By the end of the first year, after the first 'away days' had brought some of the problems of working in teams to the surface, there was evidence of nurses asking each other about their workloads and helping each other out. Team leaders, in particular, were thinking ahead about their team members and taking steps to make sure that they were adequately supported. For example, a team leader worked a '10 till 6' shift so as not to leave a new nurse alone with a heavy caseload for a whole evening, and another team leader stayed on to do a double shift when there was staff sickness. In the second year of the project, this 'looking out for each other', both within and across teams, had become the norm and often the nurses showed considerable sensitivity.

> *I have a lady with a brain tumour, Mary . . . It's been very difficult actually to cope with her . . . I think that other people recognize that she has been difficult to cope with . . . On Tuesday night and Wednesday night I had a lot of time taken up with her, trying to keep her comfortable and free from stress. Rosemary was aware that I hadn't seen much of my other primary patients and so she offered to take Mary for me on Thursday, which was great . . . Obviously, I was asked if there were any decisions to be made for her, but I just knew someone else was caring for her.* (Sharon)

Barbara recorded how, as a new staff nurse, consistent support from her colleagues helped her to cope with the initially daunting task of managing her team's caseload.

I already feel as though I've come a long way. At first, the thought of having all the Oak Team patients for a late shift was really scary . . . However, I'm already finding that an OK prospect. It's hard work, but it's good because you really know what's happening with each patient and can keep on top of things . . . I am quite surprised at how quickly I have come to this level of feeling comfortable with things. I think that can be largely attributed to the support I constantly receive from colleagues. (Barbara)

Barbara, like Kathryn, was a bright young graduate, recruited by Alison because of her commitment to the idea of patient-centred practice. But her experience of support in the ward team contrasts strikingly with Kathryn's earlier experience. By the second year of the project, newcomers were no longer considered threatening and could be welcomed and cared for, whatever their background.

While the nurses' growing concern to support each other also showed itself in their increasing willingness to bring tensions between them into the open, even in the latter stages of the project, honest confrontation could still sometimes be difficult.

A Chain Of Bad Feeling

The Elm Team members had been working well together and had become very close and supportive of each other. Then an incident occurred which made the team members angry with Sharon, their team leader. Minutes of a team leader meeting were inadvertently read by some of the team members, not realizing that the minutes were confidential. The minutes made reference to some problems in the Elm Team, about which Sharon had sought advice at the team leader meeting. The team members felt that Sharon had been talking about them behind their backs. This incident stirred up other 'niggles', such as Sharon's absence for study leave which meant that she was a little less available for the rest of the team. The team members became quite hostile towards Sharon.

Janice: '*Sharon hadn't given us a chance to air our views . . . it started a chain of bad feeling . . . it was getting quite catty and it started to drag me down. I was going home upset. No one was really talking directly to each other. It all seemed to be very glossed over and superficially mended. Nobody was coming out with those undercurrents.*'

Although the nurses were critical of Sharon and unhappy about the tension in the team, it took a few weeks before Janice raised the problems at a team meeting. The way that everyone had been feeling was then brought out into the open and the crisis was finally resolved.

In spite of such difficulties, a real commitment to try to face up to problems and to clear the air when tensions arose became a strong feature of the ward culture. It seemed that, as the demands of the nurses' practice grew, they relied on each other's support much more, so that working at maintaining healthy relationships within and between the teams became important.

During the course of the project, there was a major change in the ward culture. Greater openness, flexibility and tolerance were reflected in every aspect of ward life: in the way the ward was managed, in its intellectual life, in the nurses' approach to their work and in their relationships with each other. However, these were not changes that could be made and then forgotten about. The enthusiasm, liveliness, creativity and warmth that came with the greater openness could be dented from time to time by workload stresses and dips in the ward morale. In addition, new nurses joining the ward usually brought with them traditional expectations and some of the traditional defensiveness, and they needed help to adapt to the new culture. It was important for Alison, in particular, but also for team leaders, to build strategies for sustaining a healthy climate into their repertoire of practice leadership skills.

Chapter 6

The leadership journey

'*Primary nursing cannot succeed on any unit whose head nurse is not committed to this system of nursing care. To lead her staff into primary nursing, the head nurse must accept a change in her own role, in her leadership style, and in her function as unit manager. If she looks upon the transition as a challenge, as a means of personal and professional growth, the head nurse can make primary nursing a success.*'

Zander (1977)

INTRODUCTION

The ward sister role has long been recognized as *the* pivotal role in hospital ward life. It is the ward sister who has the key influence upon the style and quality of nursing care in a ward (Pembrey, 1980) and it has been shown that patients consider the sister to be responsible for the ward atmosphere, which they believe has a direct effect on their well-being (McGhee, 1961). The attitudes and behaviour of the ward sister have also been identified as the main determinants of the quality of a ward as a learning environment (Orton, 1981; Ogier, 1982; Fretwell, 1982). Furthermore, it is the sister who negotiates and manages the relationship between the individual ward and the wider hospital organization (Pembrey, 1980; Runciman, 1983). Even within the traditional nursing system, the ward sister role was complex and demanding, because it required a skilled integration of major clinical, managerial and educational functions (Runciman, 1983). During the course of the project, Alison had to develop a leadership role that was fundamentally different from that of the traditional sister and even more complex. The influence of the role remained, however, equally critical in the life of the ward.

There were two main factors that shaped the way in which Alison developed her role, namely her commitments outside the ward and the decentralized organization of nursing within the ward. First, while remaining responsible for running her own ward, Alison had to accommodate the additional responsibilities she acquired as one of the hospital's senior sisters and the responsibilities she had assumed by setting up this research venture, by establishing the Medical Sisters' Group and by participating in the newly devolved business management of the Medical Unit. She also had to respond to considerable external interest in her work, which brought a range of invitations to lecture in other parts of the country. Not surprisingly, this rather ambitious expansion of the traditional ward sister role was difficult to manage and, in the early days, Alison felt overloaded, while the ward staff felt neglected. Finding a way to enable her ward to benefit from her expanded role, rather than to suffer because of it, was one of her major challenges.

Whilst the precise nature of Alison's expanded role was somewhat idiosyncratic, the general idea of an expanded ward sister role has been taken up elsewhere and seems to have much to commend it, although clearly there can be problems of role overload and role conflict. For example, the lecturer/practitioner (FitzGerald, 1989a; Lathlean, 1997), the clinical lecturer (Ersser, 1992) and the head nurse/researcher (Pearson, 1985) are roles in which senior clinicians have combined the leadership of a ward or unit with additional responsibilities. In each, substantial practice development was achieved, paradoxically, both because of and in spite of the complex roles of the clinical leaders. It is not necessary for a ward sister to have an expanded role to create a primary nursing system and to develop patient-centred practice. However, the value for the development of patient-centred practice, of some senior nurses being able to lead ward teams and also contribute to management, education or research, cannot be understated. If the voice of those immersed in the daily reality of patient-centred practice is not influential outside the ward, it is unlikely that organizational and professional policy will be sufficiently informed and sensitive to support this style of nursing. Thus, while some aspects of Alison's role development are peculiar to her particular situation, the problems associated with managing a broad, clinically based, leadership role and the general approach she took to resolve these problems, will be of interest and relevance to many senior practitioners.

The second major theme in this chapter concerns how Alison developed new ways of influencing and supervising the nurses' practice within the decentralized system. The introduction of primary nursing does not change the fact that, as leader of the ward, the sister holds overall responsibility for the style and quality of the nursing service patients receive. However, by delegating the management of individual patients' care to primary nurses, the sister loses the mechanism she had in the traditional system for fulfilling her responsibility. In a primary nursing system, the sister no longer determines the routines and procedures that govern how patients are nursed and she no longer personally monitors and supervises, albeit from a distance, the care of most patients who come to her ward. Having let go of the tight, centralized control of everyday practice, in the interests of more personalized nursing, the sister has to find new ways to ensure that nurses in her ward are sufficiently supported and supervised and that patients receive competent, effective care.

The literature suggests that, with the introduction of primary nursing, many ward sisters experience the loss of their traditional controlling role as threatening and that, at least initially, they may feel insecure, devalued or even redundant (Zander, 1977; Manthey, 1980; Ersser and Tutton, 1991). Theoretical and anecdotal papers have emphasized that, in a primary nursing system, ward sisters need to create a new role as teacher, adviser, consultant, facilitator and resource person, developing the skills of individual primary nurses and validating their clinical decisions (Zander, 1977; Fradd, 1988; Lathlean, 1988; Binnie, 1989). Others have pointed out the importance of ward sisters adopting an open, democratic style of leadership and of creating a ward atmosphere in which staff feel trusted, confident and free to practise independently (Binnie, 1989; Bowman and Carter, 1990; Chilton, 1991). Some authors have reported that, as ward sisters in a primary nursing system, they were able to become more clinically involved than they had been in their traditional roles (Campen, 1988; Chilton, 1991). And the value of sisters carrying a small primary caseload, to enable them to relate to the experiences of primary nurses and as a means of teaching by example, has also been mentioned (Elpern, 1977; Singleton and Gamblin, 1989; Chilton, 1991). However, while giving some general guidance about the nature of the new ward sister role, the literature gives little indication as to how it might be developed. It is the detailed practicalities of interpreting the role that are addressed in the second half of this chapter.

DEVELOPING A CLINICAL LEADERSHIP ROLE

Alison's aim was to develop a role that allowed her to remain firmly rooted in practice, while also participating in other areas of professional and organizational life. By having direct access to forums where local policy and strategy were debated, she believed that she could serve the interests of her ward and of practice generally. In addition, because she remained in practice, she hoped to bring to these forums a nursing voice that was immediately in touch with the everyday experiences of patients and clinical staff. Alison had appreciated the value of this kind of expanded role in her previous post as a senior sister in the Surgical Unit, and she had learned there to manage her time in a way that accommodated both the needs of her ward and her other responsibilities. However, when she joined the Medical Unit, the expansion of her role was much broader and her outside commitments increased considerably.

For the nurses in Oriel Ward, the arrival of a sister who worked very differently to any sister they had encountered before was an unsettling and confusing experience. Failure to understand and appreciate Alison's role created a degree of anger and resentment amongst the nurses that had the potential to undermine the whole development.

'I can't win'

The nurses had been used to having a ward sister who, in traditional fashion, had been present in the ward for five full shifts a week. They had relied on Sister to sort out administrative problems in the ward and to deal with people from other hospital departments on their behalf. The nurses had also been accustomed to having Sister readily available to support them clinically and they expected her to be fully involved with helping them to 'get through the work' whenever she was on duty. In Alison's earlier study, she had found that ward sister roles generally were poorly differentiated (Binnie, 1988). The sisters adopted the 'in charge' role for the shift, just as staff nurses did in their absence. They rarely structured their days to make time for teaching, staff development or managerial work that was not directly associated with running a particular shift and, because they always immersed themselves in the ward's clinical work, they felt the9 did not have time for these other things. While, on a day to day basis, the staff nurses were supported, and to a certain extent protected, by the strong presence of their ward sisters, they were also keenly aware that no one was giving time to supporting their professional development or the development of the ward.

Because Alison had a reputation for developing ward nursing and for bringing new ideas into practice, the nurses were at first pleased about her appointment to Oriel Ward. In her initial study, Alison had found that nurses in the medical wards were eager for change. They felt that their practice was 'in a rut' and hoped that the development of primary nursing – occurring in other parts of the hospital – would come to their wards too. As one nurse put it,

It could be a major improvement. Anything would be good for a change . . . I think the sooner it happens the better, before we all stagnate and leave. (Binnie, 1988)

Data from Oriel Ward showed a similarly positive and optimistic response to Alison's appointment.

Before Alison arrived none of us were quite sure what to expect. She had been to see us which was very good. In fact, she'd explained her basic plans, but obviously until she actually started working we weren't sure what to expect. Some of us felt trepidation about change, although the feeling on the ward in general was positive towards the change. (Lorna)

Thus, the idea of Alison's arrival and of the much-needed change she promised were welcome to the nurses, but the reality of her unconventional leadership role came as something of a shock to them. Early on, as well as leaving the ward to attend meetings relating to her management and research responsibilities, Alison committed a lot of time to running and writing up a dependency study, which she and the other medical sisters had initiated, in order to bring some serious staff shortages in the unit to the attention of senior management. She initially gave this work high priority, because failure to deal with the staffing problems was likely to handicap any future development work. In the long term, Alison's investment in the dependency project proved worthwhile, because it resulted in a small, but sufficient increase in the Medical Unit funding, which placed the subsequent practice development on a much surer footing. At the time, however, all that the nurses experienced was a far too frequent absence of their ward sister. Although Alison was working long hours, which included a substantial amount of clinical time, the nurses' perception was that she was 'never there'.

Alison is never on the ward. I find her a very unsupportive sister . . . she is just never there . . . I find it very difficult that she can just pick and choose her hours . . . She likes to think she is a clinical sister, but she's not . . . she's got a finger in so many pies that her priority isn't the ward anymore, though she wants it to be. (Carol)

One of the major difficulties for the nurses was being left, much more than in the past, to deal with the everyday business of running the ward. Although they were used to caring for patients during the shifts when the sister was off duty, she had been a constant enough presence to relieve them of most of the administrative tasks on the ward. For example, the nurses were more commonly confronted with duty rota problems, with issues relating to other hospital departments, or with trying to obtain special equipment for a patient. At first, they were uncertain about their authority to deal with these matters and were often unsure about finding their way around the hospital system. Thus they resented Alison not being there to sort things out for them. In addition, when the ward was very busy, the nurses were annoyed if Alison went off to meetings or if they knew she was in the hospital but was not available to help them out with their clinical workload.

Having no experience of a sister with an expanded role, the nurses found it difficult to imagine precisely what Alison was doing when she was not in the ward and to understand that her work elsewhere might ultimately help them. Feeling that the nurses were under enough pressure already, Alison did not want to burden them further with her problems outside the ward and so, in the early days, she did not tell them a great deal about her non-clinical work. Her silence, however, left the nurses in ignorance and provided no counter to their accusations that she was neglecting the ward. Kathryn was one of the few nurses who was willing to acknowledge that the work Alison was doing was for the benefit of the ward.

The nurses often say, 'She's not here. Where is she?' They feel she is shirking and not committed to the day to day running of the ward. They don't realize the amount of background work she does. (Kathryn)

Not understanding what she *was* doing or how hard she was working on their behalf, the nurses were only able to focus upon what Alison was *not* doing to help the immediate situation in the ward. They saw themselves as carrying the constant heavy burden of ward work, while Alison seemed to flit in and out as she pleased, making, as one nurse put it disparagingly, 'guest appearances'. The nurses viewed work away from the ward as inevitably easier and probably more interesting than their repetitive daily 'slog'.

When Alison just nips in, she doesn't realize what the ward is like. She's not really in touch. She comes in full of ideas and we're feeling bogged down and that makes us feel guilty. (Sophie)

As we mentioned in Chapter 5, jealousy arose about the variety in Alison's work and about her frequent opportunities to 'escape' from the ward.

(Alison) can be involved with practice and she can be involved in research, she can be involved in lots of other things and that's an enviable position. (Mike)

Discontent about Alison's role grew and soon, even when she was in the ward, there was criticism of the way she worked. If she took a small caseload, in order to have more time to support the nurses, she was considered not to be 'pulling her weight'. On the other hand, if she took a full caseload *and* made time to sort out administrative problems to help the nurses, they complained, when she went home late, that she was setting an unrealistic example by working such long hours. Even when they saw her engaged in skilled clinical work, with these negative attitudes towards her, they were not able to appreciate her contribution or to recognize the opportunity to learn from her expertise. Instead, they felt that she was only able to do such good work because she had a smaller caseload than they had and they blamed her expert care for making them look 'second best' in the eyes of her patients.

We get feedback from the patients that Alison has looked after. They say, 'Why don't you pander to my every whim, like Sister does?' and that's not very nice. The patients don't realize that we've got seven other patients to look after. (Andrea)

Alison was feeling exhausted and overwhelmed by the amount of work she had to do, working very long hours and using holiday time to catch up. She was giving the ward as much of her time as she could, usually at least three shifts a week, but the nurses felt that this was not enough. She was also concerned about not being a good clinical role model, because she was always handing her patients on to others when her shifts were interrupted. However, while Alison sensed that the nurses were unhappy with the way she worked, it was our research data that made her face up to the seriousness of the problem. The data showed a crisis of bad feeling in the ward that clearly had to be addressed before any more progress could be made with the development work.

> They are making conflicting demands on me. It comes out very well in one statement where a staff nurse said, 'What people seem to want is old style sistership, but if we got that we'd lose so much.' Somehow we have to help them, but I can't meet conflicting demands. I can't be an old style sister and a new style sister ... Criticism of me is pretty brutal ... There's not much acknowledgement of what they've got. (AB)

> Your clinical expertise comes out strongly, but then it's straight on to the negative effect for them. (AT)

> They want me to sort out the irritating administrative hassles that bog them down – the presence thing – but if I don't take a full caseload they resent it ... 'You've only got two patients, you don't know what it's like to look after eight patients all at once.' If I look after eight patients and end up staying late, because I also have other responsibilities, I set them an unrealistic example ... Everything I do well is spoiled by some counterbalancing negative which is more important to them ... Whatever I do, I can't win! (AB)

Strategies for redesigning the role

It was clear that our most pressing task was to explore with the staff nurses what they really wanted from Alison as their leader and to negotiate a practical way of enabling her to meet these expectations, while also fulfilling her other responsibilities. We used the first 'away days' to confront the bad feeling about Alison's role and to develop a common understanding of how she should be contributing to the ward. The 'away days' cleared the air and provided a constructive starting point for Alison and the nurses to work together at redesigning her leadership role. However, it took several months of trial and error before the practical difficulties of juggling the different components of the role were satisfactorily resolved. Alison had to experiment with different time management and delegation strategies and with different ways of organizing her clinical workload.

Reshaping expectations

Making time for a thorough exploration of Alison's role was one of our priorities at the first 'away days'. Angie facilitated this session, structuring it in such a way as to ensure that both the nurses and Alison were able to give a full account of their perceptions of the problems and then work together on devising a solution.

Angie presented data which showed the deep discontent in the ward about the way Alison worked. Alison was honest about feeling hurt by the nurses' criticism and about feeling torn by their conflicting demands, but she also acknowledged that she thought some of the criticism was justified and that she needed to find a way to support and work alongside them more effectively. The nurses were shocked by the bluntness and harshness of the data, but, as a group, they owned the strong negative feelings expressed in the material. A long, intense discussion followed with everyone clearly trying to understand the problems more fully.

The second part of the session began with Alison presenting an outline of the different elements of her role and the relationship she saw between them. The nurses brainstormed in small groups about what they wanted from Alison as their leader. They produced enormously long lists, showing that they expected her to be a strong clinical presence in the ward, but that they also wanted her to devote time to their individual professional development, to steering the development of the ward and to acting as spokesperson for the ward in various ways. The nurses were next asked to make a hypothetical plan of Alison's diary for a week, arranging her time so that she would achieve all that they expected from her. These activities began to make the nurses appreciate the complexity of the ward sister role and the difficulties of balancing its various components. Comments like, 'She'll have to have another admin day to do all that,' showed that the nurses were recognizing that Alison could not work with patients every day and do all the other things that they were expecting of her.

The nurses' specific complaints about the way Alison worked were then considered and the following principles agreed:

- Alison should organize her time so that clinical and non-clinical work were clearly separated. Thus, she would try not to disappear to a meeting in the middle of a session when she was carrying a clinical caseload.
- Alison would usually carry a reduced caseload, so that she would have time in the ward to support nurses with their clinical work.
- Alison would report on her non-clinical work at ward meetings and talk to the nurses informally about it, so that they would have a better understanding of what she was doing on their behalf.
- There would be a regular review, at ward meetings, of how Alison's role was working out.

Finally, the nurses raised an issue that had not emerged previously, namely that they were unhappy about Alison wearing her distinctive blue sister's uniform. They saw the blue dress as symbolizing the traditional ward sister role and felt that it encouraged patients, relatives, doctors and other hospital staff to relate to Alison in the traditional manner. The nurses believed that maintaining traditional expectations in this way was undermining their efforts to establish themselves in their roles as team nurses and, ultimately, as primary nurses. They proposed that Alison should wear the same white uniform that they wore, using only her name badge to identify her title. They anticipated that this strategy would stop everyone from automatically 'heading straight for the blue dress' and would encourage people to ask for individual nurses. (Another sister in the Medical Unit, in a ward also introducing primary nursing, had already changed to a white uniform and there were positive reports of this symbolic gesture.) Alison agreed to the white uniform, but asked nurses to explain her new role to their patients and to relatives. In addition, a brief explanation of the ward sister role, within the primary nursing system, was to be included in the 'welcome leaflet' that patients received when they arrived in the ward.

Time management

Prior to the first 'away days', and following the dependency study, Alison increased the time she was spending in the ward in order to give more support to the nurses. She was usually able to devote the equivalent of three shifts a week to clinical work, but this time was often scattered in a haphazard way across the week, interspersed between meetings and other administrative tasks. In response to the nurses' initial complaints about not knowing when she would be in the ward or for how long, she tried to make her work pattern more organized and more predictable. She experimented with dividing her clinical time into five four hour chunks each week and working one four hour period in the ward each day, fitting it in to meet both the needs of the ward and her other commitments. Whilst its predictability meant that this system was an improvement on its predecessor, it still meant that Alison's clinical work was fragmented. She often felt that she was 'dumping' her patients or leaving the ward with 'unfinished business'. Within these constraints, Alison found that it was difficult to be a good clinical role model generally and almost impossible to demonstrate the role of a committed primary nurse. She often complained of feeling like '*an expensive bank nurse*', dipping in and out of practice, never able to follow things through and never able to use her clinical expertise to the full.

At the 'away days', a new scheme was proposed to give Alison a more substantial clinical role, while also allowing clearly allocated time for her other work. The idea was that she should alternate a month of intensive clinical work with a month of research, teaching and management work. Alison put this system into action at once. During her clinical 'month on', she wore her uniform, worked standard ward shifts which were marked on the duty rota and carried a small primary caseload. She kept up with important regular meetings and urgent management tasks by alternately taking half a day one week and a full day the next week away from the ward. But she saw the rest of her time during the month as a firm commitment to practice, and so research work and as much management work as possible was postponed until the following 'month off'. Similarly, invitations to conferences or to give lectures were turned down or deferred if they fell during the clinical month. When Alison felt pressured to keep up with additional non-clinical work, or when a meeting could not wait till the next month, she would schedule this extra work for before the start of a 'late shift' or after the end of an 'early shift', so that it did not eat into her clinical time. If she felt she had done an excessive amount of this extra work during a particular 'month on', she might allow herself an extra day off during the following non-clinical month – at least that was the theory. In practice, the 'months off' could often be almost as demanding as the 'months on'.

During her 'months off', Alison did not wear uniform and she was not included in the duty rota. However, this did not mean that she was completely unavailable to the ward, except on the occasional days when her work took her away from the hospital. Most days she visited the ward and would often join the nurses for a cup of coffee, so that they had an opportunity to talk any problems through with her. During each 'month off' Alison also made time to see a number of individual nurses for staff development interviews.

In general the 'month on/month off' system worked well – it provided some clarity for the nurses about what they could expect from Alison and when. However, learning to use the 'month on' time in the most effective way took some further exploration.

Structuring the clinical role effectively

When the 'month on/month off' system was discussed, it was agreed that during each 'month on' Alison should be attached to a different team and work as a team member, included 'in the numbers' on the duty rota. She would act as primary nurse for one or two patients in the team and as associate for the others, supporting and guiding the team members with their primary patients. By working as a member of a particular team, it was intended that Alison would be able to give focussed attention to the nurses in that team for the month, sharing her practice skills with them and giving them detailed feedback on their own work with patients. In practice, this system worked well for the team to which Alison was attached.

There are lots of positive things that are being said about your presence in the ward now. (AT)

That struck me too. There were more positives than I expected. Things that I had just taken for granted, had obviously been noticed and seen to be helpful. For example, Sophie working with one of my patients and using my care plan . . . saying how it made her think about the patient in much more depth. (AB)

However, Alison gradually discovered that being attached so closely to one team at a time also had its problems. It meant that she was not necessarily able to work with the nurses who needed her most at the time.

The reality is that when I join one team, I get stuck in that team. We have recognized that doing staff development work, in the chaos of practice, means being opportunistic. But then I've joined the Ash Team for a month and it's not a particularly good time for investing in the Ash Team members. For example, Mark is going through a bad patch personally. I had planned that this would be the time to focus on the Ash Team with Mark. Typical, you plan it, it doesn't work. He's doing some night duty, he's having some holiday and he's distracted by his personal problems . . . Ruth's on holiday for most of the month. She'll be there for the last week, but I'd like to have given her more time. Henrietta, the new staff nurse in the Elm Team, happens to have been on lots of shifts with me and she's been looking after difficult patients. I would have been better spending time focussing on her. And, in fact, I did Sharon's appraisal in my month off and I would like to be giving her attention, because she's at a time when she needs it. (AB)

In a similar way, Alison's attachment to one team made her clinical involvement inflexible and she found herself torn between trying to be a good team member and trying to be a supportive ward sister.

Clinical problems come up. It so happens the Elm Team have had several and the Oak Team the odd one. I get drawn off to help them out and I feel it's right that I should support them with difficult cases. That takes me away from being an Ash Team nurse and then I feel very guilty. (AB)

The following story shows that the consequences of this struggle – to be both a team member and a supportive ward sister – were sometimes distressing and clearly not in the interests of patients and relatives.

'I let them all down'

I was carrying a fairly straightforward caseload in the Ash Team, when I was most needed by the Elm Team nurses who were struggling with horrendous problems and, although I helped them as much as I could, it wasn't enough. For example, I was really dissatisfied with my contribution to the care of the dying patient and her family, who were very devoted but were making enormous emotional demands on the Elm Team. I was pulled between the Ash Team and the Elm Team. The family were turning to me as the sister and I feel, on reflection, that I rejected them. I kept referring them back to the Elm Team all the time. When I think about it, it was so complex. There was a role for me as the sister to be more involved, without undermining the nurses' relationship with the family. I didn't need to interfere, but I should have supported the nurses more. If I'd been able to be the second nurse sometimes, I would have been able to have a relationship with the woman, without undermining the Elm Team. It would have reinforced and supported what they were doing and made the family feel more confident. The patient and the family sensed my special skills and they kept telling me things and pulling me to be more involved, but I withdrew and so I denied them the support of the expert sister. I felt that I'd let them all down. (AB)

After an extended trial period, our conclusion was that, although the 'month on / month off' system worked fairly well, the team attachment did not. In addition, Alison acknowledged that always being included as 'one of the numbers' on the duty rota, during the 'months on', was not sensible. Nevertheless, the system had served a useful purpose in helping her to establish credibility with the nurses and allowing her to develop a comfortable relationship with them. The main reason why it was not viable in the long term was that it did not give Alison a sufficiently differentiated clinical role.

There are lots of good things about the way I'm working now . . . but I sense that I've been pulled too much in the direction of being made to be one of them, to prove that I can do what they can do, in order to be accepted. Because of that pressure, I'm not fulfilling a number of other things . . . I'm still being torn in two directions. (AB)

Like the sisters she had observed during her exploratory study (Binnie, 1988), Alison found that if she worked as the staff nurses did, she was not in a position to develop a distinct clinical role in which she could focus on guiding and supporting others rather than simply contributing to the overall effort to get the work done each shift.

Finally, it was agreed that Alison should continue to work rostered shifts during her 'month on', but mostly in a supernumerary capacity and without any fixed attachment to a particular team. She would still carry a small primary caseload and would always look after her own one or two patients when she was on duty, but, otherwise, she would be free to focus her attention wherever she felt she could be most valuable on the day.

Delegation

The final strategy for making Alison's role more effective and more manageable was an obvious one, but one that it seems many busy ward sisters fail to address sufficiently. It became apparent early on that Alison spent many hours every week attending to important, but very straightforward, administrative tasks. This work was associated with running the ward and with aspects of her expanded role and it needed to remain under her control, but it did not need to be Alison, or indeed any trained nurse, who actually did this work. It was clear that proper secretarial support, on hand within the ward, would make an enormous difference to the way Alison was able to work.

Existing funds for a part-time ward clerk were topped up with money from the ward's nursing budget and used to employ a full-time 'ward secretary', who combined the responsibilities of ward clerk and receptionist with being Alison's personal assistant. While not necessarily an ideal solution, Alison felt that it was legitimate to use nursing money to create this post, because it allowed her to give more time to clinical work.

The second important avenue for delegation was to the team leaders and, eventually, to the other nurses. The process of decentralization and the development of the nurses' roles (described in Chapter 4) ensured that nurses increasingly took responsibility for many aspects of the daily running of the ward which had traditionally been dealt with by the ward sister. The more this organizational development progressed, the more Alison felt that her expanded role and her new style of clinical role were sustainable.

The new style sister

The serious tensions that arose in the ward because of Alison's unconventional role disappeared after the cathartic, and then constructive, discussions at the first 'away days'. The positive response to the workshop on Alison's role was apparent in the written evaluations.

> The workshop raised issues which have been creating stress, ill feeling and uneasiness and we talked them over. (SN)

> (It has been) helpful to establish Alison's role and to see what we expected – the conflicting ideas. (SN)

In stark contrast to earlier material, there was an absence of complaints about Alison in data collected during the months after the first 'away days'. Attitudes to her role were much more positive and there were favourable responses to her 'month on/month off' system. Nurses talked about feeling that their relationship with Alison had changed for the better.

> We pushed her off her pedestal (laugh). We came more to the same level . . .
> I see her as more of a friend now . . . Since the 'away days', it's far more open.

I feel I can approach her about anything. It's because we know how she feels. We appreciate her role and also the things that upset her. The 'away days' cleared up a lot of ill feeling towards Alison. (Sophie)

The nurses increasingly valued their more open and comfortable relationship with Alison and talked about ways they had benefited personally from her support.

She is really reliable in that you know what to expect. She also made time for me when I needed to talk to her, because my motivation was low. She made time for me and we chatted informally in the office. She made me feel as if I had something positive to offer to the ward and I found that quite encouraging. (Moira)

I talked with Alison about (a personal problem) and that was definitely a turning point for me . . . She did something about it and that was completely new to me. I couldn't imagine that happening where I'd worked before. (Rosemary)

With the more positive relationship came evidence of a change in the nurses' attitude to Alison's clinical expertise. Rather than feeling jealous of her practice, or threatened by it, the nurses were able to acknowledge Alison's skill and to value her opinion on their own work with patients.

It's nice to know she's around . . . for advice really. It's reassuring . . . she gives you good feedback, always honest. It never puts you down. (Janice)

As Alison's clinical role became established, the nurses began to talk about her value as a strong clinical role model. Alison's firm commitment to practice, during her 'months on', enabled her to carry a small primary caseload without difficulty, so that she was able to experience for herself and demonstrate for others all that is involved in working closely and continuously with individual patients and their families. Alison valued her work with her own primary patients very highly. She felt that it 'fed' or 'nourished' every other aspect of her work, because it kept her close to the heart of nursing, involved with the intimate human experience of health and illness. It gave meaning to the rest of her work and was a great source of energy, inspiration and satisfaction. In the interpretation of her complex role, finding a *modus vivendi* that allowed Alison to be primary nurse to a small number of patients, during her 'months on', proved to be extremely important and worthwhile.

While being a primary nurse regularly gave Alison opportunities to experience the rich detail and the complex challenges of caring for individual patients, the 'trouble-shooter' role, which she adopted once she stopped being attached to a particular team each month, gave her a view of the ward's practice from the opposite perspective. Each shift she was usually only committed in advance to her own one or two primary patients, so that for the rest of her time she could look broadly at what was happening in the ward and from this bird's-eye perspective, as it were, she could focus down upon whichever patients or nurses she felt would most benefit from her attention and support at the time. The nurses appreciated this flexibility in Alison's clinical role. They felt that it made her more accessible as a resource who could '*point people in the right direction*' and they felt that she was '*willing to help out*' when they were stressed or in difficulty.

The nurses gradually came to understand and appreciate, rather than to resent, Alison's expanded role. Furthermore, as they became confident in their own new roles, their concern about the loss of a traditional sister disappeared.

The nurses are becoming more skilled at making priorities in terms of ward management. ... (There was a bed crisis, a fairly common occurrence.) The ward was to be 'on take' the next day and three nurses were at the desk – no team leader – and they were discussing the patients who were booked to come in the following day. They wanted to know the status of these patients, so they would be able to make decisions about cancelling them, if necessary, as emergency patients were admitted. (AT)

In some ways, this has grown up through necessity. They've not had me around to do these things, but I think they quite enjoy it now. In the old days, they would have blamed me for not being around to sort out these hassles. Now they just do it very competently. (AB)

Without the resentment of her absences from the ward, the nurses were able to take an interest in Alison's outside commitments and she learned to talk to them about her non-clinical work. The nurses liked being exposed to a broader view of what was going on in the unit and in the hospital as a whole and they began to appreciate that Alison could use her influence outside the ward for their benefit – '*She goes to meetings where policies and decisions are made and feeds it back to us.*' The nurses began to see Alison as a sister who was able to '*come up with the goods*' and they were impressed by the way she was able to '*juggle the budget*' to improve conditions for patients and themselves. The nurses also began to see that, by discussing management issues with Alison, they too could influence decisions that were made outside the ward.

The presence of the ward secretary made an enormous difference to Alison, relieving her of an array of administrative tasks, but her efficient and effective support was greatly appreciated by the whole nursing team as well. Her secretarial duties mixed well with the clerical and receptionist work previously done by the ward clerk, the combination providing a valuable degree of flexibility.

At the second 'away days', a year after the initial workshop on Alison's role, we formally reviewed the progress that had been made. In stark contrast to the previous year's session, the discussion was very low key. The nurses had little to say about Alison's role, except that they were quite happy with it now. They made it clear that the sister role was no longer an issue in the ward, confirming what our data had been indicating for some months. From Alison's point of view, she was pleased to have developed a role within the ward and a method of organizing her work that allowed her to practise in a satisfying way, that seemed largely to meet the needs of the staff nurses and that enabled her to provide an appropriate and effective style of leadership within the decentralized system. However, there were some aspects of her role that Alison never felt satisfied with. Her 'months off' filled rapidly with meetings, lectures and administrative work and there never seemed to be any free stretches of time to think, to write and to focus on the research in the concentrated way that she felt this kind of creative work required. Towards the end of the project, Alison was still talking with some feeling about her almost overwhelming workload.

> *Looking at my diary now, this week is full of meetings – people who want to see me, people I've put off because I didn't want them encroaching on my clinical time. So, there's the infection control nurse after I've seen you and there's a ward meeting this afternoon and then there's the medical forum. So that's today gone. Tomorrow is the same – the resuscitation officer wants a meeting with me and somebody else and there's a senior sisters' meeting ... On Friday I've got the morning to myself, but then a meeting with (a service manager), then the accountant, then there's another medical services meeting at 5.00 which will go on till late ... I feel terribly weighed down by outstanding things and terribly guilty and inadequate really.* (AB)

From the ward's point of view, Alison's expanded role eventually worked well. Patients and nurses were able to benefit from her clinical expertise, there was strong leadership in the ward from an experienced senior nurse, and the ward and its staff benefited from Alison's influence and contacts around the hospital and beyond. Thus, in principle, it appears that, with a decentralized system and a well-developed nursing team, some kind of expanded sister role is not only sustainable, but can also be highly advantageous for a ward. Where Alison personally got into difficulty was with the scope and volume of her non-clinical work. Not only did she have a major research commitment, which in itself could have been enough to fill much of the non-clinical part of her role, but she also had a substantial managerial role outside the ward and, being seen as a leading figure in the field of practice development, she was frequently called upon, both locally and nationally, to advise, to teach and to contribute her expertise in various other ways. Juggling all these commitments, while also leading the complex and sometimes turbulent practice development programme in the ward, was enormously demanding.

It seems that Alison's experience was not unique. Practice development work does not occur in isolation, so that clinical leaders inevitably become involved with managerial issues in the wider organization, in order to support and secure the newly emerging style of practice. Research or evaluation often accompanies new work and, even if outside researchers are involved, this adds to the clinical leader's commitments. Pioneers in any field tend to attract attention and others want to learn from them and to use their expertise, and so again more work comes their way. Other clinical leaders have reported finding themselves overloaded (see, for example, FitzGerald, 1989a; Lathlean, 1997) and it seems common for people in these positions to leave their posts after four or five years, or to give up its clinical component.

Our project has shown possible solutions to only some of the problems faced by nursing leaders who recognize the value of maintaining a substantial practice commitment. It leaves the question of the long-term viability of such roles unanswered. However, we are convinced that continuing to search for answers to these problems is crucial for the future of nursing practice. We see personal involvement in the reality of practice life as the essential foundation of clinical leadership.

INFLUENCING AND SUPERVISING PRACTICE

We have focussed so far in this chapter on the organizational or *structural* elements of Alison's role as ward leader – how she divided her time, to whom she delegated work, whether she was attached to a team, how big a caseload she carried, even what she wore. Here, we go on to consider the ways in which she developed the *process* element of her clinical work, that is, what she actually did when she worked alongside the nurses in the ward and when she cared for patients herself.

Alison always believed that it was important for ward sisters, or indeed any other senior nurses engaging in practice, to be clear about why they were practising and to try to use their practice consciously and intentionally for that purpose. One of a ward sister's key responsibilities is to support the professional development of her staff nurses. This is particularly important in a primary nursing system, where individual staff nurses are given the freedom and the authority to manage their own patients' nursing care. Only by investing sufficiently in each nurse's development as a practitioner can the ward sister be confident about entrusting them with a primary caseload (Manthey and Kramer, 1970). Furthermore, having established a basic level of competence amongst the nursing team, a ward sister needs to be monitoring regularly that the best possible standard of practice is being maintained in the ward. She also needs to have effective methods for continuing to help nurses increase their confidence and expertise, so that their practice matures and they, in turn, are able to contribute to the development of their junior colleagues.

Alison used the action research process to reflect upon how, in her own practice, she functioned as a role model, teacher and supervisor. By becoming more conscious of her behaviour and her interactions with staff, and by conceptualizing effective strategies that she could intentionally use during the course of her daily work, Alison was gradually able to contribute, in more powerful and focussed ways, to the development of the nurses as patient-centred practitioners.

Traditional ward teaching

Analysis of our early data revealed two methods that Alison used to teach and influence the nurses working alongside her. We labelled them '*Sitting by Nellie*' and '*Try this*'.

'Sitting by Nellie', or allowing a novice to observe and copy an expert role model, is a widely recognized way of enabling an individual to develop practical knowledge and skills. It is commonly used where some form of apprenticeship precedes the novice's admission to a trade or profession. Both nursing and medicine have traditionally used and valued this form of teaching and learning. Alison could recall the important influence on her own early development of experienced nurses whose practice she had admired and respected, particularly expert ward sisters. She was well aware that her own practice now, in turn, had a powerful influence upon the nurses working with her and this was strongly supported by the data we collected throughout the project. The nurses themselves were aware of using Alison as a role model. They found that, by observing her, they could develop a tangible vision of the kind of practice they aspired to and found that they could learn by evaluating their own performance against Alison's work.

> *It was good to see what she was doing. I've learned things from how she writes her care plans . . . They're always very individualized . . . I've learned from that and try to do the same . . . and I noticed that she communicated a lot with the doctors.* (Ruth)

> *Working with Alison is very challenging – it makes me think. I observe her care and then note the omissions in my own and think, 'I wouldn't have thought of that'.* (Rosemary)

The power of role modelling in nursing has been documented before (e.g. Marson, 1982). However, like Lathlean and Farnish (1984), we found that role modelling alone, that is, simply allowing nurses to observe and draw their own conclusions from the practice of an expert, has its limitations. Unless the expert takes the trouble to explain the thoughts, feelings, observations and intuitive hunches that inform her decisions and actions, the novice can easily misunderstand what the expert is doing, or simply fail to appreciate the subtlety and the complexity of apparently smooth, almost effortless work.

The second way of responding to the nurses' learning needs, with the 'Try this' method, was similarly limited in its effectiveness. Learning opportunities frequently arose when nurses approached Alison with queries about their patients' problems or with uncertainties about their own practice. As the story below illustrates, Alison's automatic 'Try this' response enabled nurses to deal with the situations immediately confronting them, but failed to exploit their full educational potential.

'I was trained to be slick'

Janice approached me for advice. She had a patient who was breathless and she just sensed he wasn't so good and she wasn't sure what to do. He was a man with cor pulmonale who was having a blood transfusion. He'd been given an oral diuretic with it, but he was more breathless, according to Janice, than normal. I went to see the patient myself and made a simple clinical assessment which indicated that he was overloaded. I went back to Janice and told her what was going on. Now she, in fact, had made a mistake. She had let the blood go through two hours too early. She had misread the prescription chart, so she had, to some extent, caused his overload.

I talked to her and said, 'I think he needs some frusemide. Would you like to call the doctor?' She had a patient in the loo and said, 'Would you do it?'. So I did, but I had given her the opportunity to deal with it herself, which was fine. However, reflecting on it, I can see where I might have improved the process of getting the right answer. I should have got her to work out what was going on to see if she could spot the error. It was partly pressure of time. The man was breathless, it was an acute situation and she was tied up with another patient, but it wasn't a dire emergency. I could have helped her to reflect on what was going on. The first thing you think of is overload and I didn't really establish whether she had thought of that. What I need to learn is to be more conscious of the process at the time, of facilitating the nurses' decision-making and building their confidence. The problem is that I was trained to be slick, to make a decision, get on with it, sort the problem out. (AB)

Reflecting upon this story, Alison recognized that she had responded as a traditional teacher, by simply explaining the problem and telling the nurse what to do. She had missed an opportunity to help the nurse to reflect upon her practice, to use her own knowledge and to think the problem through for herself, in a way that would increase her self-reliance and clinical confidence. Alison became aware that she used the 'Try this' type of response often and automatically. She felt that she was still influenced unconsciously by the traditional ward teaching she had experienced herself.

> *I don't recall ever, in eighteen years of nursing, a senior person taking me aside and reflecting with me on how I performed as a nurse with a patient, never ... I've never experienced it built into a proper work relationship, except with you (i.e. Angie).* (AB)

Nurses too used Alison in a traditional way, namely by asking her for clinical advice or by asking her to take over when they were in difficulty. They seemed to expect, from their ward sister, the kind of didactic responses that Alison was most often inclined to give during the early days of the project. There was no evidence in our early data, for example, of nurses asking Alison to critique their care plans, or of asking her to support them in working through a new experience.

The research literature suggests that traditional teaching approaches are commonly used by ward sisters. Studies by Fretwell (1980), Marson (1982) and Lewis (1990), for example, found that ward sisters perceived teaching as demonstrating practical procedures to learners, or transmitting information to them through formal instruction. The sisters adopted an autocratic style of communication and often identified nurses' learning needs for them. Both students and qualified nurses have also been found to think of teaching in this traditional way (Marson, 1982; Binnie, 1988; Ogier, 1989).

Our data showed the extent to which traditional approaches to developing and supervising nurses' practice initially influenced Alison's behaviour. She had to find a new method of supervision which enabled her to monitor the standard of care that nurses were delivering, but which, at the same time, supported rather than undermined their independence as primary nurses.

Strategies for facilitating learning from practice

Initially, we focussed upon developing Alison's ward teaching and supervisory skills, in a way that would promote and support patient-centred nursing. Later, as she became clearer and more confident about this aspect of her work, Alison concentrated on helping the team leaders, and other experienced nurses in the ward, to develop in a similar way, with a view to establishing the habits of facilitating clinical learning and of a supportive style of supervision as the norm in the ward.

Enhancing role modelling by articulating expert clinical knowledge

It has been suggested that ward sisters, and other experienced nurses, can be more effective as role models if they are able to identify and articulate the details of their expert clinical knowledge and skill. For example, Ogier (1989) recommended that experienced nurses should talk through their decisions, so that '*less experienced nurses can begin to identify the rationale for various nursing prescriptions and actions.*' Similarly, specifically in relation to supporting the development of primary nurses, Zander (1977) suggested that a head nurse/ward sister '*can use her own experiences to help her staff through the phases and emotions of primary nurse–patient relationships.*' Prompted by these suggestions in the literature and by the limitations of what one might call '*laissez-faire* role modelling', Alison began to use her own practice more consciously as a means o& teaching her staff. She tried to become more alert to opportunities that arose for her to talk about her own primary patients and for her to explain her thinking and behaviour to the nurses working alongside her.

Working closely with Angie enabled Alison to develop the skill of articulating her practice expertise in a way that made it accessible to others. During the fieldwork, Angie's frequent questions – 'Why did you do that?' and 'What were you thinking of when you said that?' – forced Alison to explore and describe aspects of her expertise that she had formerly taken for granted. Similarly, reviewing and analysing dozens of clinical stories (her own and those of other nurses) made Alison acutely aware of the fine details of nursing practice that make a difference to patients (see especially Chapter 7). Working with this material, and particularly writing about it, enabled Alison to put into her own words many of the subtle, yet very powerful, features of a patient-centred style of practice. She became more sensitive to the details of practice and she learned to talk, in everyday language, about what had previously often been hidden within the smooth flow of skilled nursing. Alison hoped that, by listening to her and by engaging in conversations about their practice, the nurses would develop their own expertise and would, in turn, become more thoughtful and more articulate about what lay behind their own clinical decisions and their own interactions with patients.

Guiding reflection and promoting independent thinking and action

Having identified the limitations of the 'Try this' type of response to nurses' concerns and questions, Alison began to watch out, during the course of her everyday work in the ward, for opportunities to respond to the nurses in a more constructive and facilitative manner. She began to turn their questions back to them – 'What do *you* think might be the problem?', 'What other possibilities do you need to explore?' – to help them draw upon their own observations and feelings, to weigh up different options and to work things out for themselves. Furthermore, she made an effort to be proactive in creating opportunities to stimulate the nurses' thinking and to encourage and guide their reflection on clinical situations.

Informally, we both encouraged story telling, taking an interest in the clinical stories that the nurses told spontaneously and listening to them carefully. By asking probing questions, and by helping them to interpret what was happening, we tried to show the nurses how they could develop their own knowledge and confidence through reflection upon their everyday practice.

When Alison became confident about her new style of practice supervision, she began to talk about what she was doing with team leaders and other experienced nurses. She encouraged them to think about the way they helped their junior colleagues to learn and she offered them feedback when they began to experiment themselves with more facilitative supervision strategies.

Calling nurses to account

There is a view that educational supervision is best separated from managerial supervision. Undoubtedly, this approach is wise in situations where the manager's style is intimidating and punitive. Employees would be afraid to expose their weaknesses and to admit their ignorance, and so there would be no honest basis for beginning the educational process of exploration and growth. However, if the manager sees that it is in the interests of the service to support and develop employees, and if this is successfully conveyed to them, then there need be no conflict between educational and managerial supervision. Indeed, we would argue that the sister's supervision of nursing practice in her ward is most helpfully seen as having both educational and managerial elements. Johns' model (1993a) of clinical supervision indicates that he takes the same view.

Once Alison had begun to establish a comfortable, open relationship with the nurses, and an appreciation of critical debate and enquiry had become part of the ward culture, it became possible for her to overlap her educational and managerial supervision functions in a complementary way. For example, by observing the nurses and questioning them about their practice, Alison could identify their learning needs and stimulate their thinking. At the same time, as a manager, she was effectively sampling the quality of their work, calling them to account for their practice and identifying where she needed to help them improve their care of patients. Because both activities were conducted in the context of a trusting and respectful relationship and because both activities had the same goal, namely that of helping nurses to give of their best to their patients, they were not in conflict. Nurses knew that there was a 'bottom line', that Alison could advise them to leave or even discipline them if their practice was unsatisfactory, but they knew that these were last-resort measures, which would only be used in exceptional circumstances or if all constructive developmental measures had failed.

New style supervision

Adjusting to a new style of practice supervision was not easy for either Alison or the nurses. It was difficult, at first, for Alison to remember to hold back when clinical problems arose and to make time, in the midst of a busy shift, to help nurses think things through for themselves. When Alison did question them and pushed them to explore practice issues more thoroughly and thoughtfully, the nurses were inclined to be defensive. Spotting or creating clinical learning opportunities for the nurses was also difficult for Alison in the early days of the project, because of the huge number of other considerations she was having to address simultaneously. However, when she eventually made this facilitation work the central focus of her attention for several consecutive 'months on', and used the action research process to help her, she began to make progress.

Gradually, Alison developed three distinct patterns of supervisory behaviour, which she subsequently called her 'supervision strategies'. They proved to be especially practical and effective in the ward setting, because they could be used opportunistically. Each strategy is illustrated in the following pages by way of a story.

'What I was trying to do here was . . . '

The first supervision strategy was the method that Alison used to make her expert practical knowledge accessible to other nurses. Practical knowledge is distinct from theoretical knowledge in that it is acquired primarily through experience. It is usually considered ordinary and unexceptional by experienced nurses, because it is tacitly embedded in their practice and often difficult to talk about (Schon, 1983; Benner, 1984; Titchen, 1995b).

'Did you touch him?'

Henrietta was a first year staff nurse. In a staff development interview with Alison and her team leader, she had expressed feelings of inadequacy when talking with bereaved relatives. Six weeks later, a young woman called Mary was admitted to the ward with a severe subarachnoid haemorrhage. She had had one ten years before which had left her quite disabled. Over the years, Mary had developed ways of dealing with her disabilities and had managed to lead a happy and successful family life.

Mary was unconscious when she was admitted and her husband, Peter, and twelve year old son, Richard, were with her and were very distressed. Henrietta was looking after Mary that evening. Alison and Henrietta discussed talking with Peter. They agreed it would be better for Alison to talk with him on her own, as it might be too intrusive for Peter if Henrietta were there as well. They decided that Alison would tell Henrietta what happened immediately afterwards, so that she could learn how Alison talked to a distressed relative. An hour or so later, the following conversation took place in the staff room. Throughout, we could hear Mary's stertorous breathing.

Alison: *First of all, I established some kind of sense of Mary's life and their life together.*

Henrietta: *And how was he?*

Alison: *When I first went into the office, I wanted to let him decide what he wanted to talk about. We sat down and I was silent. I wanted to let him talk and then pick up any cues. He started off by talking about practical things. He said he wouldn't be able to sit at the bedside all the time, but he didn't want the nurses to think he wasn't a caring husband; he was. He felt that he wanted to retain memories of Mary as she had been, not as lying in the bed dying. I told him there would be absolutely no pressure from the nurses and that he should decide the best way for him.*

Peter's mother died recently of motor neuron disease and he told me that he had spent many hours at her bedside watching her die and that this had coloured his memories of his mother. He found he wasn't able to remember her the way she used to be, but only as a body dying in the bed. I told him that I could understand how he wanted to protect himself against distorting memories of his wife.

Henrietta: *Did you touch him?*

Alison: *I sat close enough so that I could touch him if it was appropriate and I did, at one point, when he was crying, I did touch his knee.*

Henrietta: *Did he benefit from the talk?*

Alison: *Yes, enormously – he said that he did. He told me how he had been through all this ten years ago, when she had had the first subarachnoid haemorrhage. He had stayed at the bedside then, because he found that he was useful to the nurses. I asked him, 'Was it helpful for you?' He replied, 'No'. What I was trying to find out was whether he wanted to participate in her care. I established that he didn't want to be involved in the practical things, that it wouldn't be helpful for him.*

Henrietta: Did he mention Richard?

Alison: Yes, I encouraged him to talk about all the family. I wanted to establish his support network. I found out that her family were not very close. I asked him whether there was somebody around for him to talk to and he said, 'Do you mean somebody around to talk to like I'm talking to you now?' I felt that indicated that he was finding our conversation helpful. He said that there were friends who lived over the road and that he had used them before for support. What I was trying to do here was to help him establish, in his own mind, what support he needed, what his support networks were and how he would use them.

This informal debriefing session took place at about seven o'clock in the evening, when there was an opportunity to withdraw from the ward for a few minutes. Henrietta looked intensely interested in what Alison was saying. The immediacy of the situation and her own involvement with the patient and family made the discussion highly relevant for her. Furthermore, the supervision session was a response to a specific concern Henrietta had voiced in the earlier staff development interview. Aware of Henrietta's learning needs, Alison had been alert to the kind of clinical situation that she might learn from and created a supervision opportunity when a suitable situation arose.

With this supervision strategy, Alison used a number of skills to make her practical knowledge accessible to Henrietta:

- Negotiating a practical means of setting up a learning opportunity for the staff nurse, while remaining sensitive to the husband's need for privacy.
- Telling a story in fine detail and picking out the salient issues for the individual staff nurse (Titchen and Higgs, 1995).
- Describing, in detail, how and when she did things (for example, '*I did touch his knee*').
- Uncovering and articulating her own logic and intentions.

The key attribute that Alison displayed, by making time to share her practice expertise, was a genuine commitment to the staff nurse's personal and professional development.

For the nurse concerned, this supervision strategy provided an opportunity to:

- Learn about an aspect of practice in which she had expressed a particular interest.
- Access practical knowledge that is not usually talked or written about.
- Ask the expert focussed questions about a specific event, rather than generalized questions which stimulate a generalized response.
- Probe to find out how the expert made her judgements and decisions (an opportunity not really taken up by Henrietta in this example).

'Tell me about . . .'

The second supervision strategy provides a means of helping nurses to think more deeply about their own patients and to explore alternative ways of managing real clinical problems. The focus of the supervision is on the individual nurse's practice, rather than on what the expert does. But the supervisor brings a broader perspective or greater insight, which helps the nurse to think about a situation in a new way and, perhaps, to identify a way through a difficult problem.

Saying the word 'cancer'

Fieldnote: 5.15 p.m. – in the staff-room. *'While I made tea, Alison asked Moira to tell her about her primary patient. Moira's patient, Florrie, had just been diagnosed as having ovarian cancer and Moira was having difficulty helping Florrie to use the word 'cancer'. She wanted to help her to talk about and explore her diagnosis and to help her adjust and cope with her illness. Florrie had been giving out cues that she wanted to talk about it, but Moira didn't know how to help her. She was not blocking Florrie from talking about it, but she was just not able to ask the right questions to help the discussion.*

Alison helped Moira to express why she was finding it difficult to know where to go next with Florrie. She summarized and reflected back what she was saying and helped her to explore the problem fully before giving feedback or making suggestions.

Moira looked as though she enjoyed the session and, at the end, said, 'That was good, thanks' (smiling).

Five days after this discussion, Angie interviewed Moira.

Moira: *During the session with Alison, I realized that I was being tentative in the situation and that I am often tentative in similar situations. Alison talked about creating opportunities for helping patients to talk about their diagnoses, and the next day there was a chance for me to do it. I asked her whether she had any idea of what they might find when they operated on her and the patient said the word 'cancer'. She didn't say much more. She changed the subject quickly, looked out of the window and said something about the view. I felt that it had been enough for her for that day and I felt really pleased that I had provided an opportunity for Florrie to say the word and to talk briefly about it.*

When Alison asked me about it the next day, I told her I was really glad that she had encouraged me to help the patient talk. I felt I had really made progress.

Again, this supervision strategy is used informally – here, over a cup of tea in the staff-room. Alison simply invited the nurse to talk about her primary patient and then skilfully used the ensuing conversation. The key skills associated with this strategy are listening and facilitation and articulating practical knowledge.

As a facilitator of learning, Alison helped the nurse to reflect upon her practice and to identify her own learning needs. Her aim was not to make judgements or to point out weaknesses, but to help the nurse to articulate her own perceptions and intentions. Alison was then able to share her own practical knowledge in a way that was specifically relevant to the nurse's work with her patient. Additional skills and attributes that she displayed included:

- Sensitivity.
- Knowing when the time was right to initiate a discussion.
- The ability to challenge a nurse's practice without being threatening.
- Sharing ideas without being patronizing.
- Valuing the nurse's performance and ideas.
- Asking for feedback on her own performance as a supervisor.

Although her primary motive in asking the nurse in the story to talk about her patient was to create a learning opportunity, Alison was also effectively calling the nurse to account for her management of the patient's care. As the nurse talked, Alison was able to assess her level of understanding of the patient's problems, the nature of the relationship she had established with the patient and the appropriateness of the decisions she had made so far. Thus, this strategy provided a means by which Alison could sample the quality of care nurses were providing for their patients while, at the same time, stimulating their clinical development and helping them to improve their practice. Once the nurses realized that Alison would respond constructively to the weaknesses and limitations in their practice, they were rarely anxious or defensive.

The fieldnote below records Alison talking to the team leaders about the 'Tell me about . . .' strategy.

'I want to get into their heads'

I ask them to tell me about their primary patient. This is better than starting from the care plan because, if you do that, you get into technicalities and issues about style and what I want to do is to get into their heads. If you focus on the care plan, you talk about what they have grasped, not about what they haven't. I say, 'Tell me about what kind of relationship you have built up.' That really helped Moira to get into the bit that was difficult for her. Or I say, 'Tell me about your first conversation.' I use open questions to try to get a description of the nurse's and the patient's feelings. I'm careful not to make a judgement too early. I'm ten steps ahead, but I hold myself back, I slow myself down. For example, I knew there was a problem for Dave (staff nurse) with Rose's daughters, but I had to shut my mouth (put hand over her mouth) and just wait for him to bring it up. When he eventually did, I asked him if he thought he had a role to play there. I don't deny what they say, I ask another question to help them to explore the area until they make an evaluation of their own performance.

I ask the person to describe where they were sitting, how they felt, how long the conversation was, who was in control of the conversation. I ask, 'Why?', 'What makes you think that?', 'Who broke the silences?', 'Who asked the questions?' It's important to get at the nurses' long-term planning as well. Each day, I say, 'Tell me about your patient. What do you think will be the outcome for your patient? What about the family? How much have you found out?' I get them to think right at the beginning, 'What does this patient need for going home?'

When you have been asking all these questions, people then ask you what you would have done, what other options there were. (AB)

Alison's probing, exploratory questions helped the nurses to articulate their perceptions of clinical situations and the reasoning behind their decisions and actions. This process enabled nurses to identify gaps in their own understanding and it made them curious about other ways they could use to deal with a particular situation. Alison was then able to share her own knowledge and expertise without appearing too critical or patronizing. When she was able to suggest new perspectives or approaches which were relevant to nurses' current clinical work, they were able to use them immediately to devise strategies for helping their own patients and thereby incorporate them into their own practice repertoire. Seeing patients benefit at once from this learning process could be very stimulating and rewarding for nurses and could greatly increase their confidence in working through clinical problems. Meanwhile, Alison was able to assess in some detail how nurses were performing and she could guide their practice for the benefit of patients.

'Not just an observer'

The third supervision strategy involved helping a nurse to learn from a shared clinical experience. This strategy was the hardest to manage. Not only were opportunities for working alongside another nurse for any substantial period of time quite difficult to arrange in the busyness of ward life, but also comfortable roles had to be created for both parties within the clinical situation. Alison did not want staff nurses to feel that she was checking up on them, or interfering, or pushing them out of the way, when she became involved in a clinical situation with them. She did not want to stand and watch nurses work, nor did she want to push them into an observer role. She aimed, instead, to join a particular situation and to work collaboratively with the nurse involved. Alison would find time to reflect with the nurse upon what they had both experienced and how they had handled the situation.

The Two Daughters Story

AB: *Rachel and I were both on duty together when Mrs Williams was dying. We were washing her and comforting her when her daughters came in. It was a busy morning, but towards the afternoon, we had got our team reasonably sorted out and Rachel and I sat with Mrs Williams and the two daughters. We sat with them for about an hour, just talking gently with them and being with them while she died. Rachel and I were both involved together . . . I didn't feel she was just an observer . . . she was supported, but involved.*

AT: *Was it the first time she had ever done that?*

AB: *It wasn't the first time she had sat with someone when they died, but I don't think she'd done it in that way before. It was a very nice experience. We talked about it afterwards and how pleased we were at being able to manage it like that.*

AT: *Did you talk about why you felt it was an appropriate way to help the daughters? Did you theorize about what you were doing?*

AB: *(pause) Not in great depth. We talked about the daughters' relationship and how they each had a different view of what was going on, and how we were able to manage the situation slightly differently for each of them. So when she actually died, for example, the one who was most emotional about it all, we let her stay with her mother on her own for a while, whilst the other one came away. So we didn't bundle them together as 'the daughters', we talked a bit about that . . .*

AT: *How did you sense that the daughters were happier with you being there, than with you not being there?*

AB: *Because they said so. They were anxious if we went away. You could sense they were worried about the situation. But some people might have liked to have been left on their own. I did think about that, that I knew it was the right thing to do . . . When Mrs Williams actually died, one daughter obviously recognized it, while the other one didn't, or didn't want to accept that she'd gone. Now it was much easier for me to say, 'She's died', than for the one who knew, the more realistic one, to say it to her sister. There was a tension between the two daughters. They had told me they actually didn't get on very well with each other, except in their relationship with their mother. They both had a good relationship with her. So the fact that I was able to manage the situation made it easier for both of them. They seemed to need a third person to help them to come to terms with what was going on, probably like mother had done herself.*

> AT: *And did you talk like this with Rachel?*
> AB: *Not in that much depth, no . . . but we did talk about the situation and about the daughters' different needs. And about how it felt right sitting there and how nice it was that we had been able to make the opportunity, even on a busy day.*

The 'not just an observer' strategy combined the processes of the first two strategies, namely articulation of the expert's practical knowledge and exploration and extension of the nurse's practice, and added two extra processes, those of role modelling and directly observing a staff nurse's work. The skills that Alison demonstrated with this strategy were:

- Working alongside a nurse in a non-threatening way.
- Making time in a busy ward for a reflective conversation with the staff nurse.
- Role modelling how she could use her presence in a therapeutic way (in this case, acting as the 'third person' to help the daughters).
- Theorizing her practice (here, about how she was using her presence in the situation).
- Opening up new possibilities for the staff nurse by involving her in the experience.
- Evaluating the effectiveness of their care (their 'being with' the daughters).

This supervision strategy offered the staff nurse an opportunity to:

- Observe an expert's practice and the way she theorized about it.
- Receive feedback on her own performance and her attempts at theorization.

Sharing a clinical situation can be a powerful experience for both parties. It provides an excellent starting point for discussion and analysis of therapeutic practice, because both parties can consider the situation from an experiential and an intellectual perspective. Nurses reported that the combination of role modelling, articulation of expert practical knowledge, reflection upon practice and giving feedback was a very effective way of helping them to learn. Differences in the nurses' care planning, in the depth of their relationships with patients and families and in the detail and range of their work were noticed as a result of this synthesis.

Considering the three supervision strategies together, there was a strong emphasis on the interpersonal aspects of supervision, with Alison adopting the role of facilitator of learning, as described by Rogers (1983), and helping the nurses to develop their own practical knowledge by consciously learning from their experiences. She helped them to reflect, theorize and evaluate and to direct their own learning. She focussed on helping nurses to acquire knowledge that was relevant and, therefore, meaningful to them at the time (Ausubel *et al.*, 1978).

Clinical supervision with both supportive and educative functions is being advocated in nursing as a way of helping nurses to improve their practice (Butterworth and Faugier, 1992). It is being promoted as a model that has relevance throughout a nurse's career (NHSME, 1993; ENB, 1994). However, despite such urging, there is evidence that clinical supervision is not widely practised or understood by clinical nurses (White *et al.*, 1993). Furthermore, there appears to be no empirical evidence, so far, that provides practical details of how clinical supervision can be managed in a busy hospital ward, or of how expert nurses can be helped to become effective supervisors.

Kohner (1994) suggests that a valuable preparation for becoming a clinical supervisor is to be supervised oneself by a skilled facilitator. Our action research partnership served this function for Alison, for Angie was constantly facilitating her efforts to unravel and reflect upon the complexities of patient-centred practice. As Alison's own facilitation skills and her general approach to clinical supervision developed, the three opportunistic strategies provided a framework for incorporating into her practice an appropriate style of supervision. And because these strategies could be used flexibly and as an integral part of her clinical work, they could realistically be employed within the constraints of busy ward life.

Johns (1993a; 1994) has shown the value of offering nurses formal, scheduled discussions about their practice, where they are challenged and encouraged to think in new ways, much as post-graduate students are helped by their academic supervisors. Our three opportunistic supervision strategies are valuable ways of complementing the more formal, off the ward supervision that Johns described. Moreover, our strategies have the particular merit of having been designed for use as an integral part of the supervisor's practice repertoire. They need to be employed consciously and intentionally in an appropriate situation, but they are used as the supervisor and the person supervised go about their work and do not require either party to take pre-planned time away from their practice. In a busy ward setting, the three supervision strategies emerged as realistic, practical methods for influencing and supporting the development of nurses wishing to practise in a patient-centred way[1].

---

[1] Building on these findings, Titchen (1998a; 1998b) conducted an in-depth investigation of how she had helped Alison to develop the supervision skills and strategies presented here. She created a framework of 'critical companionship' to describe a relationship in which a 'critical companion' accompanies less experienced practitioners on their own very personal experiential learning journeys. Readers who want more information on how to help clinical leaders and expert nurses to develop effective supervision skills may find Titchen's work useful.

Chapter 7

The practice journey

'... there is a convergence between what I feel I am supposed to do and what I want to do ...'

Mayeroff (1971)

INTRODUCTION

Our experience of changing the 'system' in hospital nursing is that it does not necessarily produce change in the way that nurses practise. Decentralizing ward nursing gives nurses freedom to work more independently. Developing an open, caring climate and a constructive, facilitative style of leadership gives them the permission and support they need to work closely and creatively with patients. But these changes in the organization, culture and leadership of ward life provide no more than a framework for patient-centred practice. They promote patient-centred practice by providing favourable conditions, by giving nurses *opportunities* to practise differently. Helping nurses to develop the confidence and the skills to use these opportunities is another matter and was, for us, to a certain extent, a journey into uncharted territory.

In this chapter, we trace the way nurses learned to use the new opportunities open to them in their daily work and present a picture of the more patient-centred style of nursing that began to emerge in the ward. The task of developing and supporting the nurses' practice became an increasingly central element of Alison's contribution as ward sister. Many of the strategies she learned to use in this endeavour have already been described in the previous chapter, as part of the 'leadership journey'. Here we include some additional, more focussed strategies which complemented, or overlapped, the general approaches to supervision and staff development.

It is difficult, and probably fairly meaningless, to attempt to define the term 'patient-centred nursing' in any precise way. Generally, it refers to a style of practice that reflects a commitment to working with each patient as a person. By its very nature, at a detailed level, it is a style of practice that is infinitely variable. As no two people are exactly alike, so their nursing care will never be identical if it is truly patient-centred. However, from the beginning of our work a number of guiding principles influenced the way we interpreted the notion of patient-centredness in day to day practice.

Our initial understanding of patient-centred practice was formed from a mixture of gut feeling and incompletely articulated or analysed experiences of practice, combined with a range of fairly abstract concepts gleaned from the literature. For Alison, reading the work of Carl Rogers in the late 1970s was particularly influential. Rogers' (1967) insights into the nature of 'the helping relationship' gave her a new perspective on relationships with both patients and colleagues. The simplicity and the practical utility of his theory captured Alison's imagination and proved much more valuable than any of the nursing theory she was exposed to at around the same time. It was probably Rogers' work, more than any other single influence, that helped Alison to recognize and articulate her dissatisfaction with the individualized style of nursing she had initially embraced with enthusiasm. Practice that drew upon apparently holistic theories and focussed upon what were intended to be individualized care plans, but in the absence of close, continuous relationships, was clearly never going to be either holistic or individualized. Rogers' work identified for Alison the therapeutic potential of the nurse–patient relationship and brought home the message that it is not the model or the care plan, but primarily the nurse's ability to be warm, open, accepting and empathetic towards a patient that determines whether practice can become truly patient-centred.

Mayeroff (1971) and Jourard (1971), writing also from a humanistic perspective, helped Alison to apply Rogers' ideas to nursing. Mayeroff, a philosopher, presented an analysis of caring which is not specific to professional relationships, but which inevitably offers food for thought to nurses, who often claim that caring is the essence of their work. Mayeroff's depiction of a caring relationship is very similar to Rogers' helping relationship, in that both have the intention of promoting the growth and development of the other person and, like Rogers, Mayeroff sees personal involvement and commitment as fundamental elements of caring.

Jourard (1971), critical of professional training generally, suggested that it *'encourages graduates to wear a professional mask.'* He described nurses as commonly hiding behind a stereotypical 'bedside manner' to protect themselves from their patients' feelings, which may be distressing or disturbing. At the same time, he suggested that, by denying themselves access to their patients' experiences, nurses cut themselves off from an important source of information about the personal support their patients need to achieve an optimum response to treatment and care. Jourard advocated dropping the 'professional mask' and affirmed, specifically in nursing, the importance of the maturity, self-knowledge, openness and genuineness that Rogers and Mayeroff consider essential characteristics of the effective helper or carer.

Some years later, Alistair Campbell's (1984) concept of nursing as 'skilled companionship' became very important for Alison. Though approaching nursing this time from a theological perspective, again the simplicity, clarity and humanity of the writing were attractive. Campbell dismissed the outmoded notions of the nurse as 'doctor's handmaiden' or 'ministering angel' and suggested that,

'What is required is an account of nursing which is not caught in sexual stereotypes, which is professional without being distanced and manipulative, which is close to the realities of bodily care, yet also sees the personal potential of the patient, which protects the nurse from overwhelming demands, yet which

gives every patient full consideration. In short, to understand nursing correctly we need to understand the tension implicit in all human acts of care – the "teach us to care and not to care" of Eliot's Ash Wednesday.' (p. 49)

As the 'skilled companion', Campbell described the nurse accompanying her patient on a journey, using her bodily presence and practical expertise to help the patient onwards. He sees their relationship as close and open, like a friendship, and involving some risk for the nurse. But the companionship is also limited, because both parties expect to go their own way when the particular journey is completed. Campbell's image of the 'skilled companion' captured much of what Alison was intuitively trying to develop in her own relationships with patients. She used his ideas often when teaching nurses and we shall refer to them again in this chapter when we analyse clinical stories.

This chapter shows how the experience of observing and reflecting upon practice throughout the project enabled us to build upon these general ideas and to develop a richer and more detailed understanding of the nature of patient-centred nursing and the relationship upon which it is founded. We also show how this style of nursing gradually emerged in Oriel Ward and the impact it had upon nurses, patients and families.

EXPERIENCING THE CHALLENGE OF NURSING

In the traditional nursing system, personal care of patients, such as bathing, dressing, toiletting, turning and feeding, was classed as 'basic care' and was considered appropriate work to delegate to junior student nurses or auxiliaries (Goddard, 1953). This 'basic care' was seen as requiring only elementary skill and acquired a low status in the hierarchy of nursing tasks. Each aspect of 'basic care' was perceived purely as a practical procedure. Bed-bathing, for example, was described as a series of manoeuvres with towels and sheets that would allow each part of the body to be washed in a particular sequence. Seen in these terms, 'basic care' *is* fairly simple and is potentially dull and repetitive.

From a patient-centred perspective, the personal care of patients is seen quite differently. If the recipient of the bed-bath is viewed not as an inanimate body, but a vulnerable person, deprived of normal independence and struggling to cope with being ill, then the business of helping him or her to wash is transformed. The practical task becomes an opportunity for the skilled nurse to achieve much more than just a clean patient. The unusually intimate contact associated with 'basic care' affords the skilled nurse not only the opportunity to make detailed observations of the patient's physical well-being, but also a privileged opportunity to address his or her feelings and concerns. Attending to patients' personal needs becomes the medium through which a complex, highly skilled form of caring can be delivered. Seem in this light, 'basic care' becomes important, interesting and challenging.

The attitude of modern nurses to 'basic care' is ambivalent. Many nurse theorists highlight the importance of a personal relationship with patients and, increasingly, interpersonal skills training is emphasized in nurse education. When asked what they like about their work, nurses will almost invariably cite contact with people and the opportunity to help people at the top of their list. Yet, in everyday ward life, it is common for nurses to regard the intimate care of patients as menial and boring. This mismatch between what nurses say they value and what they actually experience can leave them with feelings of guilt, frustration and dissatisfaction, and a vague sense that their nursing is not what it ought to be (Binnie, 1988). A major theme in the 'practice journey' was the discovery of the hidden potential of 'basic care' and the restoration of this intimate care of patients to its rightful status as the very heart of nursing.

The daily grind

When our project began, the medical wards had a reputation in the hospital for being heavy, unglamorous places to work. The nursing was perceived to be an exhausting, unstimulating routine. Nurses in the Oriel Ward complained of getting *'bogged down and depressed'* because of all the *'chronic patients and strokes'*. They talked of *'just washing patients'* and *'slogging, not achieving anything'*. They were unhappy and some felt guilty that they felt this way about their work. Indeed, there was a strong sense that this was not how nursing should be, that this was not what they had trained for and that the patients deserved something better.

> *Sometimes I get bogged down by tasks. I feel anyone could do what I am doing. When I'm down, I only see the basic care as tasks and not about thinking, 'how can I help this patient with incontinence?' I only see the wet bed to change.* (Moira)

Nurses frequently expressed feeling overwhelmed by their workload and frustrated that the heavy, basic, practical work left them no time to talk with their patients and to address their personal concerns and worries. The nurses seemed to feel that they were victims of the system, trapped on a treadmill.

> *I don't have control over our situation. All I am asking for is to be able to provide the basic care and nobody cares.* (Mike)

Moira described her ideal way of nursing as *'having time to sit with patients and chat with them'*, but she found she was rarely able to do that because *'there is always so much pressure on you; it's always so stressful.'*

A consultant, looking back to the time when the project began, recognized the impact on the nurses' motivation of the daily grind of medical nursing.

> *There was a time when they looked so damned harassed that they had almost lost interest.* (Consultant)

The nurses themselves complained about their work not being intellectually stimulating or challenging. Many felt they should be able to motivate themselves to learn and to develop professionally, but found they could not because their work was too tiring and draining. They wanted to be lifted out of this professional inertia and, when Alison joined the ward, they looked to her to help them. Sometimes her encouragement stimulated them to become interested in a clinical issue or prompted them to start some project work, but frequently, because their nursing provided no intrinsic motivation, they got sucked back on to the treadmill and then had no energy left to sustain their new interest, so that projects remained half finished.

Strategies for uncovering the potential of basic care

When discussing the nurses' perceptions of their work in a reflective conversation, Alison commented upon how differently she felt about everyday practical nursing. Although at times experiencing the same exhaustion as the nurses and the same frustration at not always having time to do everything she would like for patients, for her, basic nursing was 'never boring'. On the contrary, it was always an opportunity to get close to patients and to discover how they were feeling, and to convey caring through the gentleness and sensitivity of her touch and through the careful attention to detail that can make so much difference to patients (a perspective that has been well documented in a study by MacLeod, 1994). Articulating these personal perceptions made Alison aware of the possibility of sharing them more explicitly with the nurses during the course of her everyday work, with the intention of helping them to see the challenges and opportunities hidden beneath the surface of 'basic nursing'. In due course, overtly valuing basic care and being explicit about what could be learned or achieved by approaching it in a more alert and imaginative way, became a major strategy for raising the status of practical bedside care within the ward and for helping nurses to see this aspect of their work in a more positive light.

The bedside handover provided a particularly useful opportunity for Alison to talk about her work with patients and for her to help the nurses to reflect upon what they had been doing. The story about George, from the early days of team nursing, illustrates Alison's approach to working with a 'heavy' patient and the kind of things she was able to explain and discuss with the nurses during the handover. Alison reflected upon the way she had been able to make a real difference to George by approaching his 'basic care' thoughtfully and creatively, while, in contrast, the other nurses in the team had been passively bathing, turning and 'humping George about', making little progress from day to day.

George had had a stroke which had left him unable to speak and unable to move his right side. He was a tall, solidly built man and extremely heavy to lift now that he was disabled.

Humping George About

AB: *George is the sort of patient where people tend not to use as much imagination as perhaps they need to. He is the kind of patient whom it is very easy to see as just 'humping around'. I feel I've been more like his primary nurse, because all the improvements in his care have come from me. I was the one who got him dressed in his own clothes. When I first nursed him he was in a hospital gown. I know Rosalyn had had a busy day, but he was unshaven too. I found out that he could shave himself, if I set things up for him. I organized the hoist so he could be lifted in a more dignified way, and so it wasn't such a burden for the staff. I got his Roho cushion.*

AT: *You suggested the physio, the standing in the parallel bars, the self-propelling wheelchair.*

AB: *I got him his regular newspaper to read. I initiated getting his medication changed as well. I even spotted his necrotic haemorrhoid when I gave him his enema yesterday. I was cleaning him up and I saw a funny looking something and I couldn't wash it off. When I examined him properly, I found a necrotic pile. Everyone else has been giving him enemas and not seen it. So all these subtle little things add up and really make a difference. I asked Brenda to take him to The League of Friends Cafe too.*

> *AT: It's all improved the quality of his life and the result is that smile on his face and the joke at handover. Still that almost mask-like face, but he does react now, he doesn't look so down.*
>
> *AB: It's interesting, reflecting on it, that there are so many things I did that made a difference, but it's shocking really that they were all my initiatives ... But if I hadn't been there, George could be being humped around, a big heavy lump and being very depressed and waiting a long time for anything to happen. His medical investigations have taken ages and it's quite possible that nothing much would have happened, on the nursing side, till now, when the medical stuff is finished and people start agitating to get him home. Then they might be thinking about getting him dressed.*
>
> *AT: The sense I get at handover is that the nurses feel very positive towards him and very caring. They are fond of him. Even though he is slow to respond, they do include him in the handover.*
>
> *AB: Yes, they see him differently now.*

While at this early stage in the ward's development, the nurses were often following Alison's lead with patients like George, by participating in this proactive style of work, they were able to experience first-hand some of its challenges and satisfactions. For some nurses, simply watching Alison carrying out 'basic' tasks for patients opened their eyes. They suddenly saw, for example, just what a sophisticated activity washing a patient could be, in highly skilled hands. Rosemary's story of Alison bed-bathing Ray provides another example of 'basic' care being used as the medium through which the nurse–patient relationship can be developed and a whole range of nursing concerns addressed. The story also illustrates the power of role modelling and shows the value of an expert continuing to participate in the day to day personal care of patients and of learning, where possible, to make this aspect of her work visible to less experienced nurses.

> **Washing Ray**
>
> Care Plan Project data: *We observed Alison help Ray, an elderly gentleman, to have a wash in bed. She took the opportunity, given by the wash, to let him talk about his life. There was no discussion about the wash itself, it flowed smoothly and was incidental to their conversation. The total attention that she gave to him, rather than to the task of washing, allowed her to tune in to him quickly.* (Rosemary)

This simple story carries the central message that Alison tried to convey to the nurses about 'basic care', namely, that the psychological aspects of caring – the listening, explaining, reassuring, encouraging and supporting – that they wanted to offer their patients, need not compete for time with essential practical tasks. On the contrary, the tasks themselves – the bathing, the turning, the enema, the walk round the bed – provide often the best opportunities for this truly patient-centred work (Taylor, 1992; MacLeod, 1994). The moments of privacy and the intimacy in so much of this work allow the nurse immediate and close access to the patient's very personal world. The closeness to the physical body and to its discomfort, its dysfunction or its deformity, can bring the alert and sensitive nurse equally close to the patient's feelings and concerns.

Being open to each patient's emotions, at every bedside encounter, is potentially overwhelming, so nurses have to learn the difficult trick of prioritizing and focussing their use of time and energy. Socialized in a 'getting through the work' culture, the nurses in Oriel Ward were not used to making decisions about what to do now and what to leave till later. The traditional system had rewarded them for completing specified tasks to a specified timetable and, to a certain extent, it had protected them from the anxiety associated with sometimes having to omit the finer niceties of caring. One could always blame the system for what was left undone, rather than face up to it being the consequence of a personal decision. However, once team nursing was established, nurses were free to manage the care of their own caseload of patients for the shift, in whatever way they felt was best, so that decisions had to be made about what to do and when. Beginning to recognize that physical and psychological care could be integrated rather than necessarily separate activities, was a step towards making a patient-centred style of practice more manageable. But it could not entirely change the reality that there was rarely time to give everything one would like to every patient. Initially, many of the nurses found taking personal responsibility for prioritizing their work both difficult and stressful. In response, Alison made a conscious effort to role model and articulate her own management strategies in this area. Rachel's comments illustrate how nurses learned from observing the way Alison managed her time when she worked with patients.

> *Alison wasn't rushing around worrying about everybody all the time. She can sit down and spend time with her patients, while I'm running around trying to get things done. If I start to talk to someone, I'm constantly thinking I should be doing this or that ... The other day, I spent three quarters of an hour talking to a patient and when I started thinking 'I must do this.' I thought, 'Well, Emma will deal with anything that comes up.' It was quite important to talk to that patient. It's the first time I have felt like that ... I'm getting into the habit of thinking, 'Is this really going to make a difference to this patient?'*
> (Rachel)

Alison used handover time to provide concrete examples of the way she prioritized her work. For example, she would tell late shift nurses that because she had needed to spend extra time with Mrs Jones, she had not done A, B and C, and she would explain why she had made that decision. The fact that Sister did not always finish everything that needed doing by the end of the shift, and that she was quite comfortable about handing work on to colleagues, gave a clear message that it was acceptable for others to do likewise. Further 'permission giving' was achieved by Alison looking out for nurses who were harassed or overwhelmed by their workload. She would talk through with them what they had to do, helping them to decide what was important and what they could leave out, and reassuring them that this was a perfectly reasonable course of action in the circumstances.

Using these various strategies during the phase of team nursing, Alison was able to help nurses to approach the 'basic care' of their patients in a more flexible and imaginative way. However, it was not until the new nursing roles had been negotiated that her efforts to establish the importance of 'basic care' really bore fruit. Primary nursing made it easier for nurses to prioritize their time. Instead of feeling pressure to be all things to all the team's patients, primary nurses could legitimately focus upon the special needs of their own few patients, confident that someone else was doing the same for others. In addition, being personally responsible for primary patients encouraged nurses to be more interested in the fine details of their nursing. It provided a stimulus for them to use the opportunities that they were discovering within the apparently simple tasks of their daily work.

Nursing is exciting

Formalizing primary nursing produced a marked change in the nurses' attitudes to their work. The strong sense of personal responsibility associated simply with having one's name attached to a patient was, in itself, very challenging for the nurses.

> *People now say, 'Oh speak to her, she's the primary nurse.' I find this very daunting.* (Janice)

But the responsibility seemed to initiate a snowball effect. It made the nurses feel that they should know more about their own patients. As they became better informed and more involved with their patients, the more complex were the issues they uncovered and the more interesting their work became. Furthermore, as individuals were helped to take up the challenge to manage their own patients' nursing, and to assert their authority to get things done, they became more confident and more able to make the decisions required to take control of their workload.

The motivation that came from the sense of being visible and exposed as a primary nurse was very clearly expressed by Janice.

> *I felt challenged. I had got something to get my teeth into. It gave me the interest to go and look things up, because I felt responsible. Being a primary nurse made me feel I had to be able to argue my case. I felt I had to be able to answer questions from patients and relatives . . . I had to be prepared . . . I didn't want to look stupid after I had introduced myself as the primary nurse.* (Janice)

After a particularly demanding but successful experience as a primary nurse, Rosemary reflected upon the personal contribution she had made within the multidisciplinary team and the real difference she had made to her patient.

> *It backed up my self-worth, really, feeling valued as part of the team . . . I realized the power of nursing practice and just how much I personally believe in that, being able to experience this type of thing and actually how much it motivates me to go on . . . What suddenly struck me was how much I really believe in what I am doing now . . . I undervalued my contribution before, but now I could argue for hours about the complexities and the skills that are needed and how not everybody could do it.* (Rosemary)

Rachel's story of nursing Daphne shows how the nurses were discovering that even simple tasks could take on a new meaning and be used with particular therapeutic effect, when understood in the context of the particular patient. Daphne was frail and confused and showed no sign of recognizing her nurses from one shift to the next.

Making Things Familiar For Daphne

I spoke to her daughter in Rome quite a lot about how she was and I put Daphne on the phone to her. The daughter must have said something along the lines of, 'Rachel brought you to the phone' and Daphne said, 'Who's Rachel?' I just thought to myself, 'Never mind!' I said, 'It's me,' and she said, 'Oh yes.' She didn't have a clue who I was . . . I don't think she feels anything different about me than anyone else at the moment. She hasn't that ability with strangers. Yet on the phone to her daughter, about three or four days ago, she was quite lucid and quite warm. On several occasions I haven't been able to have a sensible conversation with her and I've said to her daughter, Sarah, 'I'm not promising that she'll be able to say anything back to you because she hasn't said a word to me for days.' I carried her to the phone and she wasn't as articulate as she was the other day, but she said, 'Hello darling, yes I'm OK thank you' and I was gob-smacked because she had not managed to say anything like that in this unfamiliar environment. As soon as she recognized Sarah's voice, she was OK. Also, when her friends have visited, she has been a lot more able to speak and interact with them. I'm sure a lot of her problem is where she is. I think a familiar environment would be a lot better . . .

One day, after I had looked after her for a couple of days . . . she had been incontinent, so I thought I'd put her in the bath. As soon as she got in the bath, with water all around her and in that little space, she seemed to improve ever so slightly. She used the cloth and actually washed a bit of herself, whereas before if I had given her the cloth she wouldn't have known what to do with it. So, I felt that maybe it was because the bath was familiar to her, because I mean a bath is a bath, and that bit of familiarity seemed to help her. I've given her a few baths because it is something she can actually relate to. Also, I get her dressed in her own clothes, because that's familiar and it seems to give her an idea of what time it is.

I think the lack of familiarity is one of her biggest problems and I recognized that and although there wasn't much I could do about it, I did the little bit I could. If I hadn't worked with her for quite a few days, I suppose I wouldn't have recognized the little changes. (Rachel)

Rachel was stimulated and challenged by a very difficult patient from whom the feedback and rewards were small. By paying careful attention to detail and by thinking intelligently about Daphne's situation, Rachel was able skilfully to use the opportunities of 'basic nursing' to make a difference to her patient and this was a satisfying personal achievement, of which she was justifiably proud.

Having clearly defined personal authority and experiencing making decisions that made a difference to patients seemed to make nurses feel generally more in control of their work. The fact that they could be personally influential in managing their patients' nursing seemed to make them feel more confident and assertive in managing their workload as a whole.

The rewards for discovering the excitement and challenge of everyday nursing, and for learning to use it in creative ways, lay within the work itself; it was intrinsically motivating. However, there was often the additional satisfaction of appreciative feedback from patients or relatives, which became more specific and more personalized as the nurses' patient-centred approach developed. 'The Lavender Story' below shows just how gratifying that feedback could sometimes be. It also shows how profound and far-reaching the impact of exquisitely sensitive 'basic nursing' can be for those who receive or observe it. The story has an added richness too, when one recalls the views that Janice had expressed about her work in the ward early in the project:

> *The chronic cases really get you down. It's very basic nursing. One doesn't have time to put in the psycho-social side of care. Many of the patients are so ill they wouldn't notice anyway.* (Janice)

A year later, Janice reflected upon her experiences since primary nursing had been established.

The Lavender Story

I like looking after terminal patients, the sort of patient who is unconscious . . . I just feel you can put a lot into it if you want to.

The daughter was feeling a bit rejected because nobody was coming in to see her mother and that had happened on the previous shift. I think people were assuming that because the daughter was in there, she would just come out and get someone if she needed anything. She was very open about this fact that she was very cross with the people who had been on the previous shift. So I went out of my way to call back regularly to see if she was alright and to sit down and talk to her about how her mother had been. I remember her saying that her mum was a very proud lady and she would have hated to have smelt as she did, because she was leaking all the time.

Her skin was very dry, so I just started to use some lavender oil. I knew she liked lavender because she had some lavender eau de cologne. I started rubbing it in and I used to just sit on the stool and talk to the daughter while I was massaging her mother's arms and legs. I don't know if it made any difference to her, I like to think it did. But it made a difference to her daughter because she really felt that her mum was being cared for and she said that she really smelt nice. She wrote a lovely letter. (Janice)

The letter thanked all the Elm Team nurses, but included a few special words for Janice: *'Lavender will always bring my mother back to me.'*

The letter was passed around the ward with great delight. The nurses were deeply touched by it and shared Janice's satisfaction. Letters like this one reinforced the nurses' commitment to the new style of nursing they were all developing. They provided tangible evidence that everyday nursing tasks, when seen and managed in a patient's personal context, can be transformed from tedious chores to skilled acts of caring.

BECOMING A PATIENT-CENTRED NURSE

The developments in Oriel Ward brought nurses much closer to their patients than they had been before. The team system meant that relationships could develop without the threat of sudden interruption. Nurses could say to their patients, 'We can follow that up tomorrow' or 'We can work on this together', confident that they could keep their promises to see things through. Learning to value the contact of 'basic nursing', and to use it to observe and listen to patients, heightened nurses' awareness of their patients' experiences of illness and suffering. In addition, the primary nursing system placed the onus on individual nurses to respond to their patients and to achieve the best they could for them. The nurses found themselves entering into a new kind of relationship, with new demands and responsibilities. The relationship often provided extraordinarily privileged access to the patient's private world and the nurses recognized that this closeness called for a personal, as well as a technical, response. Patients in distress were trusting them with personal disclosures and, while some of the distress may have been relieved with practical measures, the trust itself demanded a human response. It meant that nurses were involved as people and were called upon to give something of themselves.

Getting close to patients made the nurses' work infinitely more interesting, but they approached the new relationships with caution. They were concerned about their own lack of skill and anxious that they might get out of their depth and let a patient down. An increasingly central part of our work, as the development progressed, was helping nurses to manage therapeutic relationships with patients and their families.

Passing acquaintances

While traditionally nurses were taught not to get involved with their patients, the modern ethos is quite the reverse. The Oriel Ward nurses had learned during their training that the individual nurse–patient relationship was important and that providing information, teaching and counselling for patients and their families was part of every nurse's role. They believed what they had been taught, but their experience of practice was that this kind of 'psychological care' was difficult to provide and their skills in this area were not well developed.

> *I always think of them as a whole because that was really drummed in during our training. But . . . it never really gelled together. With the approach we're using now, I think I'm beginning to see the whole entity.* (Janice)

Before team nursing was introduced to the ward, lack of continuity and fragmentation of care made it difficult for nurses to form or sustain close relationships with patients or families. In addition, the 'in charge' role took experienced nurses, with the most skill and confidence, away from the bedside and reduced their contact with patients even further. Alison's initial study recorded nurse–patient interactions in the medical wards as mostly brief and superficial (Binnie, 1988), findings which reflect those of earlier communication studies in similar settings (Faulkner, 1979; Macleod Clark, 1984). However, an exception to this pattern was noted in Alison's study in relation to some young haematology patients who were admitted on a recurring basis and who, over time, became much closer to the nurses than was usual. A similar example in our own data shows that this closeness, when it did occur, was not necessarily accompanied by self-awareness and skill.

'He couldn't talk about dying'

One haematology patient who was eighteen, all the nurses had become very fond of him, so much so that they were going out with him socially. I knew him very well, but not as well as some members of staff. I think we cushioned him in many ways from his illness. He couldn't be cured, we couldn't get him into remission. I think he found it very difficult to open up and talk to the staff because he saw them as friends and he didn't want to hurt them. It would have been a good opportunity for good continuity of care, because they knew each other so well. But he ended up speaking to somebody very frankly, a doctor he had never seen before . . . We felt that we wanted to speak to him about it, but that he couldn't, or he didn't want to hear . . . it's difficult. (Moira)

Throughout the period of team nursing, and during the early days of primary nursing, the nurses continued to experience difficulties in handling their relationships with patients. Sometimes they felt unable to develop the relationship in the way that was most helpful for the patient. Alternatively, a degree of trust and openness would develop and the nurse would become involved in supporting a patient in some way, but then get stuck.

Quite often I feel there is more behind what they are saying and I feel like getting them to explain what they mean and being helpful, but I can't. I'm not sure what I am saying is the correct thing. (Moira)

Like participants in Johns' (1993b) study, the nurses were sometimes unintentionally clumsy in their handling of relationships, beginning to work openly with a patient, developing the kind of working partnership they believed in, but then, unaware, falling back into a more traditional mode of behaviour which undermined what they were doing.

'I'm not mad, am I?'

Jenny came in her own time to a ward meeting to present a problem she had come across with a patient's care plan. The patient's wife had read his care plan and burst into tears. She showed her husband and he was very angry and upset about what had been written.

Jenny had developed a good rapport with the patient and he told her the story, after first breaking down and crying. He said that what had been written about him was untrue, 'lies'. He was also very distressed because the care plan stated that he had been referred for a psychiatric opinion and he had not known about this (he was depressed after a long illness). He said, 'I don't want to see a psychiatrist. I'm not mad am I?'

The patient asked to have the offending comments about him removed, because he did not want what was written to jeopardize his care in another ward where he was due to undergo surgery. Jenny said she would talk to the nurse who had written the care plan, which she did.

. . . Afterwards, I asked Jenny why she had raised this matter at the ward meeting. She replied that we all needed to think more carefully about what we write . . . 'I didn't want this kind of thing to be repeated.' The incident prompted a discussion in the ward meeting about the nature of partnerships with patients and Alison helped the nurses to identify what had gone wrong in this case. (AT)

Caring for and supporting patient's families was another area of 'relationship work' that was initially undeveloped within the nursing team. Traditionally, relatives and friends were largely excluded from the care of patients. They were allowed into wards only during short official visiting hours and dismissed by the ringing of a bell when their time was up. Nurses tended to withdraw from the ward during visiting hours and relatives wishing for information normally had to take the initiative to approach the sister or nurse in charge. When staff wanted to discuss an important issue with family members, they were usually invited for an interview in an office away from the bedside and, again, this was the job of the sister or her deputy. The practical care of patients more or less stopped during visiting hours – nurses tended to regard relatives as interrupting their work and often saw their presence as something of a 'nuisance' (Anderson, 1973). Bereaved relatives were comforted and offered tea in the ward office, but otherwise actually caring for relatives was not seen as part of the traditional nurse's remit.

Individualized nursing challenged this virtual exclusion of relatives. It emphasized that patients were part of a family and social network which did not disappear when patients were admitted to hospital. Nurses were encouraged to find out about their patients' home circumstances, and the idea that carers too may need looking after, and may sometimes find it helpful to be involved in their relative's nursing, was generally promoted.

The attitude to relatives in Oriel Ward was fairly relaxed and welcoming, even at the outset of the project. Visiting hours had been extended and were not rigidly enforced. Bedside nursing inevitably had to continue during this time, so that nurses often had the opportunity to talk informally with relatives when they attended to patients. However, there was little evidence of nurses purposefully setting out to establish a relationship with a family or of actively negotiating their involvement in a patient's care. In the early days of team nursing, Alison observed that, although nurses were finding out about their patients' family situations, they were not doing very much with this information, unless the problems were very obvious. She herself was often the one to address family issues that had not been picked up by the team. At this stage of the ward's development, there was no one nurse within the team who was personally responsible for working with the family and Alison suggested that this might account, at least in part, for the reluctance of individual nurses to take the initiative in this sphere of their work.

The challenge of involvement with patients and families prompted the nurses to reflect upon the ways in which they needed to develop. They became more alert to the way Alison managed her relationships with patients and recognized, by comparison, their own lack of skill and confidence. For example, Rosemary described Alison working with a young man who had a malignant tumour and who was not coping at all well with his illness. She described how, in managing the man's pain, Alison had also skilfully confronted a major psychological problem. Rosemary said, '*I wouldn't have been brave enough to do that.*'

In the early part of the study, it appeared that all the staff nurses had some difficulty in managing close relationships with patients and their families and they felt underconfident and unskilled at dealing with the psychological or emotional issues that confronted them in the course of their work. Consequently, they tended to maintain a distance, which led us to characterize their relationships with patients and families as more like those of passing acquaintances than those of the skilled companions that Campbell (1984) described. Our findings mirror those of Lathlean *et al.* (1986) in a study of newly registered nurses (NRNs), where it was found that '*many of the NRNs had difficulty noticing, understanding and responding appropriately to certain psychological or emotional needs of the patient, including those which appeared to be fairly clearly identifiable from the patient's condition or verbal or non-verbal communication*' (p. 36).

Strategies for developing skills for patient-centred nursing

In the previous chapter, we explained how, in a primary nursing system, the sister's key role was to influence the quality of care in her ward by supporting and developing her staff. We described some of the strategies that Alison used for providing clinical supervision within the unpredictable environment of a busy ward. A central element of her supervision work inevitably focussed on the nurses' relationships with their patients and so the general supervision strategies should be seen as complementing the more specific strategies that we highlight here.

Another crucial factor in the development of nurses' relationship skills was the presence of the open, supportive ward climate described in Chapter 5. The importance of nurses feeling that they could comfortably seek guidance and share emotional burdens is worth reiterating in this context. The role of the ward sister in creating that climate and being herself a key source of support and expert advice was critical.

Being there in the background to give confidence

We found that by consciously 'being there' for the nurses, Alison could help them to extend the boundaries of their practice. When they could see what needed doing for a patient, but were tentative about asserting their view or anxious about taking a calculated risk, being able to check it out with Alison first gave them confidence. Recognizing the value of being present for the nurses in this way, Alison tried to be more alert to situations where the nurses might be experiencing difficulty. She would unobtrusively indicate that she was available, perhaps simply by asking a general, open question ('How are you getting on with Mrs Smith?'), in a tone that invited discussion. She also learned to spot opportunities where she could gently push nurses forward by suggesting something challenging, but also making it clear that she would be there in the background to guide, advise and perhaps even take over, as a last resort.

Giving a Gentle Push

Quite often I gently push people when I think they are ready to take the next step . . . and then I try to be around to give them some support and feedback. An example is the recent work with Janice, where I encouraged her to be primary nurse to Neil, a very complicated patient with an extraordinarily difficult wife, both of them requiring an enormous amount of time and care. I pushed Janice into taking on a primary nurse role, reassuring her that I would be there to supervise her. I really did make an effort to make sure that I was giving Janice enough leeway to take on the primary nurse role, but also to be there when things were difficult . . . (to ask) her when she would like me to intervene to support her.

It worked really well. I was delighted with the way Janice matured through taking the responsibility of this patient. She was fantastic. She put an enormous amount of time and energy into working with these people and handled it well. The other day, I sat down with Janice and asked her what she felt she had got out of being involved with the situation. She talked about how much she had enjoyed the responsibility and feeling that she had something to offer. I was able to feed back to her how I had observed her practice maturing and how impressed I had been. She was delighted and I think the whole experience has helped her to grow in confidence and to enjoy the primary nurse role. (AB)

To extend their clinical skill and confidence in this way, Alison had to work closely with nurses when they were near the boundaries of their present capacity. If she were to take them further, they needed to feel comfortable exposing to her their doubts and uncertainties in a situation and to feel confident of being accepted, understood and helped. Being consistent in her approach was crucial here. The slightest threat of condemnation or ridicule could make nurses reluctant to show their limitations and Alison would then be denied access to their 'growth points'. Rosemary, in the next story, could have been made to feel stupid for feeling anxious and timid, but by taking her experience seriously and talking it through with her, Alison was able to confirm her decisions and her behaviour and strengthen her confidence to assert herself on behalf of her patients in future.

'He doesn't want to sit down. He wants to walk in the corridor'

I went to a lady who arrested before my very eyes and her husband was with her. Alison came and dealt with the arrest situation and I went to the husband and took him away. He was looking very shaken ... The lady died and there were a lot of complicating factors ... I told him that she had died. I can remember, he didn't want to sit down, he wanted to wander in the corridor. Another senior sister came past and said, 'Take him in the office and sit him down.' I said, 'He doesn't want to sit down, he wants to walk in the corridor.' ... It was the first time that as a qualified nurse I'd come face to face with having to deal with the family in a situation like that and Alison supported me so that I was still making the decisions, but she was always there. We decided to phone the son and we talked about what we should say over the phone.

... And after it was all dealt with she gave me feedback on how I'd done. She said I'd handled things really well and that I'd been right to tell him when he asked me ... and she reassured me that I'd been right to stand up to the senior sister ... It was really nice to have somebody there to support you through difficult issues. That incident gave me so much confidence for subsequent things. (Rosemary)

Role modelling and articulating practice

Nurses learn the skills of patient-centred practice through experience, by observing and listening to role models (Estabrooks and Morse, 1992; Savage, 1995), and by discussing clinical situations with others who can articulate the detail of their practice (Benner, 1985). Throughout our project the power of Alison's role modelling to influence the nurses' practice and behaviour was very evident, but in the area of developing and managing close relationships with patients and families, the presence of an effective role model for the nurses seemed to be particularly valuable. Sometimes the nurses learned consciously from observing Alison.

Last night, Sophie and I were sitting at the desk – it was fairly quiet – and Alison was with a patient, sitting on the bed, engaged in a deep conversation. We asked ourselves, 'Why are we sitting here at the desk, while Alison is out there listening and talking with the patient?' She had been off duty for a couple of days and yet she had very quickly established a deep, comfortable relationship with the patient. I asked myself, 'How does she do it? How does she develop the relationship so quickly and home in exactly on the problem?' I thought it might be her concentration. She sits on the bed, near the patient, and she seems to be totally absorbed in that conversation. She doesn't seem to get distracted at all, totally concentrating on the patient. She just seems to have the ability to go straight in to being close. (Rosemary)

The nurses also learned unconsciously, automatically copying effective patterns of behaviour. For example, when the bedside handover was first introduced, nurses could be seen standing in a huddle at the end of a patient's bed, looking at charts, talking to each other and more or less ignoring the patient. Although the nurses knew that the intention of the handover was to involve the patient, they had no previous experience to guide them. Their nearest model of this kind of bedside interaction was the medical ward round, and its influence on their early behaviour was obvious. On the other hand, Alison behaved quite differently, sitting down close to patients and actively involving them in the discussion, whenever this was possible. Gradually there was a change in the nurses' behaviour. The formal, brisk, information sharing between nurses at the end of the bed was replaced by warm, often lengthy, conversations with the patient, with the nurses sitting or kneeling at the patient's eye level, or perching comfortably on the bed.

Despite the strong influence of role modelling, it was a haphazard way of teaching on its own, with limited power to increase nurses' insights into the nature of expert practice. Alison therefore tried to reinforce what she demonstrated in her practice by explaining what she was doing. Reflective conversations helped her to put into words the formal and informal theory that informed her practice. By responding to Angie's probing questions, she learned to articulate her practice know-how and thus to make it more accessible for the nurses. For example, she described to Angie, and then later to the nurses, her way of 'talking through the patient' – a strategy she had developed for involving patients in the bedside handover.

You start a sentence talking to the nurse you're handing over to . . . and you say, 'He's not been feeling so well today.' and then you turn to the patient and complete the sentence saying, 'Have you?' So that's actually a grammatically incorrect sentence, but it works, if you switch halfway like that. (AB)

Thinking ahead, taking things further

Working in a patient-centred way challenges nurses to think ahead. Getting close to patients brings with it a responsibility to respond in some helpful way. It means making a commitment, not only to share some of the patient's experience, but also to use one's skill and expertise to make that experience more successful or more comfortable. Nurses have to think ahead about the possible consequences of their strategies, about who will continue them when they are not there, about how they will communicate their intentions and gather support from colleagues, and so on. However much the patient is involved, nurses need to take charge of their own contribution and to plan and manage it as effectively as possible.

Before team nursing began in Oriel Ward, the nurses had not been used to thinking about their patients' care, in any detail, beyond the end of their shift. Without predictable continuity of contact and without real authority to prescribe nursing care beyond the shift, there was little incentive for nurses to worry about tomorrow, or to make longer-term plans with patients.

I used to feel that I made a difference to the patient for the shift and for the days that I was on duty, but I didn't think forward. . . . I only used to think one or two hours ahead. (Sophie)

Alison had to help the nurses to develop the habits and skills of planning ahead. Simply probing and prompting, in a timely, sensitive and supportive manner, was usually all that was required, but it could be very effective and could make a significant difference to the way nurses managed their patients' care. As in Rosemary's story below, nurses could get a little carried away with their success at just getting close to patients and discovering what was troubling them. A gentle prompt might be needed to remind them that they had a responsibility to do something with the important insights they gained into their patients' problems.

'She asked me what I was going to do'

I went away to lunch feeling we'd really achieved something and that I'd been able to give her reassurance and had relaxed her. We talked about it a lot at lunch and Alison asked how the morning had gone and we told her the story and she asked me what I was going to do . . . She said that it was marvellous, that it was really good nursing, a therapeutic nursing relationship. I was feeling quite amazed that I could be having this relationship, but she actually did bring out to me that I needed to act on the information that I had acquired.

. . . I felt quite guilty that I hadn't really gone on to thinking about (a strategy), but I realized that was the next thing to do. (Rosemary)

Gradually, thinking ahead became incorporated into the ward's style of nursing and nurses would ask each other future-oriented questions.

Now I'm thinking ahead sometimes two weeks. Alison used to question me to make me think ahead and now I'm doing that with my team members. (Sophie)

Skilled companions

As the nurses' confidence in managing the care of primary patients increased, so their relationships with patients deepened. They began to attend more carefully to each patient's point of view and so became more able to address the things of greatest concern to them and to deal with these issues in a very personalized way. They became more aware of their patients' social circumstances and support networks, and so families became more important to them. Indeed, their patient-centred work could often more accurately have been described as family-centred care. Closeness led to greater understanding and we also found impressive evidence of difficult patients, who would previously have been classed as 'unpopular' (Stockwell, 1972), coming to be liked, or even loved, by their primary nurses.

Within the qualitatively different relationships that developed between nurses, patients and families as the project progressed, we were increasingly able to identify the characteristics of Campbell's (1984) skilled companionship.

Therapeutic relationships

Initially, the nurses found forming close relationships with some patients very difficult, particularly with those who were depressed or distressed, and this limited both the practical and emotional support they were able to offer. Often, nurses referred these patients to Alison. Discussing her own work with patients in reflective conversations helped Alison to analyse and articulate the elements of her own kind of 'skilled companionship'. The insights gained in this way helped her, in turn, to help the nurses develop their practice.

The following story – just a tiny vignette from everyday practice – is an early example of patient-centred practice.

Tim and the Orange

The patient had been in hospital feeling unwell and with rather vague symptoms – profuse sweating, fevers, vomiting, diarrhoea – and had had a whole battery of tests that hadn't produced an answer. Not surprisingly, he was in rather low spirits. He was so fed up that he wasn't feeling like getting up in the mornings. I remember, about eleven o'clock one morning, a nurse asking me if I would spend some time with him because she didn't know what to do with him, he didn't want to get out of bed. I went into his single room and found him lying dishevelled, unshaven, hot and sweaty, in a very crumpled bed. He looked lethargic and miserable. I sat on his bed with him for a few minutes, not saying very much at all, just with my hand on his hand. I could feel inside of me quite a strong desire to get him out of bed, get him in the bath and get his bed freshened up and I knew if I could do all that, he would feel better. I also knew that if I suggested such a line of activity he would resist strongly because it wasn't at all what he was feeling like. So I sat and waited for some initiative to come from him.

After a period of silence he said, 'Do you know what I've been dreaming about? I've been dreaming about a fresh orange. I want to suck on a fresh orange.' He asked if there was any way, if he gave me some money, I could go and buy him a fresh orange. I told him that it wouldn't cost him anything, that I could get him one from the kitchen. I did so and brought it back, peeled and nicely presented, cut up into segments. He said he thought he was allergic to oranges and that it would probably make him sick, but he wanted it more than anything else. I thought it wouldn't matter too much if it did make him a bit sick, if he enjoyed it at the time and if he felt that I was trying to respond to his needs, as he saw them.

So I sat on the bed with him while he sucked away on his orange. He told me that he hadn't eaten anything for four days and that he thought it had something to do with why he was feeling so weak and lethargic. There were very few things that he fancied to eat that didn't make him feel sick or have diarrhoea. While I listened to him and we talked together gently, he did come up with a few suggestions of things he might be able to tolerate . . . I wrote them down on a care plan, so that other nurses would know what to offer him.

Having done this work with him, having started where he was, wanting an orange, I had gently built up some trust and confidence with him and felt able tentatively to suggest that he might like to have a bath. He said he felt he couldn't cope, that he didn't have the energy. So I suggested taking him in a wheelchair and sitting him on a seat in the shower. He said he would try that. So I did exactly that, wheeled him down to the shower, sat him down, washed him all over, really freshened him up, helped him shave, brought him back to his room and put fresh sheets on his bed. He was very weak and he did find it very tiring, but he was just so much better afterwards. He really felt better, he was much more positive and really pleased he had made the effort. (AB)

Carefully analysing the detail of this story, and many others like it, helped us to articulate some of the key characteristics of the therapeutic relationship, which was always at the heart of nursing practice that was truly patient-centred.

Addressing the patient's experience

The simple story of 'Tim and the Orange' illustrates a very important feature of patient-centred nursing and something that became the focus of much discussion and exploration in the ward, namely, the value of addressing the patient's experience and of seeing it as the starting point for a nurse's work with a patient. This principle was referred to colloquially as 'starting where the patient is at.' The nurses discovered that this was often not where they had started before, and that they had commonly made assumptions about what patients were feeling, based perhaps on medical diagnoses or experiences with other patients. Consciously starting afresh with each patient, and listening attentively to their personal stories, was a new experience, which sometimes took the nurses off in unexpected directions. Although connected with the concept of 'knowing the patient as a person' that others have described (e.g. May, 1991; Appleton, 1993; Tanner *et al.*, 1993; MacLeod, 1994), this specific notion of 'starting where the patient is at' appears not to be documented in the nursing literature.

Drawing upon Campbell's (1984) idea of the nurse joining her patient on a journey, Alison recognized that to accompany her patient in a helpful way, on what was inevitably a very personal journey, she must understand the patient's starting point and the patient's perceptions of what might lie ahead. Benner and Wrubel's (1989) concept of illness was useful here too, since the journey that the nurse and patient share is usually a journey through a period of illness. These authors have defined illness as '*the human experience of loss or dysfunction*', emphasizing the subjective nature of illness. If nurses are somehow to influence this experience, they need to address their patients' interpretation of what is happening to them and to appreciate the meaning it holds for them. The concepts of 'the journey' and what came to be called the patient's 'current experience' (i.e. how a patient perceives the situation now and what he or she feels about it) were helpful for the nurses and became absorbed into their everyday language. It took time, however, for them to develop the skills and the confidence they needed to enter another person's personal world and to embark upon an unpredictable and possibly risky journey.

> *The idea is to find out about them and help them move on, something I hadn't really recognized before . . . There have been cases where I have been able to do that, but I think it is quite difficult. I need more experience.* (Ruth)

It is important to emphasize here that, when talking of discovering a patient's starting point, we refer not only to a nurse's initial assessment of a new patient, but also to the nurse's general approach to every encounter with a patient. If nurses want their nursing to be truly patient-centred, they need to be open and alert to patients' experiences and ready to follow their lead, 'to journey with them', whenever they can. In the following extract, Alison is trying to put into words, for nurses who have been watching her work, how it is that during the course of a simple bed-bath she managed to engage her patient and uncover, in a very short space of time, his feelings and concerns.

What I feel is important, is total focus on the patient, total attention. That's quite difficult sometimes with all the distractions and you're busy and thinking of lots of things . . . except it becomes a way of practising . . . to give that full attention . . . I think it is quite powerful for the patient, the patient senses this total attention. It's this business of starting where the patient is, but in order to discover that, you've got to be with them, you've really got to engage with the patient. Although other things are going on in my mind sometimes, there's still part of me that really just attends to the patient and that is very accepting and listening, quite still if you like. I try to put over a kind of stillness . . .

Although it sounds a bit of a luxury to do, it's a very cost-effective use of time, because you're using all your senses at the same time to absorb what's going on with this patient. Even when you're busy, you can make little portions of high quality time when you really focus in and you can get so much out of it, even in just five minutes. (AB)

The story of 'Tim and the Orange' provides a good example of Alison 'focussing', 'giving total attention' and using 'stillness'. Her behaviour conveyed respect and valuing of the frightened, vulnerable man and made him feel safe enough to disclose his dream. By entering her patient's personal world in this way, Alison was able to move on with him, not to the wash she had initially planned, but to address the more important issue of his difficulty with eating.

Early on in the project, Angie noticed the distinctive focussed attention that Alison gave to patients. She recorded specific behaviours, such as sitting on the bed, listening, eye contact, touching the patient's hand and allowing silences. But gradually, this kind of behaviour became commonplace amongst the other nurses too. It was most obvious, at first, during bedside handovers when nurses were seen huddled in little groups around their patients, intently involved in conversations in which the patients took a central part. Once primary nursing became established, seeing individual nurses involved in deep conversations with patients, at any time of day, became the norm. The interactions often occurred in the open ward in full view of other staff and patients, yet they had a sense of the nurse and patient being surrounded by an invisible wall. Their intimacy, their concentration and total absorption in each other separated them off, momentarily, into their own private world. As a business manager commented, *'The nurses are always in little knots with the patients'* – this was not something she had observed to the same degree in other wards.

The nurses themselves began to recognize that they were approaching their work with patients in a different way.

I discuss things a lot more with patients, their plans, worries . . . I open up with them and find that they open up with me and this leads to more trust. (Sophie)

The nurses' stories showed how they were using this new closeness and trust in responsible and highly creative ways. Their willingness to travel with their patients in unanticipated directions was transforming their nursing. Rosemary had talked to Angie about the way Alison related to patients and wondered if she would ever be able to work with the same expertise. Six months later she told a story about nursing a young woman who was severely disabled with multiple sclerosis. A short précis of it follows.

A Fear of Needles

Susan was nineteen, wheelchair-bound and able to do very little for herself. She had been admitted with a deep vein thrombosis and was receiving anticoagulant therapy.

Rosemary met her first at breakfast-time. She fed her and then stayed to chat with her, to find out how she managed at home and generally to establish an initial relationship. Susan asked how long the heparin pump would stay in and Rosemary explained the course her anticoagulation would follow. Suddenly, Susan felt sick and her breakfast came straight back up.

Rosemary: *She said she thought it was the coffee and I guess, on that first encounter, I didn't really pick up much more ...*

Later, when I sat down on her bed, she started to cry. She said that she was frightened about being in hospital, she really didn't like hospitals and was frightened by all the long words they used. I said that was part of the reason I was there, to be able to fill in those things that she didn't understand. She was obviously relieved by that and held my hand again. I felt that she did trust me and that we were already establishing a good relationship ... She talked about how difficult it was having the drip put in, how it hurt and how it was all a bit of a shock ... I began to gather that being in hospital was much more of a problem to her than her leg.

The next sort of real encounter was at lunchtime ... she'd eaten about half her dinner and then said she wasn't really hungry. Then she said that she was really nervous about the blood tests ... She went on to talk about her fears when she was in hospital when her illness first started. She said that everyone was having secret talks and they weren't talking to her. She'd had loads and loads of blood tests and nobody explained anything and she thought she had cancer and was going to die. So when they told her she had MS, she said it felt like a relief. But obviously she has terribly painful memories and she associates that time with blood tests. And her fear of needles was making her sick ...

I told her that we would draw up a plan together to face tomorrow morning when she had to have her blood taken again.

Rosemary went on to arrange that the same doctor, whom Susan trusted, would take the blood each day. She asked him to make sure that either she, or an associate nurse, was there to hold Susan's hand and support her. She also obtained some anaesthetic cream to apply to Susan's skin before the blood was taken (though this was not actually needed).

Rosemary: *The next morning she said to the doctor, 'I am going to have my blood taken, but Rosemary's going to be with me; she's going to be my ally.' ... She kept saying to me, 'You've got to tell him to be nice to me,' and I was saying OK, but she was actually quite relaxed. It was brilliant. It was over in a flash ... she was just so visibly different ...*

Later, Alison came into the room and I introduced her to Susan. She said, 'I hear Rosemary has been working with you this morning.' Susan looked at her and said, 'Yes, we get on really well. Rosemary has helped me to overcome my terrible fear of having blood taken'. That made me feel so emotional, tears were coming up in my eyes. It was brilliant. It was just an amazing experience.

Attending to the patient's point of view and focussing upon his or her concerns reflects a practice that Jourard (1971) described as reading the patient's 'phenomenal field'. He used this term to refer to,

> *'the sum total of a man's conscious experience at any given moment. The phenomenal field includes an individual's perceptions, beliefs, imaginings, and memories ...'* (p. 191)

Jourard argued that, while doctors and nurses have traditionally learned to take measurements of physiological indices, such as temperature and pulse rate, as a means of assessing a patient's overall condition, they have neglected to take readings of the patient's subjective experience, which is an equally significant indicator of well-being. He suggested that by adopting this one-sided approach, professionals *'are ham-stringing their diagnostic and therapeutic endeavours.'* He proposed that,

> *'this complex perceptual-cognitive system – the phenomenal field – is the variable which, when 'integrated' into medical and nursing curricula and practice, will bring about the outcomes which educators have sought, (namely) more personalized care of patients, more apt diagnoses, and more effective therapy.'* (p. 191)

The stories nurses shared about accessing 'the phenomenal field' of their patients show how much more rounded, how much more pertinent and how much more effective their practice became, when this neglected dimension of caring was integrated into their daily work.

Presence

Addressing patients' personal experiences of illness and hospitalization opened up the possibility of nurses offering the kind of companionship that Campbell (1984) described as *'being with and not just doing to'*. Once nurses developed the confidence to embark upon a 'journey' with a patient, we observed them learning to use their personal presence, as well as their practical skill, to convey support and caring. This 'active presence' (Paterson and Zderad, 1976) was communicated not only by the attitude and attentiveness of the nurses, but also, less consciously, by the way they used their bodies. Nurses' posture, their use of touch and the sensitivity of their movements powerfully influenced the quality of their physical presence at the bedside. (Similar observations have been reported by Wallace and Appleton, 1995, and Ersser, 1995.)

In the early days of the project, nurses consciously observed Alison's skilled use of her body as an instrument of caring and compared it to their own awkwardness.

> *I usually stand leaning against something. Perhaps standing on one leg and feeling very uncomfortable and that distracts your concentration, but Alison always sits on the bed looking very comfortable.* (Rosemary)

Alison's role modelling undoubtedly influenced the nurses, but, as their confidence in relating to patients grew, they became more relaxed in their patients' presence and their physical gestures began spontaneously to reflect and reinforce their genuine commitment to their patients. When Rosemary told her story about Susan, she mentioned a number of times, quite unself-consciously, how she had used her body to create intimacy and to reinforce the understanding and sharing she wanted to communicate. She talked about a ward round, which Susan had found frightening.

> *That was when I sat on the bed, facing her with my back to the rest of the team, and I held her hand. I wanted to be able to make eye contact with her and keep us together as a unit, if you like. I felt that if I sat the other way that I would be like the team, which was not what I wanted. And she held my hand really*

tightly . . . and she stroked it with her thumb. It was a very close gesture. We talked in quiet whispers while they were there. (Rosemary)

In contrast to their earlier 'rushing about', nurses learned to convey a sense of 'having time' for patients, even when they were actually very busy. Again, it was the combination of appropriate body language and careful attention that made the nurses seem very much present with their patients or, as Ersser (1991) put it, 'available' to the patient.

Warm, spontaneous gestures of affection exchanged between nurses and patients seemed to be tangible evidence that, when nursing becomes the truly patient-centred, skilled companionship that Campbell described, it is indeed a form of love.

Sharon gave her a big hug . . . she just needed it. (Janice)

The hand-holding, the soothing caresses, the gentle massages, the hugs and cuddles, and the simply 'being there' are all part of '*a closeness which is neither sexual union nor deep personal friendship. It is a bodily presence which accompanies the other for a while*' (Campbell, 1984, p. 49). It is a physical and emotional love with limits, a '*moderated love*'.

Working with

The nurses ability to 'be with' their patients seemed greatly to enhance their ability to 'work with' them. The notion of partnership has been frequently advocated in the nursing literature and was something the nurses aspired to, although, as the stories 'Removing the Charts' (Chapter 5) and 'I'm not mad, am I?' (earlier in this chapter) illustrate, they initially found it difficult to realize in their practice.

Being able to involve their patients in the bedside handover was an early example of nurses 'working with' their patients. In addition to developing the verbal and non-verbal skills required to make patients feel able to contribute to the handover discussions, the nurses learned to present themselves as fallible, open to being questioned and corrected and as not always having the best solution to a problem. A relative commented upon this openness.

This was another thing I found helpful. I would read the charts and the care notes and I was encouraged to do so . . . I would look at the temperature chart and the water and what he should be taking and all these aspects of it. In fact, on one occasion, it wasn't frightfully important, but something had been forgotten or left off. I mentioned that this was incorrect and there was no apparent animosity . . . The whole point was sharing care, finding out what was really happening, what our hopes and fears were, what the treatment was. All this was very open and helpful. (Relative)

A genuine invitation to a patient or family to work in partnership with a nurse has to be accompanied by an acknowledgement that the patient and family will have their own opinions and suggestions, which may challenge the nurse's view. The nurse has to be confident enough to expose her expertise to scrutiny, to admit her limitations and to welcome the contributions of patients and relatives as valid and potentially valuable. Partnership means exchanging the traditional 'nurse knows best' and 'tell the patient what you are going to do' approaches for something nearer to 'this is what I suggest; what do you think?'

Genuinely working with a patient begins with negotiation of the relationship (Morse, 1991). While the nurses in Oriel Ward learned to offer closeness, and often found that it opened the way to a therapeutic way of working, they were equally able to respect a person's desire for privacy when it was indicated. Some patients and relatives made it clear that they preferred a more formal, less open relationship with staff and the nurses were able to respond to this without withdrawing their care. The silent acknowledgement of the person's wish for privacy seemed in itself to convey a kind of closeness and caring, a sharing that was achieved without words.

> *Whenever the wife came in, I made an effort to go up and speak to her and ask her how she was. She wasn't a particularly open kind of person, but I think she appreciated my going up to her . . . I felt quite pleased that I'd been able to do that for her. Quite a simple thing really.* (Moira)

A striking feature of the nurses' behaviour, when they became involved in real partnerships with their patients, was their integrity. They went to great lengths to keep promises and they were not prepared to collude with doctors or relatives in keeping secrets if the patient was indicating a wish for the truth. They recognized that being trusted by a patient was a responsible and privileged position to be in and they were not prepared to abuse that trust.

> *Her son didn't want her to know the diagnosis, which he had guessed, but Violet began to ask more questions about what was happening and what the tablets were for. So one evening, I told him what was happening and that if she asked me about it I wouldn't be able to lie to her . . . He said, 'Couldn't you tell her you don't know yet,' and I said, 'No, it's not really fair.'* (Sharon)

This integrity was linked to a sense of commitment. Once nurses discovered what was really important to their patients, and that there was something they could do to make a real difference, they felt challenged to do their best for their patients, to stay with them and see things through with them. This feeling of obligation to see 'the journey' through to a conclusion led the nurses into some difficult territory and it drew from them some sensitive and highly creative nursing. Sharon's story of how she helped David to negotiate a reconciliation with his daughter before he died is a fine example of a therapeutic partnership.

The Reconciliation

I think we were very close . . . I was special to him. I was certainly very protective of him . . . I think people saw David as an 'unpopular patient'. He was very fussy and demanding and he drove people mad. What I was trying to get them to see was that if you just appreciated the person he was, and the way he liked things done, then there was no problem.

He was so slow. It took him ages to answer a question and he hated being rushed . . . It took him a long time to take in what the doctors were saying (about the three options for treating his cancer) without getting muddled up. So he wrote them down and I wrote them down on his care plan, so that other people could follow through and see what his options were . . . We weren't rushing him to make a decision . . . He told me about his fears of dying . . . and about how he had divorced and left his wife and how he had always felt that Marjorie (his daughter) resented him for it. With his permission, I talked to Marjorie about how he was feeling, how worried he was. After that, they had a chat and there was a reconciliation . . . I think that it helped David before he died. (Sharon)

Being able to work with a patient as a primary nurse can be an immensely rewarding experience, especially when there is both a shared struggle and a shared achievement. Kate's story of nursing an elderly carpenter gives a flavour of the intensity of feeling and the joy that can be experienced on both sides when nurse and patient see a journey through together.

All he could say was 'Yes'

He had a stroke and all he could say when he arrived on the ward was 'Yes' ... From the things I'd read about him and from what his daughter had said, he was very independent, lived alone, did a lot of carpentry, made a lot of beautiful things ... I really worked hard on him to try and get him to speak. I referred him to the speech therapist and all the usual things and I spent an awful lot of time just going out and sitting with him and structuring questions so that he would not be able to say 'yes' or 'no'; so that he'd have to say something a bit different. Very, very gradually, over the weeks that he was here, he started to get his speech back. Then he was telling me this story which just cracked me up. This was a real crunch point and I thought, yes, I really like him and get on with him. It was all very disjointed the way he said it, but I got the gist of it, that his neighbour cooked cakes for him and, if he wasn't in, she'd leave them in a bag hanging on the garden gate. I asked what they were like, if the cakes were nice. After quite a while he said, 'Bloody awful!' I remember we were both laughing our heads off – he was nearly crying. We got on really, really well. He always remembered me and when he went home, he squeezed me to death and he's come up to the ward loads of times to see us. (Kate)

Receiving and learning from patients

While the professional partnership between nurse and patient is established specifically for the benefit of the patient, it is nonetheless a partnership and that implies a degree of giving and receiving on both sides. Traditionally, the dedicated nurse has been portrayed as all-giving and professionally obliged to shun personal gifts from patients. In patient-centred nursing the code of practice relating to substantial material gifts does not change, but the concept of 'gift-giving' widens and the notion of reciprocity becomes important (Muetzel, 1988).

Campbell (1984) points out that the act of professional caring brings its own rewards. Professional carers are able to use their gifts of intelligence and personality in ways that are fulfilling and in ways that may satisfy their own need to be needed. As the nurses in Oriel Ward began to form relationships with patients in which they were free to use their own personalities and their own creative talents to express themselves professionally, they began to experience their work as vastly more rewarding than it had been. But they also became more open to sharing part of themselves with their patients. They were able to respond to any interest patients showed in their lives outside of work and to concerns about them being busy or tired. They learned, in return for the closeness and care they offered to patients and relatives, to accept little gestures of intimacy and kindness. This reciprocity enhanced the sense of partnership, because it acknowledged that it was not only the patient who had needs and not only the nurse who could care – each had something to give the other.

Alison became conscious of the importance of reciprocity in patient-centred nursing when reflecting upon an intensely demanding, but enormously rewarding relationship that she had with an extremely sick primary patient and his wife whom she nursed for a month. The following story illustrates the kind of small gesture that the sensitive nurse can recognize as a meaningful and generous gift from her patient.

Paul's Recipe

Yesterday I had planned to take the dressing off Paul's head because it had become matted and uncomfortable and I wanted to soak it off, but I didn't have time. I had to dash off to a seminar. I came back specifically to do that and to write up some care plans. After half an hour, I realized that I was exhausted. It was seven o'clock and Rebecca, the wife, came in to see me. I said I had promised Paul that I would do his head and that I must do it before I went home. She said, 'Don't worry.' She went to see him and came back and said, 'He couldn't bear you to do it. You're too tired. He said no, he didn't want you to do it'. I gave up writing and I went to his room and we sat and chatted for half an hour. He asked me about the seminar and I told him and then he said, 'What are you having for supper?' I told him I had some green beans in the fridge and he said, 'Well, I'll tell you what to do with them,' and he gave me this little recipe and I went home and cooked it. Today he wanted to know how it was. (AB)

Being able to give to a nurse in this way, in this case releasing Alison from her promise, taking an interest in her seminar and offering the recipe, enhances the patient's separateness within the relationship. He is taking the initiative, making his own independent contribution. Whilst the therapeutic nurse–patient relationship is characteristically close, the closeness is between two separate human beings who have their own identity and destiny and who will, in due course, go their separate ways. By accepting gifts of care and concern from their patients, nurses are respecting this separateness and guarding against the unhealthy imbalance of dominance and dependence that can occur when caring travels in one direction only.

Professionals are usually regarded as people with expert knowledge that is used for the benefit of others. Drawing upon their expert knowledge, nurses spend time explaining health problems and treatments to patients and teaching them skills that they need to care for themselves. That the patient may be a teacher too is less often acknowledged. Nurses certainly recognize that they learn from working with patients, but it is usually what they observe or what they have to do for patients that counts as a valuable learning experience. As the nurses in Oriel Ward learned to listen to their patients more carefully, they became more interested in their views and some of them discovered that here was a rich new source of wisdom. For Alison, the experience of caring for Paul and his wife extended her understanding of the 'skilled companion' relationship and increased her sensitivity to the needs and perspectives of the close relative. Joanna Hedges' experience of nursing a retired clergyman during his recovery from a serious illness was a similarly rich source of learning for her. She had long discussions with him about the spiritual aspects of caring and healing, which influenced her profoundly. In an article developed from her reflective diary entries, Joanna described how the encounter with this patient crystallized a number of ideas she was becoming generally aware of in her work.

'The conversation with this patient helped to:
- *clarify, for me, the concept of nursing as a journey;*
- *demonstrate the power of nursing through the nurse–patient relationship – how we enable someone to move forward by drawing alongside and journeying with them;*
- *highlight the two-way nature of this relationship – through this man's insight I was able to grow as a person and a nurse.'* (Hedges, 1993)

Patients bring with them rich and varied life experiences and they have enormously varying perspectives on what it means to be a patient. Recognizing and valuing patients themselves, and not just their illnesses and treatments, as potential sources of learning helps again to bring some balance to the nurse–patient relationship. Sharing their own knowledge and insights with nurses is another way in which patients can assert themselves and reciprocate for the care they receive. This is another kind of gift that nurses can accept gratefully and, in so doing, enhance the sense of partnership.

Unpopular patients

Nurses commonly ask the question, What happens when the primary nurse and patient do not get on? Nurses are only human and inevitably find some of their patients more likeable and easier to relate to than others. The prospect, for nurses who have not experienced primary nursing, of being obliged to work closely, day after day, with some of the less likeable patients, is not attractive. Similarly, it is recognized that there is sometimes a patient who takes a dislike to a particular nurse and it is suggested that the patient might justifiably feel aggrieved if this nurse were to become his primary nurse.

Stockwell's (1972) study, carried out in traditionally organized wards, showed nurses judging and classifying patients according to whether they enjoyed caring for them or not. Nurses were observed to discriminate against the less popular patients in various ways, but particularly by simply ignoring them. There was no evidence in the study of nurses seeking to explore or understand what lay behind behaviours they found irritating, such as grumbling, complaining, attention seeking or malingering. Indeed, it is clear that talking to patients, other than when performing a specific task or seeking some particular information, was not considered to be part of the work of these nurses. The study pre-dates the introduction to British nurse training of concepts like 'psychological care' and 'individualized nursing'. However, it shows vividly the origins of the fear of being 'stuck' with an unpopular patient as a primary nurse.

In theory, if a nurse and patient cannot work together effectively, then the relationship should be terminated and another primary nurse should take over. In practice, however, after watching many different nurses work with many extremely 'difficult' patients and families, often over quite long periods of time, we never found it necessary to change the primary nurse because of a 'personality clash'. It appears that the primary relationship can transform the way nurses and patients feel about each other and, consequently, the way they are able to work together. It seems there are a number of factors that bring about this transformation, as shown in Figure 7.1.

While this sequence represents the essence of what we observed time and again, it is a somewhat simplified version of what actually happens in many

- When a 'difficult' patient is admitted to a team, nurses may feel some reluctance about accepting the role of primary nurse. But there is also a sense in which they are challenged – 'Are my nursing skills up to this?', 'Can I show that I can get somewhere with this difficult patient?' There is potentially the reward of publicly visible success, if a primary nurse can make real progress with a 'difficult' patient.

- Once a nurse accepts the challenge and makes a commitment to do her best for the patient, she gives the patient time and tries to get to know him. Once she hears the patient's story, perhaps uncovering fear or loneliness, or some tragedy, she begins to understand the behaviour that was previously regarded as irritating or objectionable. She starts to feel sympathetic towards the patient and genuinely wants to help.

- The patient responds to someone who is prepared to give him time. He may feel relieved at having shared his fears or concerns and appreciate being accepted for what he is. Complaining or attention-seeking behaviour may be modified, or even cease. He may be able to accept help and advice from a nurse whom he feels understands him. He may begin to respect the nurse and be prepared to work with her, so he is no longer seen as 'unco-operative' or 'difficult'.

Figure 7.1 *The challenge of the unpopular patient*

cases. Ruth's experience of working with Leonard provides a fairly straightforward and typical example of the transforming power of the primary relationship.

'I just basically got to know him'

I met Leonard the day after he'd been admitted. He was still confused then. He was in quite an acute condition. The next day, his diabetes was more under control and he'd had things disconnected, so he could walk to the bathroom. He was being incontinent of faeces and I felt he was just being lazy . . . there wasn't any need for him to be incontinent. So our relationship wasn't that good to start with. I suppose I was a bit annoyed with him because he didn't seem to want to take care of himself . . . I used to find it quite frustrating looking after him. Then it was found that he had renal failure which was making him tired and he was quite poorly, so I recognized that he had a reason for not being motivated. Once I'd recognized that, I started to treat him differently, in that I'd say to him, 'Do you want to do it yourself?' and if he didn't want to then I'd help him . . . once I showed that I was willing to do things for him, we started to get on very well and he started to be quite willing to do things for himself as well . . . I just basically got to know him and to understand him. (Ruth)

Having started from a rather prejudiced, judgemental position, by staying with this patient and being involved with what was happening to him, Ruth came to understand what lay behind his behaviour and began to work 'with' rather than 'against' him. Not all the 'difficult' patients responded to an understanding nurse as readily as Leonard did to Ruth. However, because the primary nurses were committed to their patients and 'stuck' with them, there was an incentive to face up to confronting them and to negotiating some ground rules for working together. Sensitive but frank discussion could increase respect and understanding on both sides and greatly improve working relationships.

'I just went straight over'

Eve was critically ill for a long time. She was just one of these ladies who didn't say please or thank you and you just could not do anything right . . . She quickly picked up that I was her primary nurse. In some ways that created problems, because she couldn't accept that I had to look after other people at the same time. She said to Sophie, 'She's my nurse and she's only meant to be looking after me'. I confronted her about this quite early on and she said, 'You should sit with me, you are my nurse' and we talked about this. She knew I couldn't be with her all the time, but then she started telling her relatives that we were neglecting her . . . I just went straight over – I've changed in that sort of way. I said, 'You've been telling your relatives that I've been neglecting you' and she said, 'Yes, I have. You don't sit with me enough.' But she was completely unrealistic. I said, 'You would like me to sit with you all the time, wouldn't you?' and she said, 'Yes I would,' and we talked about it . . .

There were some days when she was just so horrible to me, she used to say some really horrible things and you couldn't do anything right for her. Some days I found my patience a bit more thin than others. She'd turn to me and say, 'Well, I only tell you off because you're my best friend,' and I used to think, mmm. But I liked her and I think, again, because of being her primary nurse I found out things about her, sort of deep things from the past, that explained why she behaved as she did . . . She didn't ever take up discussing things at length, but I think we got on better for each knowing the other knew. (Rosemary)

Some primary nurses found that skilful and sensitive use of humour was a way to reach through to patients who were difficult to relate to, or to break into what lay beneath a bout of grumbling and complaining.

'Just arrange an appointment with my secretary'

He was quite an intellectual chap really. He was a scientist when he was younger, so he was very intelligent, but he had the sort of sense of humour that was very dry . . . The rest of the team didn't get on with him at all . . . they found him awkward and a difficult patient, whereas I just couldn't see it myself . . . He used to make quite a few little jokes and I caught on to his sense of humour . . . I tuned in to his sense of humour. The doctors came round one morning to see his leg and he was on the bedpan and he pointed to me and said to them, 'If you could just arrange an appointment with my secretary and come back later.' They just looked at him and I was trying not to laugh, and they went out and he winked at me, it was so funny . . . But you had to tune in to him or you would think he was a bit strange. (Kate)

While primary nurses were often able to develop comfortable relationships with 'unpopular' patients, and even came to like them, as Kate's comments above show, this did not always influence the views of other nurses in the ward. Learning to like patients could make it easier for nurses to cope with the intensity of working with them for some time, but it was not essential for being effective professionally. Increasingly, as they took up the challenge of working closely with 'difficult' patients, nurses learned the skill of separating out their feelings about a patient from their understanding of the patient's situation and their duty as professionals to help.

So long as associate nurses were able to support the work of the primary nurse with an 'unpopular' patient, and deal kindly and tolerantly with the patient when the primary nurse was away, it seemed enough that there was one nurse who was special to the patient. Indeed, the idea of too many people becoming too close and involved did not seem helpful. However, there were occasions when the whole team had to tackle the problems of an 'unpopular' patient together, as in the case of Gerald and his wife Agnes who presented an enormous challenge.

Gerald and Agnes

Gerald is the schizophrenic chap who lost his leg. The psychiatrist described his wife as having a paranoid personality. She has delusions about there being a drug ring in the ward and she wanted all the doctors' blood taken to check they weren't on heroin and she has a whole lot of other obsessions . . . it's incredibly complex. She phones up MPs, the Community Health Council, the Health Authority, psychiatrists, consultants in the middle of the night . . . She phones up the ward endlessly and keeps people talking for ages. She is abusive to the nurses, constantly threatening litigation, and then the next minute she's totally charming – incredibly difficult to deal with. It's very difficult to have a logical conversation or come to any agreement with either of them. They are both highly manipulative and the energy it demands from me and the nurses is enormous.

Gerald first came to us four months ago with very complicated problems. He was in another ward for a while and when he came back, interestingly, the Elm Team took him on again. I thought that was very impressive, because they knew what they were in for and it's a horrendous experience. There was no question about it, it was never suggested that he should move from the team. Nurses in the other teams say things like, 'I don't know how they cope. I can't stand that woman. I'd hate to have to look after them,' but you don't hear the Elm Team saying things like that. (AB)

Stockwell (1972) found that patients with a psychiatric disorder were among those most likely to be classed as unpopular in general hospital wards. The reaction of the other teams to Gerald and Agnes shows that this can still be the case, but the patient-centred approach of the Elm Team ensured that their patient was not the victim of unwitting prejudice or intolerance and that he and his wife received the best nursing possible. The patience, tolerance and support that both primary and associate nurses provided for them, over a long period of time, was outstanding. While at times stressed or exasperated by the tremendous demands of this couple, the team nurses remained open to them, trying to accept them, listen to them and relate to them and, within the boundaries they tried to negotiate with them, to give them all the care they could.

The 'difficult' patients put patient-centred practice and the primary nursing system in the ward to the test and the results were very positive. Patients who would have been labelled 'unpopular' and discriminated against within the traditional system came to be liked, and even loved, by their primary nurses and those whom it was difficult to like became a 'challenge'. We saw nobody being ignored.

Family care

Once primary nursing was formalized in the ward, there was a marked difference in the nurses' behaviour in relation to patients' families. For example, Sophie was observed sitting on a chair at a patient's bedside and seated with her, in an intimate little circle, was the patient and three or four relatives. They were deeply engrossed in a serious conversation. Angie was struck by the scene because it was not something she had seen before. In an interview, Sophie confirmed that, as a primary nurse, her relationship with patients' families was changing.

I'm getting to know the family much earlier on . . . I'm really looking forward to involving the family a lot more. (Sophie)

Other nurses made similar comments and, increasingly, were seen with family groups at the bedside or, if it were more appropriate, inviting them into the office. They also began to take a more active role in organizing and co-ordinating communication between family members and other health professionals involved in their patients' care. This new work could be complex and, initially, primary nurses sometimes had to learn from their mistakes.

Nurses began to involve family members in bedside handovers when this was appropriate, encouraging them to offer suggestions, to ask questions and to contribute their observations on the patient's progress. There was also a qualitative difference in the telephone conversations nurses held with relatives. The traditional, formal, rather guarded condition report became rare and reserved for strangers. More commonly, there were warm, friendly exchanges between people who knew each other, with the nurses passing on information or messages that were likely to be reassuring to the recipient. The nurses noticed this change themselves and felt good about their more personal contact with families. As Janice commented, '*It's nice when they phone and ask for you. It gives you an ego boost!*'

A condition of the greater openness with families was always that it was acceptable to the patient concerned. Respect for a patient's right to confidentiality was not new to the nurses and being conscientious about checking out to whom, and to what level of detail, disclosures might be made, before getting involved with a family, was something they managed without difficulty.

By getting to know patients and their families well, nurses became more alert to the impact family tensions and communication problems could have on both the patients' well-being and the relatives' ability to be supportive. Primary nurses sometimes found themselves acting as a 'bridge' between patient and family. When they felt they had the skill and confidence to accept this role, they were able to open up communication and greatly reduce anxiety on both sides. Sharon's story above, about facilitating the reconciliation between Peter and his daughter, is a good example of this kind of work.

By this skilful 'bridging', or 'mediating', nurses were sometimes able to help patients and families to reach mutually acceptable decisions about treatment or aftercare. Primary nurses made a great effort to be sure that both parties were properly informed, that they had time to discuss their concerns independently and, then, that they could talk through the consequences of a decision together. Rachel described work of this kind with a patient who had to decide whether to go through with a risky heart operation. The family were naturally anxious and wanted to be able to understand and support his decision.

I got really involved in this whole debate about whether he should or shouldn't have it done and I was talking to him and his family about it. I was helping to relay information to enable him to make the decision and I got quite involved in telling his brother and son what the pros and cons were. The doctors had spoken to them about it, but I sat down with the son in the office, and we had a cup of tea and we really talked about why he should have it, or why he shouldn't have it. Obviously, he felt his father should make the decision, but I felt I was able to expand a bit on the facts the doctor had given him. It just gave him a bit more of an opportunity to talk about it. (Rachel)

When Alison reflected upon the way she had helped a daughter to discuss a delicate subject with her father, she tried to articulate what it was that made her effective as a mediator.

'I asked the questions she couldn't ask'

I facilitated Mr Stone and his daughter talking about the possibility of selling his house. It was a delicate situation and she was reluctant to bring the subject up. She talked it through with me first and then I sat with the two of them. I asked the questions she felt she couldn't ask. She told me at the end that she was very grateful to me for bringing the discussion into the open. (AB)

There are times, of course, when patients are too ill to participate in making decisions about their care. It then falls to the health care team and family members to act on the patient's behalf and to make decisions in accordance with what they believe to be the patient's best interest and what they believe the patient would wish. Decisions are often not clear-cut and the responsibility of trying to make the best choice for a loved one can be an enormous burden for relatives already distressed by the patient's illness. The nurses' skilled balancing of choice, advice and support was greatly appreciated by relatives.

We also really valued the honesty and patience with which you discussed the available possibilities of medical intervention with us. You showed great skill in approaching these issues in a way that neither interfered with our choices nor left us feeling alone with the decisions we took. We felt happy with the eventual choice that allowed Harry a peaceful and dignified death. (Letter from a relative)

Learning to see patients as belonging to a family, rather than to the hospital, and acknowledging the needs of relatives for care and support led, gradually, to nurses involving many relatives in the practical care of patients. Whether and how involvement was achieved was always a sensitive and individualized decision. Some patients did not want their family involved in the intimate, personal aspects of their care, whereas others found it a great comfort. Similarly, while some relatives, long over-burdened with home nursing, were desperate for a rest, many were pleased to have something useful to do when they visited. Others needed to learn and practise practical skills they would have to continue when the patient was discharged to their care at home.

A policy of open visiting gave a clear message to relatives that they were welcome in the ward at any time. An open ward can be potentially threatening for nurses, because their work is much more exposed to the critical scrutiny of relatives. As Alison discovered, nurses who genuinely wish to welcome and support relatives have to learn not to be defensive about their work and to be willing to explain their decisions.

> **'One might have pushed her out'**
>
> *Mrs Jones had just had an amputation and I had found her early in the morning in quite severe pain. I gave her a strong analgesic injection, made her comfortable and left her to rest. That was carefully planned, that she would probably sleep for a while and that, when her pain was controlled, I would be able to move her without difficulty. I got on with my other patients and later, when I was behind the curtains of the patient in the opposite bed, I heard Mrs Jones' daughter arrive. She said, 'Oh, you haven't had a wash yet and you've still got that gown on,' slightly critical remarks. As soon as I had finished with my patient, I was planning to go to bath Mrs Jones. So there was this feeling of the daughter criticizing everything I had planned so carefully. I heard the daughter get out the wash things and fill a bowl of water to wash her mother. I went out and greeted the daughter and joined in and gently took over, but got her to help me and gave her a clear role in it. I didn't want her to feel put out. You can see how, in the traditional role, one might easily have pushed her out of the way.*
>
> *I went in and explained, in a very gentle voice – not critical of her – what I had done that morning and why . . . I had to do that for my own sake, but also because it was important that the daughter didn't feel that I had just left her mother all morning. It turned into a very nice activity – getting her mother washed. The daughter did everything with me apart from changing the sheet.* (AB)

As nurses responded to Alison's constant prodding, 'Have you met the family yet?', and as they became more confident and more flexible in their own practice, there were more examples of nurses sharing practical care with relatives, supporting and guiding them when necessary, but also encouraging and accepting their suggestions. Sometimes nursing activities were planned around when a relative could be present to participate and, increasingly, messages were left on the care plans about what relatives liked to do for patients and how they needed to be supported. For some relatives, the opportunity to be involved in the practical care of a patient was tremendously important and, for the patient, it could mean that an important relationship remained very much intact and accessible at a time when it was particularly needed.

Acceptance, by the staff, of an active role for a visitor was something that stood out for Rebecca, the wife of Alison's patient Paul, who was critically ill for over a month. After Paul had been discharged, she commented,

The other brilliant thing was the way they allowed me to be there, going in and out like part of the staff. I loved it, a redeeming feature of the whole thing. The fact that they allowed it and had confidence to allow me to participate was wonderful for me . . . Their extraordinary acceptance and how they used to let me bath him and so on . . . They would support what I was doing. (Rebecca)

Her husband drew a comparison between this experience and what they had known in hospital previously, *'This is very new isn't it? Remember the old system!'* The couple went on to explain why the welcome, acceptance and support of the family, as well as the patient, were so important to them both.

I felt my life at home stopped virtually . . . I had transferred all my energies to the hospital. (Rebecca)

Alison and the team realized that, which was important. They realized that we actually lived there. Our home was now the hospital and they made it our home and made us feel at home . . . (Paul)

When Rebecca wrote to Alison after Paul's discharge, she described how the opportunity for her to be practically involved in her husband's nursing transformed her experience.

Rationally I could obviously not have welcomed Paul's illness but, despite the strains and stresses, it actually became quite a positive situation in which I had a tangible role – not just as a dutiful visitor . . . I hope it will be an encouragement to you to know that what could have been a very traumatic experience had a very fulfilling side to it. (Rebecca)

A group of relatives with whom nurses worked much more intensely, and in highly sensitive and individualized ways, was the families of patients who were dying. It is not unusual for families of dying patients to be given special attention, and they have often had privileges in hospital wards, such as the waiving of visiting restrictions or the provision of overnight accommodation. But it was not the bending of organizational rules that struck us, instead it was the warm human bond that developed between nurses and families. This bond seemed to grow out of a willingness on the part of the nurses to share, as best they could, in another's sadness, a willingness to be open to a family's pain and loss and to be there for them. Continuity of involvement and the personal responsibility of primary nursing seemed to reinforce a certain pride in the care of dying patients. Nurses were deeply concerned to make a patient's death as comfortable, peaceful and dignified as possible and this became as much, if not more, for the sake of the family as for the patient.

The value of the nurses' love and support at such a critical time was reflected in letters from relatives. The example that follows came from a man whose young wife died after being in the ward less than twenty-four hours. The letter was addressed to the Elm Team, but mentioned the individual nurses who specially cared for the couple by name.

Such a long journey we travel and so many meetings along the way. We touched for just a few moments, but you will remain in my heart forever . . . I shall never forget the love and tenderness that you gave one sad traveller . . . (Letter)

Even over a short space of time, the companionship that skilled nurses can offer during some of life's most profound crises can indeed, as Campbell (1984) suggested, be experienced as a form of love.

The personal cost of patient-centred nursing

We have shown that when nurses learned to practise in a genuinely patient-centred way, their work became more challenging, enjoyable and satisfying. However, we also found that patient-centred practice does have a down side for nurses. We have already alluded to the stresses and strains associated with making the complex journey from one style of nursing to another, but these are essentially the traumas of major change and they are of limited duration. What we wish to address here are the tensions that remained once a stable, patient-centred style of practice became established in the ward.

Interrupted relationships

A recurrent problem for the nurses was the sudden interruption of their relationships with patients. It was quite common for patients to be transferred on from Oriel Ward to a specialist or rehabilitation ward, or to be returned to the care of community services. When this occurred in a planned way, there was no major problem. However, the need for the general medical service to respond to a large number of emergency referrals created an intense demand for beds and the pressure to discharge or transfer patients was considerable. At times, planned discharges or transfers had to be brought forward unexpectedly, to make space for the next emergencies. This is the reality of many similar hospital services throughout the country. Such arrangements are clearly not ideal for patients and their families, but they also create difficulties for nurses trying to practise in a patient-centred way.

Having invested time and energy in getting to know patients and their families and in making careful plans to work together, nurses felt deeply dissatisfied when their work was unexpectedly interrupted in this way. They experienced frustration at not being able to complete interesting or challenging work that they had begun, guilt at not being able to fulfil promises they had made to their patients and also, sometimes, a sense of loss because a warm relationship had been broken off without an opportunity to close it comfortably. They felt angry at 'the system' for causing the problem and were sometimes left with a disheartening sense of 'why do I bother?'

> There have been a couple of occasions recently when the nurses have been disappointed because their patients have been moved suddenly. They are left feeling that they have put a lot of effort in for nothing. They haven't been able to follow things through, or they feel a failure, or deprived of job satisfaction. I have been trying to reframe the way they see these situations, because it is the reality of hospital life that people get moved on . . .
>
> There was a lady who was in with a very serious skin condition and other problems, but she was only with us for twenty-four hours. Rosemary looked after her and she contacted the dermatology nurses and she spent an hour or so sorting everything out so we could look after her properly. She set it all up brilliantly and then, an hour later, the dermatologist appeared and said the lady could be transferred right away. We knew that might happen in a few days, but not quite so quickly . . . Rosemary was quite angry. (AB)

Situations like these can be frustrating for nurses however they practise, but we found that with commitment to a patient-centred approach, the frustrations seemed to be more acutely felt.

The endless demand

In the traditional system, nursing was fairly predictable and its boundaries were clear. Essentially, the nurse had certain tasks to perform and when they were done, the nurse's work was complete. With patient-centred practice, obvious boundaries are far fewer. With every patient there are different possibilities and nurses have to make judgements about where they can most effectively focus their limited time and energy. The openness of this approach allows for sensitive and creative work, but we found that it can also put nurses at risk of feeling overwhelmed.

You can see what could be achieved, and you can see what you want to achieve, and it's distressing when you can never quite match up. There are always things that you can't do that you want to do. (Mike)

As nurses became more aware of their patients' individual concerns, there was more that they wanted to do for them, but their ideal of perfect nursing for every patient was not always achievable. The realities of time, staffing levels and workload pressures meant that each day they had to set priorities and negotiate what was possible with their patients. Within these limits, they often managed to achieve outstanding work, but sometimes, when they were closely involved with patients, they lost sight of all they had done and could think only of what more they might have done. As Mike continued,

You think, 'Have I done this, have I done that?'. It might not do them any harm (i.e. not doing absolutely everything possible), but you want to make sure you do the best at all times and you just can't. (Mike)

This sense of not being able to do enough for primary patients was common, especially when the ward went through a particularly busy phase, and Alison had to encourage nurses to recognize and value what they did achieve and help them to accept the realities of working conditions in the health service. More specifically, nurses sometimes found themselves feeling overwhelmed by the demands of a particular patient. Having made a commitment to a primary patient, they might find they had taken on more than they had bargained for. There were no examples of nurses giving up their patients in these circumstances, though there were occasions when it was seriously considered. It seemed that the commitment to the patient and the challenge of seeing things through to a conclusion always finally outweighed the difficulties.

Letting go

Relationships between hospital nurses and their patients and families formally come to an end when the patient is discharged, transferred or dies. Usually this is what both parties anticipate and relationships are terminated with comfortable 'goodbyes', expressions of appreciation from the patient and family, and good wishes from the nurse. Sometimes lasting friendships do develop from the professional relationship, but this is rare.

As a patient-centred style of practice emerged, there was no major change in the expectation that the nurse–patient relationship must inevitably be of limited duration, but some of the nurses did become aware of subtle pressures that sometimes made separation more difficult than they had experienced before. It seemed that it was more difficult for both parties to withdraw from the intensity of the primary relationship, than from the more formal, conventional nurse–patient relationship.

It's the idea of knowing where your involvement stops . . . Should I be doing more? I don't know. Should I be following them up when they go home? Letting people know that you are still thinking of them. (Janet)

Often, when a relationship had been particularly close, nurses and patients or families made one follow-up contact and that was usually sufficient to acknowledge the significance of the relationship and to bring it to a close. Also, on several occasions, nurses were given, and accepted, an invitation to a funeral.

These brief extensions of an important hospital relationship seemed to be comfortable and satisfying for both parties, but there were a few occasions when, perhaps from loneliness, extreme gratitude or a continuing need for support, patients seemed to want to cling on to their nurse indefinitely. Nurses were not always sure about the extent to which they should or wanted to sustain a relationship.

Jim is the only person I see. He phones me two or three times a week and when I go to see him he makes me tea and I have to stay two hours. I only see him because he has been in here three times. But it is difficult, I'm not sure what to do . . . no, I don't think it happened so often before primary nursing. (Sophie)

As time went on, and through discussion of such problems among themselves, nurses became more aware of the need to manage the closure of their relationships and, like Sharon, they became more confident and skilled at setting boundaries.

I visited Edith because she was on her own. But as I give so much of myself at work . . . and I don't give enough time to my own family, I made the decision that I would not set up long-term relationships with patients. I feel it's not really my job to give continued support. (Sharon)

An open ward climate and a supportive ward sister can do much to limit the kinds of stresses we have identified, but because they seem to be intrinsic to patient-centred nursing, they will not disappear. Thus they need to be honestly acknowledged as the personal cost of becoming a patient-centred nurse.

Making a difference

This final section of the chapter highlights the ways in which a patient-centred style of practice had a significant impact upon both the experience and the well-being of patients.

Patients find it healing

The central feature of the patient-centred nursing that we observed was the warm, human bond that developed between nurses and patients. The relationship was not in every case tremendously close. Some patients neither welcomed nor needed the opportunity to share their innermost feelings. But, regardless of closeness or distance, there was a profound respect for the individual – a sincere acknowledgement and acceptance of the patient as a person. In addition, nurses brought themselves as people into their relationships with patients, conveying the message, 'I am here for you as a person, open to your feelings and concerns.' They showed that they were willing to negotiate a relationship which was not predetermined or stereotyped, but which was comfortable and helpful to the individual. Thus nurse and patient worked person to person, rather than in a technical or traditionally distant professional relationship. For many patients experiencing the fear, isolation and helplessness so commonly associated with hospitalization, the genuine human care and concern of the patient-centred nurse was deeply comforting.

The nurse gets to know your problems and you get to know her. I think it helps. You feel as though you know the person you are talking to and it helps you relax. When you need something you know she'll help you if she can. In the old system, you had perhaps seven or eight nurses and you didn't really know any of them. (Patient)

If it hadn't been for Rosemary, I think I wouldn't have calmed down so much. She's more like a friend I've known for years. She sits on the bed and has a little chat. (Patient)

They make me feel I have something to live for. It's the way they talk to me, the time they take to explain, being nice to me. (Patient)

You feel more secure, more relaxed. It's like a family. You get to know the nurses. (Patient)

Many patients talked about their experience of nursing making them feel more secure and relaxed than they had expected. A style of nursing that relieves patients of undue worry seems worthwhile in itself, but it is also likely to have a beneficial physiological effect. For seriously ill patients, a style of nursing that promotes peace of mind, rest and relaxation is also making a valuable contribution to physical recovery. Alison's patient Paul had no doubt that the quality of his nursing had been the critical factor in his recovery from a life-threatening illness. The recurring, committed presence of his nurse, even during his terrifying period of confusion, made him feel safe, gave him something to hold on to and gave him the will to struggle for survival.

He's a very clever surgeon and if it hadn't been for him I wouldn't be here now. But I wouldn't have got to surgery if it hadn't been for the others – so, in a sense, Alison and her team saved my life. You see me here today and you can put that down, ten out of ten, to Alison and her team. (Paul)

When nurses shifted the focus of their work towards therapeutic relationships with patients, there was an associated beneficial change in the atmosphere of the ward. Although there was no reduction in the nurses' workload (if anything, it increased because their care of patients became more comprehensive), the pervasive sense of rush and hurry to get through the work gradually diminished. Patients and relatives were sensitive to the focussed attention they received from nurses and commented upon its value.

She never gave the impression that she was too busy or too hurried to talk. She would sit on the bed and chat and just give us her time and herself . . . She was clearly an important role model for the other nurses. I could see the same characteristics coming through in the other nurses. (Patient talking about AB)

Another patient commented that nurses often said they were busy, but she had never felt it – '*There is always a sense of calm and of people having time for you.*' A patient, who was a senior figure in the church, talked at length with his primary nurse about the spiritual dimension of caring and told her that he felt there was '*a community of healing*' in the ward. It seems that the nurses were successful in fostering the kind of healing relationships that have been reported by Benner (1984) and by Lewis and Brykczynski (1994).

Attention to detail

When patients and relatives described what was different or special about their nursing, they frequently mentioned attention to some fine detail of their care as illustrating what really made a difference to them. In 'The Lavender Story', it was the thoughtful use of pleasant smelling oil that left the patient's daughter with a precious memory. In the 'Fear of Needles', the primary nurse's astute and sensitive observations transformed the course of her patient's stay in hospital. There were other examples too, such as the relative who was deeply touched by a nurse playing tapes of favourite classical music for her dying mother, and the wife who was delighted because her aphasic husband's passion for Foxes Glacier Mints was recorded in his care plan. Attention to details of this kind may sound trivial, but to patients and their families it was not only a source of material comfort, but also an important acknowledgement that their personal wishes and concerns were being taken seriously.

Alison's patient Paul pointed out, with a colourful analogy, just how much worry and energy could be saved when one was cared for by a familiar nurse who paid attention to detail.

> *It's like when you are with your mate on the golf course. You say to your mate, 'Oh, I had a bad shot on the fifth and the bunker on the seventh is a real so and so.' If the guy knows the course, he knows what you mean, you don't have to explain. It's like that when Alison comes on. I don't have to explain; she knows the course. I've been so ill, nearly dying. I don't want to make new relationships all the time, it's just too exhausting. It saves so much energy because she knows what I need.* (Paul)

A similar story concerns one of Janice's primary patients, a woman with a terminal illness, who asked to come back to Oriel Ward if she were readmitted. Janice heard that her patient was coming into hospital again, but this time under the care of a surgeon, so she was due to go to another ward. Janice went to considerable lengths to negotiate having her back in Oriel Ward, so that she could continue her nursing where she had left off. The woman was immensely grateful and said that, knowing she had so little time left to live, she did not want to waste it explaining everything to new nurses. As her time was so precious, she wanted to be with nurses whom she knew and who understood all the details of her care. (See Janice's story 'I pulled out all the stops' in Chapter 8.)

It has always been the case with good nursing that attention to detail could make a significant difference to the course of a patient's illness. Observant nurses have been known in the past to alert doctors to subtle changes in a patient's condition in time to avert catastrophe. With primary nursing, however, nurses in Oriel Ward found that it was much easier to recognize small changes in a patient's appearance and to detect tiny nuances of change in behaviour, because they knew their patients so well. As Alison put it, they were 'attuned to their symptoms'. Sometimes nurses could intuitively sense a change before there was anything tangible to notice – 'I just had a feeling something was wrong'. Knowing their patients well gave them confidence to report these hunches and often doctors were able to investigate and treat new problems early as a consequence.

Thus it seemed that concern for fine detail in nursing practice was enhanced by continuity of care and a close nurse–patient relationship. As a visiting sister observed,

The nurses' relationships with their patients are much more intimate than I've seen before. It means both nurses and patients can ask intimate questions and discuss things in detail.

The relationship between closeness and attention to detail was particularly evident in the bedside handover discussions observed during the latter months of the project. These interactions were of a consistently high quality, with the nurses listening carefully to their patients and considering minute details of care. The responsiveness of patients and families to these discussions and their active participation, adding information, offering suggestions and making choices, clearly indicated that these were valuable exchanges and that they made an important difference to their experience of being in hospital[1].

---

[1] Titchen (1996; 1998a) developed a conceptual framework for the kind of 'skilled companionship' described in this chapter. She also shows how 'critical companionship' (mentioned in the footnote at the end of Chapter 6) can be used by a clinical leader or expert nurse to help others to become skilled companions, that is, patient-centred nurses (Titchen, 1998a; 1998b). These frameworks offer useful adjuncts to the leadership and practice journeys.

Chapter 8

The doctor–nurse journey

'But where do the majority of nurses stand in their relationships with doctors? Will it be possible for all nurses . . . to bridge the gulf which at present exists? Do they wish to participate in such a change, and make the necessary investment of time, energy, and probably personal suffering which are demanded in any such exercise in self-determination? Or are they content to take the line of least resistance, and play the game as it now stands, replete with dishonesty and exploitation?'

Dingwall and McIntosh (1978, p. 108)

Introduction

In the traditional hospital ward, the relationships between doctors, nurses and patients mirrored those in the patriarchal Victorian family (Carpenter, 1977; Gamarnikow, 1978). Male doctors played the dominant father role, assuming authority to make any significant decisions. Female nurses, like dutiful wives, were expected to support and assist doctors while, in the background, also ensuring that the domestic sphere and the personal care of patients were properly managed. Patients meanwhile, like obedient children, were 'seen but not heard' and were expected to accept gratefully the wisdom of their betters.

The superior education provided for doctors and the fact that many of them came from upper class backgrounds reinforced the gender inequality in the traditional hospital world. The historical literature documents the degree to which the subservience of nurses to doctors became institutionalized during the first half of this century (Dingwall and McIntosh, 1978; Gamarnikow, 1978; Keddy *et al.*, 1986), while research in recent years has shown that an unequal and problematic balance of power still remains in modern hospital wards (Mackay, 1993; Meyer, 1993; Sweet and Norman, 1995).

Stein (1978) described a highly ritualized pattern of indirect communication which he had observed in doctor–nurse interactions and which he labelled 'the doctor–nurse game'. The game allowed nurses to use their initiative and to make significant recommendations about patients' treatments, but they were only to do so in a subtle, veiled manner, so that doctors could reproduce the recommendations as their own instructions. Playing the game meant that nurses' valuable knowledge and experience were used for the benefit of patients, without there being any threat to the apparent omniscience and omnipotence of doctors. Stein described how the socialization and training of both nurses and doctors taught them the rules of the game and their respective roles within it. The doctor–nurse game worked because both parties were willing to play and because both parties accepted the hierarchical relationship upon which it was based.

In a later paper, in which the doctor–nurse game was reconsidered, Stein *et al.* (1990) observed that many contemporary nurses were no longer prepared to participate in the traditional game. New diploma and degree programmes were teaching them that they had their own professional contribution to make to the work of a health care team, in which the doctor was just another member. This view was being reinforced by declining public esteem for doctors, arising from increasing recognition of their fallibility. Furthermore, the growing numbers of women in medicine and men in nursing were making roles based upon gender stereotypes less tenable. Stein *et al.* (1990) described nurses, in their struggle to assert themselves, as behaving like '*stubborn rebels*'. Meanwhile, doctors were puzzled and confused by changes in their relationships with nurses, and they sometimes felt angry and betrayed.

> '*Physicians for the most part did not perceive nurses to be subservient in the first place and are thus confused by their efforts to gain equality. It is, of course, not unusual for those in power to be oblivious to the fact that those under them may feel oppressed.*' (Stein *et al.*, 1990, p. 548)

At the beginning of our study, we found doctor–nurse relationships much as Stein *et al.* (1990) had described them. The nurses in Oriel Ward resented being cast as handmaidens and believed that they should work in a collaborative partnership with doctors. However, it seemed that it was their own lack of confidence and skill within the relationship, as much as the doctors' reluctance to change, that denied them the status they wanted.

Two broad themes emerged from our data. The first concerns the doctor–nurse relationship generally and includes the perceptions and feelings each party had about the other, as well as the practical problems of working together in busy hospital wards. It shows misunderstanding, and sometimes overt hostility, being gradually replaced by at least a reasonable degree of mutual trust, respect and co-operation. The second theme focusses upon the nurses' role in the medical ward round. It traces the nurses' struggle to find ways of making an active and useful contribution to ward rounds, without having to resort to the humiliating pretences of the traditional doctor–nurse game.

EARNING RESPECT

Mutual respect is a prerequisite for any healthy, successful human relationship. In the traditional hospital ward, where the hierarchical nature of the doctor–nurse relationship was accepted by both parties, each could win respect from the other by playing the role assigned to them in a skilful manner. The problem with the modern hospital ward seems to be that nurses have unilaterally decided that they no longer wish to be respected for hiding their expertise behind a facade of obedience and deference. We found evidence of the tensions caused by nurses adopting this modern stance and by trying to change their own style of work, while doctors continued to work much as they had always done.

Reluctant handmaidens

A fundamental problem for the nurses was that they felt doctors did not understand or value their contribution to the care of patients. They considered that doctors were only concerned with the management of patients' medical problems and that they did not recognize the often complex issues of care that nurses were dealing with, or that they tended to trivialize them. When Janice was interviewed about the experience of nursing her first primary patient, she told a story about coming up against this narrow medical view.

'Let them have a bit of dignity'

I felt quite upset when I couldn't get anywhere with the doctors, when he was very ill. I found that the doctors wouldn't take the nursing point of view about his care or consider the psychological care . . . He had end-stage cardiac failure and was very, very short of breath. They kept giving him frusemide and he couldn't wee into a bottle, so he kept having to get out onto the commode. He was just getting more and more tired and more and more upset about this. I suggested why couldn't we catheterize him? I said I appreciated the risks and I had weighed up the risks against the benefits . . . I got a lecture from the registrar, who was very much against the catheterization, and he made me feel really very small, as though I was suggesting it for my own good and not for the patient's good . . . Later the house officer came back and said, 'Can you get me the equipment for doing a catheterization.'

. . . I'm not sure whether, as a nurse, you tend to think more of their quality of life. Why don't we just let them have a bit of dignity, instead of this incredible suffering? The doctors are always striving for cure . . . If I actually talk about it with the doctors I'm just shut out, as if it's not part of my decision. (Janice)

This problem of differing perspectives was often compounded by nurses feeling intimidated by doctors, or lacking the skill and confidence to present their own case convincingly to them. For example, in an early interview, Carol talked about how she felt much more confident in her work since the introduction of team nursing, because she knew her patients so much better, but this was not yet enough to overcome the awe of doctors that had been instilled into her during a traditional training.

I've not asserted myself with people like that (registrars and consultants). No. I would be too frightened! (Carol)

Later in the project, when nurses were more willing and able to discuss their patients' management with doctors, there was still frustration because so much of their work was not seen or acknowledged by doctors.

I think that's what the medical staff think our main role is – to carry out the medical procedures to support their work. I don't know why I bothered the other day, with Daphne. All they wanted to know was what her pulse and weight were . . . Her main problem had been her heart failure, which had probably contributed to her confusion. But now her confusion is the main problem, but they didn't even speak to her. This great revelation that I had had that she had made a massive improvement, that I was so excited about, they weren't interested in that. They just wanted to know what her weight was . . . They see . . . my input as weighing her once a day and taking her pulse. I'm sure that's all they think I'm here for, and maybe they think she needs a bit of a hand with a wash. Yet I think that is only a tiny little bit of what I'm here for. (Rachel)

Evidence of some doctors continuing to think of nurses as subordinates and of not respecting their independent contribution to patient care came not only from nurses.

There are medical staff who aren't prepared to treat nursing staff in a reasonable manner. They just expect them to fetch and carry the whole time and don't treat them as human beings. (Registrar)

But overall, the picture that emerged from doctors was a mixed one. Some doctors spoke appreciatively of the benefits of being able, in the team system, to work continuously with nurses who knew their patients well.

We have got a lady at the moment who is quite unwell . . . and there's one nurse who has been looking after her for the whole two weeks, stayed with her on and off during her shifts. I've come to rely on her to give me an update, if I'm too busy or whatever, to tell me how she is. It's been great, because when we thought her infection was getting better, it was the nurse who first prompted us that there was something else going on. And it was the nurse who very quickly was aware of other problems, in both her life and in her general state. She had other problems developing that we weren't aware of . . . I was really grateful to that one particular nurse who really knew the patient and her family. It made a tremendous difference. (Consultant)

A newly qualified house officer, for whom '*this was really my first real experience of nursing care,*' also spoke positively about working with the nurses and acknowledged the value of their close relationships with patients.

Most of the things we are doing for patients have to go through the nurses . . . So I do tend to work very closely with the nurses, because they explain things to patients that sometimes patients don't understand from doctors. Maybe we explain things in too complicated a way, or in too jargon a form. Also I find that patients often tell nurses things that they don't tell us, because they are frightened to, or whatever reason. The nurses come and tell you, which I find very helpful. (House Officer)

This kind of appreciation of nurses who knew their patients well was not, however, matched with any recognition that developing close, therapeutic relationships with patients demanded any special skills or presented any great challenges. Indeed, some views to the contrary were specifically expressed.

It sounds like common sense, rather than a novel thing. I think what it boils down to is a great deal of emotional support and understanding for the patient . . . but I don't know that one has to sort of dress it up. (Consultant)

I think a lot of looking after people is just common sense really. If you are polite to them and sensitive to them, whether it's this primary nursing system or the old system, then people will appreciate the fact that you're caring. (Senior Registrar)

Given the doctors' failure to see the complexity and the therapeutic potential of skilled interpersonal work, it is perhaps not surprising that they found it difficult to grasp what nurses were trying to achieve through the changes occurring in the wards and in the profession generally. They believed that improvements in their education, for example, would give nurses more of a technical/medical bias, which would inevitably take them away from the bedside. They seemed to find it hard to imagine that a graduate nurse would want to remain involved with the intimate personal care of patients.

If nurses are going to become well qualified, they are going to know all these things and they are going to want to do more in the way of interesting nursing, not just clearing up diarrhoea and vomit and so on. Who is going to be doing the basic nursing? Because it is all the time that they spend with the patient that builds up their role and if all of a sudden they are not going to want to get their hands dirty in that kind of a way, they will actually no longer have the kind of rapport and relationship with their patients that they have now. (Consultant)

This doctor, of course, was making an important point. It is precisely the close, daily, physical contact with patients that gives nurses such privileged and valuable access to their patients' experiences of illness. But, to be fair to the doctor, as we showed in Chapter 7, it took the nurses themselves some time to recognize that 'basic nursing' was no longer 'basic' when they approached it with intelligence and with a genuine openness to their patients' suffering. Then, the 'dirty work' of nursing was transformed into a powerful medium for the kind of therapeutic work that could challenge and stimulate the brightest of educated n5rses. As the nurses were only just beginning to discover for themselves the potential and the satisfactions of approaching their everyday work in this way, it is not surprising that, in the early days of the project, they had not managed to communicate these things to doctors.

Another doctor saw the changes in nursing as primarily a bid to enhance the status of nurses. Like the physicians that Stein *et al.* (1990) referred to, this doctor did not seem to see anything wrong with the old ways of working and he was uncomfortable with modern nurses trying (perhaps a bit like Stein's '*stubborn rebels*') to make a more active contribution in the ward team.

As I understand it, there is a very strong desire to make more of a profession out of nursing ... I think all health care professionals should be good at their job and so on. But I sense that there has been a positive decision to go for much greater independence in decision-making about patient care and I'm not sure that isn't actually missing the point, which is really a matter of team-work. I have come across instances in this hospital of sheer antagonism from nursing staff, which has been unhelpful. That is not an atmosphere in which I care to work. You know we have always worked in the spirit of collaboration and mutual respect for the roles we are playing, which are quite different. I would be very pleased and I think it is a very good thing if nursing is developing, but I am suspicious that there is a current which is actually to take it away, to sort of split it off from medicine. That is actually quite undesirable and unfortunate. (Consultant)

During the early days of the development work, junior doctors also found it difficult to understand what nurses were trying to achieve and they too reported that relationships with nurses were sometimes strained.

I don't really know how to tell you this, but I have noticed sometimes that some of the nurses come across, the ones that are most into primary nursing, as being fairly hostile . . . actually, the junior doctors here admit that, since the primary nursing, they are not happy at all, to put it mildly. (Registrar)

In general, doctors were uncertain about the motives behind the changes taking place in nursing, they were unclear about how these changes would affect patient care and they were uncomfortable with some of the nurses' (probably rather unskilful) early attempts to participate openly in decisions about the management of patients. A crucially important relationship in the doctors' professional world was changing, in ways they did not really understand, and this was unsettling. As one consultant put it,

You would go to lunch in the consultants' dining room and they would say, 'Well, I don't know what on earth things are coming to'.

The philosophical basis for the changes in nursing and the shifting ground under the doctor–nurse relationship were rather vague, intangible entities that may have been difficult for doctors to grapple with. There was, however, one aspect of the new style of nursing that had a direct, practical impact on their daily lives, and it was not a positive one. The one significant change that every doctor was eager to report was the fact that, in the new system, communication with nursing staff had become more complicated and time-consuming. The specific problem was that when doctors came into a ward, they found it difficult to find the right nurse to talk to about a particular patient. Furthermore, if they wished to discuss several patients, they might have to seek out two or three different nurses. The following comment was typical.

In many ways (team nursing) has advantages, but it does mean that if you are visiting three or four patients on the ward, you have to communicate with different people potentially. And if they are busy, or tied up with another patient, you end up leaving a series of messages, which sometimes aren't passed on, or they're passed on inaccurately, or you get accused of not communicating with the appropriate person, even though the appropriate person wasn't available to speak to you at the time. (Registrar)

Traditionally, communication with ward nurses had been quite simple. Doctors could go straight to the nurse in charge of the ward, who was usually fairly accessible because she did not involve herself very much with 'hands on' nursing. They could receive at least a superficial condition report on any patient from the nurse in charge and they could leave instructions with that nurse. Inevitably, detailed information about patients was often missing, and the views of patients and the nurses working most closely with them were also excluded. But, from the doctors' point of view, the system had seemed efficient.

With the team system, doctors usually acknowledged that, when they did find 'the right nurse', the quality of information they received about a patient was much higher than it had been before. But unfortunately, because they were busy or because they anticipated it might be difficult, doctors often did not try to find the right nurse. Indeed, doctors were commonly observed coming in and out of the ward without making contact with any of the nurses at all. The consequences of this lack of communication could be frustrating or embarrassing for the nurses and, occasionally, potentially dangerous for patients. For example, nurses spoke of patients announcing that doctors had said they could go home, when the nurses had had no opportunity to discuss whether this was appropriate or confirm that suitable arrangements could be made. Similarly, nurses reported treatment charts being changed, or new drugs prescribed, without their being informed.

Some junior doctors coming to the study wards for their first house jobs adapted to team nursing more easily than their senior colleagues. They were more inclined to make use of the communication system that the nurses were trying to put in place, which made life easier for them. One house officer also observed that the old system had its faults too.

> We have a patient on another ward that doesn't do team nursing, and I find that I tell one nurse what's happened with a patient, and that's fine, she understands it, but it doesn't seem to be communicated. You can be down there an hour later and another nurse will ask you the same question, or someone will bleep you and say, 'What is going on with Mr so and so?' That can get very infuriating. Also I think that patients get more care with team nursing, so that's definitely its strength. (House Officer)

However, this kind of assessment was the exception rather than the rule. For most doctors, already feeling hugely overworked, the additional time that it took to find 'the right nurses' was the overriding consideration. And this practical communication problem tended to obscure the more fundamental issues, to do with power and professional respect, that concerned the nurses.

It emerged that it was not only doctors who had difficulty finding the right nurse. Nurses also often had difficulty finding the right doctor. This was not a consequence of changes in the organization of nursing, but a long-standing problem that had gradually worsened over the years as pressures on the acute general medical service had increased. Because each ward accommodated patients admitted by any of the medical teams, nurses in each ward had to relate to as many as six different pairs of house officers, who all covered for each other during 'off-peak' hours. Complicated medical rotas were available in each ward, but actually making contact with the right doctor for a particular patient could be a time-consuming and frustrating process for nurses. However, this problem was neither voiced as loudly nor given as much attention as the doctors' problem with finding the right nurse.

Strategies for promoting collaborative work

Progress with many other aspects of the development work indirectly helped nurses in their efforts to establish more collaborative relationships with doctors. In particular, being able to work closely and continuously with a small group of patients meant that nurses knew their patients well and this, in turn, made them more confident in discussions with other health professionals. Nurses could speak with the authority that came from being intimately involved in a situation, in a way that had rarely been possible when they had cared for different patients each day. In addition, when primary nursing was introduced, individual nurses had a much greater incentive to find out what the medical plan was and to make sure that their nursing perspective and their patients' views were properly communicated, for they felt keenly their personal responsibility to do their best for their own patients. Thus, all the strategies we used to help nurses become secure and confident in their new roles served also as ways of gradually transforming the doctor–nurse relationship. Nurses needed to build their self-esteem and to become clearer and more articulate about their own special contribution to patient care, before they could expect doctors to respect them as colleagues.

Role modelling and coaching

Alison consciously worked to use her own relationships with medical staff as an example for the nurses. Aware of nurses' resentment when they felt ignored or patronized by doctors, she tried to show how it was possible to be assertive, and even challenging, without appearing hostile. She believed that by initiating interactions with doctors in a positive way, rather than timidly or defensively, nurses could pave the way for constructive, open dialogue. Thus, for example, she would always acknowledge and courteously greet doctors when they arrived in the ward. It was much easier then, having established a respectful atmosphere, to say, 'While you are here, I would like to talk to you about Mrs Jones. I am concerned that ... ', and there was a good chance then of being taken seriously.

Alison also tried to remind the nurses that, in spit% of their sometimes superior manner, doctors were only human, and that they got tired and harassed like everyone else. She encouraged them to show doctors the sensitivity and kindness they would show each other, and again, in this way, *to take the initiative* to create an atmosphere in which a respectful, adult kind of relationship could develop. Alison would point out, for example, that while it was unreasonable and unnecessary for busy nurses always to be expected to lay up trolleys or to make tea for doctors, in the old subservient way, it was quite another thing occasionally *to offer* to lay up a trolley or to make a cup of tea for a doctor who was stressed.

Though they may seem rather obvious, these strategies served well in everyday ward life as 'rules of thumb' to counter the tendency of modern nurses, in their determination no longer to be handmaidens, to be haughty and unhelpful. Alison's aim was to avoid the hostile 'stand-off' in working relationships that the doctors had reported. Instead, she hoped to create conditions in which the nurses' newly emerging confidence and competence might receive at least an open response from their medical colleagues.

The doctor–nurse relationship was important to both parties and it was in the interests of neither for the relationship to remain strained. It seemed that none of the doctors really expected, or even wanted, the nurse's traditional handmaiden role to survive, however much their own habits and attitudes still reflected the influence of the old order. So it seemed reasonable to hope, that if offered a constructive alternative, they might gradually adapt to it. There was some support for this view in the literature (Hughes, 1988; Porter, 1991) and comments like the following suggested that there was room for optimism.

There is a recognition that we need to work together. There is this 'thou shalt not be the doctor's handmaiden' sort of thing, which I entirely approve of. I know exactly how doctors behaved with nurses before. I think now there has been a recognition . . . if you have worked in an intensive care or a renal unit, as I have, you begin to realize what nurses can do, and there is a lot of respect . . . There has been a young boy on the ward, very worrisome. I tell you what's been good. I know that Jane is his nurse and I know that she knows him. She has actually been to seek me out more than once, which I greatly approve of. She has said, 'Look, actually he's not very bright and there are problems'. I can't remember the details, but she has taken the initiative to put her point of view forward, which actually is rare in nursing. (Consultant)

Here, a consultant, whom some might have described as 'old school', was acknowledging the demise of the handmaiden era without regret, and his story showed him quite able to accept an overt, active contribution to a patient's care offered by a nurse in a competent, constructive manner. Our strategies were designed to make this kind of interaction less of a rare occurrence.

In specific situations, Alison tried to help nurses to work collaboratively with doctors. She would observe their interactions with doctors and give them feedback and advice (as in 'Ruth's Story' in Chapter 5, in which she observed Ruth, in a conversation with a doctor, appearing disinterested and ill-informed about her primary patient). Alison would also sometimes join nurses when they had to talk with doctors in potentially difficult circumstances. In this way, she was available to support them if necessary, but again could observe how they handled the situation and could give them feedback afterwards.

Janice and the Psychiatrist

Janice and Alison are talking in the office with a psychiatrist about Janice's primary patient. He has been a difficult case, because his wife is very sensitive and difficult to convince that the nurses and doctors can help her husband. She believes her husband needs porridge, kippers and fresh air to help him recover. She has been resisting a change in his drugs and Janice explains this to the doctor. He says, 'Tell the wife that you cannot help her with this, because you do not prescribe drugs. Refer her to the doctor.' Janice gives a considered reply, 'I think this is one that we nurses need to handle, because the problem will be the same one for the doctors, and she is already very demanding of their time.' The doctor conceded, 'Yes, you're right.'

The psychiatrist had been asked to assess the patient, but the wife was very against it. The psychiatrist wanted to come in when the wife was not there and then face her with a fait accompli. Janice expressed her concern at the deceit and felt that it would be better to be honest and talk the wife round – 'She usually comes round in the end.' Again, the doctor conceded. Afterwards, I praised Janice on her handling of the situation and for giving the nursing perspective so confidently and convincingly. Alison joined in the praise. (AT)

Nurses were encouraged to consider the management of doctor–nurse interactions a skill that they needed to develop as part of their professional repertoire and to see Alison as their mentor or coach in this aspect of their work, as in others. Alison made herself available in order to talk through difficult doctor–nurse issues, she helped nurses to plan strategies for presenting their case or for confronting a doctor and she supported them with her presence when necessary.

'Face-saving'

Moira was primary nurse to a gentleman who belonged to an outlying firm. The consultant had come on the ward round with lots of people. His body posture was dreadful, one knee up on the bed and his back twisted half away from the patient. The patient had asked what was wrong with him and the doctor said, 'Well, its cancer'. And the patient said, 'Well, is there a sort of technical name for it?' 'Yes, cancer,' in a big loud voice that all the other patients in the bay could hear, 'You've got about three to five years.' And basically that was the end of the ward round and they all trooped off. Moira said the patient burst into floods of tears and the other patients in the room were saying things like, 'Gosh, if I had cancer, I wouldn't want to be looked after by him.'

Moira wondered whether she should have confronted the consultant at the time, but wasn't sure she had the confidence to do it. She was wondering if it should be taken further, so she came to me for advice. We talked about what our options were, you know, like letting it go for the sake of peace ... but we decided to see him together.

We talked about how to conduct the meeting and I talked about the importance of face-saving. You're going to confront a senior person, with two of us there. You can't expect to humiliate him and leave him sobbing and apologetic. He has to maintain his status and we have to go on working together. So, although we shouldn't shy away from being honest and telling him what we've seen, I said we may have to accept his excuses. That didn't matter, it would allow him to save face, but he would go away with our message.

We invited him to come to the ward and we saw him together. Moira handled it very well. She looked him straight in the eye and just stated the facts, in a nice straightforward voice. She sat comfortably, with open body language. He didn't sit down at first. I had to invite him twice to sit down, and he kept looking at his watch. He did make excuses about there wasn't time and he blamed the system. He also said he had known the patient for a long time and had found that a rather curt approach was the only way to get this man to face up to what was happening. I said if that was the approach he was taking, had he thought of telling the nurse why he was taking that line, so maybe she could have supported him if she'd felt it was a sensible way of dealing with the man? ... So then I turned it into a discussion of how he wasn't using the ward rounds as an opportunity to discuss his point of view and explain to the team, more of a general discussion about communication. So it ended quite comfortably.

A few weeks later, Moira reported that the consultant had been back on the ward a few times and had been very polite and courteous to her. (AB)

Informing doctors about changes in nursing

Explaining to doctors how and why nurses were trying to change the way that wards were run was not as easy as one might imagine. Alison used the obvious strategies for conveying information with only limited success.

A short, concise paper entitled 'The Aims and Aspirations of Primary Nursing' was circulated to all twenty-two physicians who were likely, at some time, to have patients in the medical wards. A few consultants politely acknowledged the paper and said it was helpful, but it was not so well received by others.

The problem with medical staff is that they get sent bits of paper and they tend not to read them . . . I cannot bear bits of paper. I take one look at them and, if I can, I throw them in the bucket. There is so much every day. I have up to two and a half hours dictating every single day, coping with letters that have come in, so unless it is vital . . . (Consultant)

However, in response to the paper, Alison and two of the other medical sisters were invited to join the end of a meeting of the 'on-take physicians'. This gave the sisters an opportunity to explain briefly the purpose of some of the organizational changes taking place in the wards and to hear and respond to the doctors' views. Some of the physicians seemed quietly sympathetic and supportive, but, as can often be the case with formal meetings, the discussion was dominated by a few individuals who wanted to air their strong negative opinions. Thus there was little in the way of really constructive dialogue. It was difficult to assess how useful the meeting was, but the invitation from the physicians had itself seemed a significant gesture. It implied that the doctors were taking the nurses seriously and that there was a desire for better mutual understanding and collaboration. In spite of the uncertain practical outcome, the meeting did have important symbolic value.

Less formal meetings with junior doctors were also initiated. For example, a welcome meeting for each new group of house officers was valuable for establishing the tone of future working relationships. The message was conveyed that a collaborative approach to interdisciplinary work was expected and that constructive, open dialogue was welcome. Doctors commented positively on these meetings and some took up the invitation to bring problems and ideas to the nurses. In time, support from the registrars reinforced the value of these introductory meetings.

In addition, Alison arranged to see key consultants on a one to one basis, to talk about nursing developments in the wards. These meetings were well received and seemed to elicit general goodwill and support. However, Alison sensed that the benefit of the meetings was more that the consultants felt pleased she had sought them out and listened to their views, rather than that they had really understood what she and the nurses were trying to achieve. Interview data supported this perception.

My understanding of it is probably pretty primitive . . . I did know (about the changes on the wards), but really that was because . . . well I'm not sure whether Alison came and talked to me about it before, I think she did. The personal approach is more effective than sending round papers. (Consultant)

Papers and meetings of various kinds undoubtedly had their place as strategies for conveying information to doctors about our development work. However, we found that the most effective way of helping them to understand what the new style of nursing had to offer, both directly to patients and to the work of the health care team in the wards, was to expose them to it.

It is difficult to describe, in an abstract way, the complex, subtle skills of nursing practice (see, for example, Benner, 1984; Lawler, 1991). It seems that because it is so context-dependent, so rooted in experience, nursing practice cannot be adequately depicted in language that does not include rich description of actual situations. Much of the richness of nursing is lost when it is explained, rather than experienced, and it seemed that the doctors needed the full impact of the experience of patient-centred practice in the wards before they could recognize it as something of value and worthy of respect.

Practical communication strategies

The mechanics of communication in the new system needed careful attention. Figure 8.1 summarizes the aids to communication that already existed at the beginning of the project, their strengths and weaknesses and ways in which they were improved. It also indicates new strategies that were developed.

Initial strategies

The white board at the nurses' station – Identified each patient's name, bed number, consultant, primary nurse and the nurse caring for them on the present shift. Colour-coding indicated which nursing team was responsible for each patient. The white board was potentially very useful for doctors, other staff and visitors, but the information was not always accurate and reliable. Nurses agreed to check and update the board as part of their handover routine every shift. The ward secretary was asked to ensure that admissions, discharges and bed moves were included during the day.

Coloured name badges – Doctors usually knew nurses on their 'home wards' by name, but doctors from other firms were less familiar with the nurses. When nurses wore name badges in their team colour, it was much easier for doctors to spot the right nurse from a distance. It was therefore agreed that all the nurses should use this simple means of identification.

'Doctor spotting' – Because of the bed scatter problem in the Medical Unit, many different doctors came to the wards during the day. The nurses recognized that, without the 'in charge' figure who had been easily accessible to doctors, they needed an alternative way of facilitating communication. They agreed that any nurse who saw doctors arriving in the ward should respond by greeting them and offering to direct them to other nurses as necessary. This 'doctor spotting' strategy enabled them to keep in touch with treatment changes and other medical decisions that affected their work. The new ward secretary's receptionist role also entailed welcoming and directing doctors.

Later strategies

Co-ordinated bleeping – For house officers having to work across many different wards and departments, being frequently interrupted by nurses bleeping them for non-urgent matters was frustrating. Nurses agreed to co-ordinate their calls by checking with nurses in other teams to find out whether a particular doctor had already been asked to come to the ward, or whether a number of messages could be relayed in one call.

Planned ward visits – Further reduction in non-urgent bleeping was achieved by on-call house officers agreeing to do regular rounds of each ward where they had patients. Nurses kept non-urgent matters for these visits.

Communication sheets – To ensure that nurses did not miss house officers making their regular visits to the wards, a communication sheet was devised for leaving messages at the nurses' station. Simple messages alerted doctors to tasks that needed attention. When a nurse wanted to discuss a problem, she could indicate that the doctor should seek her out.

Figure 8.1 *Practical methods of communicating with doctors*

These practical communication strategies sound simple and obvious, but in the complicated organizational environment of an acute medical unit, they were not easy to establish. Alison and the team leaders had to work hard at reminding people to use the agreed strategies properly and consistently and at discouraging them from falling back into old habits.

Working as colleagues

Nurses' growing confidence in their relationships with doctors emerged clearly during the project. They were increasingly able to approach medical staff about clinical problems and to present their views in a clear and comfortable manner. For example, Janice went to great lengths to negotiate with doctors to have a dying patient readmitted to Oriel Ward, where she knew the nurses.

'I pulled out all the stops'

When she was admitted the first time and she was told the diagnosis, she actually said that if she was ever readmitted, would it be possible for her to come back here? The doctor at the time said 'yes'. And she was readmitted and I heard through the grapevine, because Medical Records phoned up for her notes. I pulled out all the stops to try to get her back up to the ward. I had a long chat with one of the surgical doctors – she'd come in under the surgeons. She needed palliative care and I said that we could do that as well as any surgical nurses, but with the added advantage that we had that long-term relationship with her. We wouldn't have to start again. We knew her attitude and her routines, knew what she liked, and she knew us. There was quite a lot of hassle about that. The chap I spoke to first of all said yes, he didn't see any reason why she shouldn't come onto our ward. Then they said no, they wanted her downstairs and I asked why. They said she's a surgical patient, but they weren't operating, so I said, 'Nursing is nursing whatever sort it is' . . . but she did come to the ward and I was really quite pleased with that. (Janice)

In Rosemary's story about Susan, the young woman who was afraid of needles (Chapter 7), there is a good example of effective collaborative work initiated by a nurse for the benefit of her patient. Rosemary talked about the experience and her response to it.

Yes, and I spoke to the registrar at that time a little bit more about why I did feel it was so important to deal with and he agreed and we had a real co-operative working out . . . Yes, he really took on that this was a problem . . . I suppose I was worried that it would be a bit of a fight and it wasn't. It went really smoothly and I think that's what led me to proclaim how 'in paradise' I was, because I had worked through something with a patient that had implications for other members of the team. They took me seriously and they were going to take action with me to try to solve the problem, and that really made me feel good. (Rosemary)

Nurses were increasingly able to be assertive and challenging with doctors, but in a calm, polite way that did not suggest hostility. They also became unwilling to tolerate unreasonable behaviour from doctors, as the following account shows.

A senior registrar from an outlying firm had come into the ward wanting to know about a patient's home assessment. Jenny had told the doctor as much as she knew, but said that the patient's nurse had just taken another patient to theatre. The doctor then started ranting and raving in the middle of the ward, saying that the nurses on this ward were useless, that his patient had been in for three weeks and nothing had been done and he was going to transfer her to another hospital. Jenny said very forcefully, 'Will you come in here,' and led him into the office, where she told him that it was very unprofessional to shout accusations and criticisms of the nurses in the middle of the ward. He looked shocked that someone should challenge him like that. Sharon then came back to the ward and told him all the things they had been doing for the patient. (AT – Fieldnote)

Generally, doctors got used to the nurses' stronger, more active contribution to patient management and began to appreciate it. Nurses talked of doctors being more inclined to include them in discussions about patients and to ask specifically for their opinion. This pleased the nurses and reinforced their growing professional self-esteem.

In the latter stages of the project, there was much less evidence of tension in doctor–nurse relationships. In contrast to their early defensiveness and hostility, nurses could be warm and generous towards medical colleagues. For example, a female doctor felt able to turn to the nurses when she was stressed and received sympathy and support.

Cheryl (SHO) is a very good doctor and the nurses respect her medicine. I walked into the staff room a few days ago and a couple of the nurses were there and Cheryl had her head on her knees and she was sobbing. She was just exhausted. She'd been on take and been up all night and had twenty-four patients to see and she'd just trailed round on a boring consultant round. She was at the end of her tether and couldn't cope. She said she had a sore throat and couldn't go home because there was nobody to cover her. She was just sobbing and I thought it was significant that she was able to break down with us, not in the doctors' office. I had quite a chat with her and the nurses were being very supportive. She talked about what a horrific life it is really and about how upset she felt because she was becoming bitter and uncaring towards patients, because she just couldn't handle it. She said she'd done three years of this job and it had ground her down and it was unreasonable. And she talked about how, if you complain, you are regarded as a wimp of a woman and how you have to go through all this to prove you are up to it . . . I thought it was quite good, because it made the nurses realize just what a hell of a time these junior doctors have . . . I was quite pleased she had been able to show her feelings with us. (AB)

The empathy between women who have experienced oppressive working conditions and relationships was probably a factor in this story, but it had the effect of breaking down traditional doctor–nurse barriers. In less obvious ways, nurses were able to be open and generous-minded with male doctors too. For example, there was a lively debate in the ward staff-room in which three doctors and a group of nurses were exploring ways of improving junior medical cover at night.

The nurses were seriously applying themselves to looking at ways of improving the doctors' working conditions (demonstrating to the doctors that nurses are not only interested in nursing issues and conditions).

AB said that the junior doctors are afraid to suggest innovations to their consultants. She thought there were opportunities for fostering partnerships with the junior doctors to help them push through changes – 'I can talk to the consultants'. (AT – Fieldnote)

Nurses began to behave with doctors less like angry, oppressed subordinates and more like mature, self-respecting colleagues. They began to see doctors in more human terms, with individual strengths, weaknesses and difficulties, rather than in stereotypical ways, and so there was more scope for genuine, constructive working relationships to emerge. At the same time, there was evidence that nurses were gaining respect from the doctors, and that doctors were more inclined to be appreciative than critical of the nurses.

Rosemary was making tea in the staff-room and she overheard two junior doctors talking. One was new to the unit and the other was telling him about the pressure and how you've got to keep up and not put a foot wrong, 'but the nurses are really good here, they really take the pressure off you.' Rosemary thought that was a very revealing statement about how the junior doctors perceive the nurses. (AT – Fieldnote)

In the later interviews, doctors generally spoke positively about the nurses and their work, but communication difficulties remained throughout the project.

I appreciate what you are trying to do and I think it is beneficial for the patient. It's good that when you do ask the nurses, they know a great deal, and it's extremely rewarding to have that. But there is no doubt that it makes our job harder, especially when you have to find four nurses on each ward. (SHO)

The doctors were left with having to make a little more effort to communicate with nurses, but received better quality information and a more active and thoughtful contribution to patient management when they did. This exchange became more acceptable when the doctors saw nurses making efforts, from their side, to facilitate effective communication with their various practical strategies. The 'doctor spotting', in particular, made the team system less problematic for medical staff.

The nurses here are very helpful. If you get a green team nurse and you actually want blue patient information, they will go out of their way to find someone, whereas elsewhere, if it's busy, you get dismissed . . . I think that's a crucial part of it. People actually respecting the system and trying to get it to work, because if they don't you get stuck. It's very nice coming on to wards like this where the nurses actually see you and come with you to go and see the patients and are interested in what you have to say. It's quite nice not always having to make the first move. (Senior Registrar)

Many of the doctors did consider that patients were benefiting from the new kind of nursing, but their comments about how and why these benefits were being achieved were rather vague. This may be because, in spite of the close interdependence of medicine and nursing in hospital wards, doctors actually see very little of what nurses do with their patients. And it was changes in the nature of the hidden, intimate work with patients that were at the heart of the development of patient-centred practice. As one senior house officer explained, doctors could only really see the *consequences* of the changes in nurses' practice, not the practice itself.

I have to go a lot by what I am told nurses are achieving, because I haven't spent a day with a nurse on that ward, so I don't see what is happening. What I'm told is that the nurses are trying to achieve a patient-centred approach and that you introduce yourself to the patient, so that on a named basis you look after that patient or your team does. Each patient is an individual and you look after that patient with their specific needs in mind. I wouldn't be able to tell you accurately whether this is being done of course. I can only tell you that the nurses appear to know a lot of what is going on with the patients. (SHO)

Doctors saw improvements in the nurses' knowledge of their patients, a greater commitment to patients and a more informed and active contribution to their overall management. They also received positive feedback from patients and families about their nursing care. Experience of these benefits of the new style of nursing brought respect from doctors and provided a basis for the development of a healthy doctor–nurse partnership.

WARD ROUND BEHAVIOUR

In general wards in a teaching hospital, much of the medical care of patients is provided by junior doctors, with senior registrars often functioning as the main decision-makers. Junior doctors make their own rounds in the wards. These rounds involve only a few people and are usually fairly brisk and business-like, their purpose being to review each patient's progress and to make decisions about routine tests and adjustments in treatment. Final decisions about a patient's discharge from hospital might also be made on these rounds.

Consultant ward rounds are rather different. They can have several functions, but primarily they provide an opportunity (often the only opportunity) for consultants to see the patients who have been admitted under their care. The conventional format for these rounds is for a house officer or medical student to present the details of the case and then for other junior staff to add their thoughts about the diagnosis and possible treatments. The consultant usually examines the patient and asks questions to clarify the history. Finally, the consultant makes decisions about further investigations and the general approach to the patient's medical management.

Through the ward round, the consultant is able to review and supervise the work of his junior staff in relation to hospital in-patients. For senior registrars particularly, the ward round can be an opportunity to access and learn from the consultant's clinical expertise and teaching, for all the junior staff, is usually part of the consultant's agenda on his round. When medical students are attached to the firm, the teaching focus of the round may be expanded considerably.

Ward rounds also provide the main opportunity for nurses and other health professionals to talk with their patients' consultants, to present their perceptions of their patients' progress and to contribute to decisions about their overall management. Thus, depending on who attends, the consultant ward round may have a multidisciplinary focus.

Traditionally, attending consultant rounds was an important part of the ward sister's role. Consultants allocated beds in a particular ward would appear to do their rounds at specified times each week. Because these rounds were predictable and few in number, the sister could plan for them and accommodate them in her work schedule.

This traditional scenario had largely disappeared in the Medical Unit before the project began. The combination of a very high bed occupancy level and an emergency admission rate of around twenty or thirty patients a day, meant that new patients had to be placed on any medical ward where there was an empty bed, regardless of which consultant firm was admitting them. A number of medical patients also ended up in wards belonging to other specialties. Although each consultant firm nominally had their own 'home wards', in reality their patients were likely to be spread across as many as eight or ten wards, sometimes more. The effects of this 'bed scatter' problem on the working lives of doctors and on the relationship between doctors and nurses are well described by Pembrey (1995) in an article based on a small study conducted in wards which included our study wards. Pembrey portrayed the house officers, who inevitably spend their time trailing from one ward to another to see all their patients, as effectively 'homeless'. Looking at the Medical Unit in particular, one could consider each entire medical team as 'homeless' because of the bed scatter problem. A consultant described what it was like doing a 'post-take round' under these conditions.

We did a round yesterday which started at nine and finished literally at twenty past one and I went as fast as I possibly could, because we had had twenty-six in and there were fifteen others to see . . . There were only eight patients on our own two wards, they were absolutely everywhere. We started in Coronary Care and went to Short Stay, then up to Level 5, up to Level 6, then all round Level 7 . . . So I end up in my own wards right in the middle of lunch, you know, it couldn't be worse. I get there about twelve thirty, whacked and intellectually blunt, to start going round my own wards. (Consultant)

From the nurses' point of view, the bed scatter meant that there were likely to be patients from six different firms in each ward and consultants or junior doctors from any of the firms could appear to do rounds at more or less any time. It was not unusual for more than one round to be going on at once in a ward. In order to discuss their patients, nurses had to keep their eyes open and be prepared to drop what they were doing when the doctors appeared. It is hardly surprising, in these circumstances, that early in the project nurses often did not manage or did not bother to attend ward rounds.

Tackling the medical bed problem was beyond the scope of this project. It is itself a symptom of complex social and economic problems which continue to challenge the combined forces of nurses, doctors and managers, both within and beyond the Medical Unit. Within the project, our aim was to work with the medical system as it was, enabling nurses to make the most effective contribution they could to the many ward rounds that occurred.

At the back of the crowd

In the early days, medical teams were observed walking into the ward, visiting their patients and leaving, without making contact with any member of the nursing staff. Sometimes the nurses were unaware that the doctors had been to the ward. On other occasions, they saw the round going on, but let it proceed unaccompanied. The nurses complained about the number of rounds, their unpredictable timing and the communication problems that inevitably arose because they did not join them. It also emerged that they had a low opinion of ward rounds.

Sometimes I think they are picking on a particular medical student or sometimes I think they are just about who can suggest the best thing and get a pat on the back. I don't have much respect for ward rounds . . . You have to listen to a lot of drivel before you get to the vital bit of information and you have usually switched off by then. (Sharon)

Certainly, a lot of the time it is not that useful from my point of view and, if I'm not given the opportunity to contribute, it seems a waste of my time and so I carry on what I was doing. I'm not going to drop everything as soon as they walk on the ward. (Rachel)

The nurses' views were similar to those of nurses in a cancer unit reported by Whale (1993), who stated,

'The meeting with patients (i.e. the bedside ward round) was seen as overwhelmingly unsatisfactory, producing barriers to communication and confidentiality . . . Some aspects reported by nurses, such as misleading patients or demeaning them, appear so extreme as to support the observations of High (1989) that professionals are not sensitive to the authority and power they possess.' (p. 159)

Nurses in our study were also critical of the way patients were treated by doctors on ward rounds. Failure of some doctors to greet patients and to introduce themselves, patronizing manners, talking over patients and use of language patients could not understand, were all features of ward round behaviour that the nurses strongly disapproved of. It appeared that for some nurses, non-attendance on ward rounds was, at least in part, a passive protest against an aspect of ward life that they considered insensitive and dehumanizing for patients. One nurse specifically stated that by joining ward rounds he felt that he was silently condoning this kind of *'appalling behaviour'* and this made him feel extremely uncomfortable.

While the nurses generally felt powerless to influence the conduct of ward rounds, many of them also felt underconfident about contributing to them at all. They spoke of feeling that doctors did not listen to them or did not value their opinion. Junior nurses found ward rounds especially difficult.

I hate ward rounds . . . I would rather not speak, if I'm not sure. It's lack of confidence. I feel self-conscious, even though the doctors are very nice. I'm never quite sure what is important and what isn't. For example, this morning one patient has back pain. It could be from a test that she had recently, on the other hand, she has a tumour in her adrenal gland. On the way out of her room, I mentioned it to (the registrar) who said, 'Oh, we would expect that.' I feel as though I should have spoken out in the room when they were all there . . . I just feel my knowledge is so much less than theirs. (Henrietta)

This nurse's perception that her knowledge was *'so much less than theirs'* echoes the finding in Street's (1992) study that nurses value medical knowledge above their own.

The ambivalence and underconfidence of nurses of all grades was evident in their body language and behaviour, particularly on the larger consultant rounds. They commonly stood at the back of the crowd of people around the bed, making no effort to participate and only answering occasional questions addressed specifically to them. Doctors often did not acknowledge the nurses or thank them at the end of a round and this made nurses complain that, '*I might as well not have been there*' or '*It's humiliating not to feel involved*', but these nurses had made little effort to contribute to the bedside discussion.

Doctors who commented upon nurses' behaviour in relation to ward rounds thought that either they were not interested or that they were too busy to attend. The more senior doctors regretted the loss of the traditional consultant round. They missed the presence of the traditional sister who had guided them around the ward, apparently having all the information that they needed about patients at her fingertips. Younger doctors, however, were less inclined to express nostalgia for the old system and were critical of the remaining features of the traditional ward round.

Most of the doctors would not conduct huge ward rounds in the way that our bosses do now, because we can see how ghastly they are. (Registrar)

Overall, during the early part of the project, the nurses had very mixed feelings about ward rounds. They were beginning to recognize that it was in their patients' interests to attend, but, at the same time, they experienced ward rounds as interrupting their work, they disliked the way they were conducted and they felt uncomfortable and underconfident about participating. These early findings have much in common with those of Busby and Gilchrist (1992), who reported that nurses played a very limited role in medical rounds and also noted that patients were largely excluded from ward round discussions. In another study, Porter (1991) observed that on consultant rounds, '*Nurses were often reduced to listening on the sidelines, only contributing factual statements when requested.*'

Strategies for influencing ward round behaviour

Creating incentives

Other aspects of the development work helped to provide nurses with some incentive to join ward rounds. As they became more involved with their patients, they became more exposed to their patients' questions and anxieties about medical problems and treatments and it was difficult to respond to them effectively if they were not fully informed about the doctors' opinions and proposals. Similarly, as nurses became more proactive and more creative in their own work with patients, they needed to know what was happening from a medical point of view, so that they could plan their contribution to their patients' care in a complementary way. As their practice perspective was lifted beyond the daily routines of baths, turns, 'obs' and drug rounds, there was an incentive for them to join ward rounds, as a means of accessing information that they now needed and as an opportunity to influence important decisions affecting their patients.

Indirectly, Alison made a point of highlighting the value of attending ward rounds when she discussed nurses' patients with them, particularly during bedside handovers. When reviewing nurses' plans for their patients' care, she would often ask, '*And what is the medical plan?*', to remind them that they were not working in isolation. Alternatively, when she saw that there was potential for nurses to influence their patients' overall management, she would prompt them to report their observations, to speak on behalf of their patients or to make suggestions on ward rounds.

Organizational strategies

Providing any nursing presence on so many ward rounds, occurring at only vaguely predictable times, was difficult enough. Ensuring that the particular nurse who could make the most helpful contribution was present at each bedside discussion was a considerable organizational challenge.

In the very early days of the project, the nurse acting as 'co-ordinator' for the shift tried to attend all the ward rounds, communicating with doctors on behalf of her or his colleagues and relaying information back to them. However, co-ordinators often felt at a disadvantage because they had not been sufficiently involved in every patient's care to make a well-informed contribution to the round. Meanwhile, other nurses became frustrated with the inadequacies of second-hand information and wanted to talk directly with doctors, particularly when their patients had major problems or concerns.

Thus ward rounds were organized 'in teams'. Traditionally, doctors had begun their rounds at one end of the ward and worked their way steadily to the other end, visiting each of the patients under their care as they went. Instead, they were asked to join a nurse from each team in turn and to see all of their patients being nursed by one team before moving on to the next. Initially, the doctors thought that this would be too complicated and involve too much walking up and down the ward. However, provided the nurses took a strong lead in steering the doctors around their patients, ward rounds 'in teams' could be managed quite efficiently and they had the added advantage that there was always a well-informed and interested nurse in attendance.

But ward rounds 'in teams' only worked well when nurses actively managed them. At first, Alison had to play a prominent role in showing nurses how this was done and in prompting them when they began to take the lead themselves. When she was working as a team member or with her own primary patients, Alison showed that by responding proactively to doctors' visits, she could ensure that the round was comfortable for the patients, efficient for the doctors and useful from her own point of view.

When doctors arrived to see patients being cared for by other nurses, Alison would often greet them and find a nurse to start the round with them. She would then tell other nurses to be ready to join the round when the doctors had seen the first team's patients. At first, Alison had to work hard at managing rounds in this way, steering them in the right direction and prompting nurses to join them at the right time. Without this strong lead, doctors would revert to their old pattern of working their way from one end of the ward to the other and nurses, deeply absorbed in their own work, could remain oblivious of the doctors' presence. Gradually, as the general work on doctor–nurse collaboration progressed and as the 'doctor spotting' strategy was introduced, nurses began to share responsibility for organizing ward rounds. Their proper management became less dependent upon Alison's presence.

When the secretary became established in the ward, her help with organizing ward rounds was invaluable. Based at the nurses' station, she was often the first to see a medical team arrive. She would greet them, check on the white board which patients they would want to see and then find the nurse most able to free herself to begin the round. She could also warn other nurses who had patients to be seen on the round, so that they could free themselves in time to take over when the doctors had finished seeing the first team's patients. When there were a lot of patients under one consultant in the ward, the secretary was asked, in advance of a round, to make a list of which of his patients were in each team, so that nurses could easily steer the doctors round the ward to see the right patients.

Role modelling and articulating practical strategies

Alison's role modelling of effective ward round management was a powerfully influential strategy. She demonstrated that, in spite of all the organizational difficulties, a nurse could have a positive influence on the conduct of ward rounds and could make a worthwhile contribution to them. In her behaviour, nurses had an example that they learned from. Sometimes they unconsciously adopted similar behaviour themselves and sometimes they consciously made comparisons between Alison's behaviour and their own.

> *I know I should have been sitting on the edge of the bed. I know what Alison would have done if she'd been there . . . she just sits at the patient's bedside and will talk to the doctors without being spoken to.* (Henrietta)

Angie observed the specific skills and strategies that Alison used to manage ward rounds.

> *AB greeted consultant and team – easy, informal, hint of humour. They had come to see her new patient. She provided information, was at bedside before everyone else. She explained what was happening to relatives, and introduced patient to doctor. She sat on the bed.*
>
> *Negotiating with HO and SHO about doing an iron infusion, AB said, 'Let's do it tomorrow – much more sensible, there are three of us on.' AB made the decision.*
>
> *Skills that AB used were:*
> * *interacting with doctors as colleagues;*
> * *putting forward precise, pertinent information at the right time, in a clear confident way;*
> * *eye contact/social exchange;*
> * *thinking ahead, e.g. getting to the patient first and explaining quickly what was happening;*
> * *reassuring manner;*
> * *picking up cues from patients and responding to them;*
> * *interpreting what the doctors were saying for the patient;*
> * *explaining the decisions made.* (AT – Fieldnote)

Becoming more conscious of her own behaviour on ward rounds enabled Alison to talk explicitly with nurses about how they might develop skill and confidence in this area of their work. For example, when she saw nurses standing at the back of the crowd round the bed, she encouraged them to try positioning themselves next to the patient, opposite the consultant, so that they were available to support their patient and to participate in the discussion. She advised nurses to sit down at the bedside whenever they could, as this encouraged the consultant to come down to the patient's level too, making the situation less intimidating for the patient. She talked of leaving space for the consultant to have his own conversation with the patient, because this was often his only opportunity, but of gently prompting or guiding the patient when necessary. Before leaving the bedside, Alison suggested that nurses should briefly recap the decisions that had been made, so that, particularly after a lengthy debate, everyone was clear what had been agreed and who was to do what.

Enlisting the help of junior doctors

Some junior doctors were critical of the way the larger ward rounds were conducted. Angie encouraged nurses to talk informally with junior doctors about their concerns, as a means of raising awareness generally about ward round behaviour and as a way of enlisting practical help to make the rounds as comfortable as possible for patients.

> *Are you getting any sense of what your junior doctor colleagues think about ward rounds? (Mike had previously agreed to discuss ward rounds with some of the junior doctors.)* (AT)
>
> *Yes. Even though I haven't actually spoken to anyone formally, the word has got around, and I had a chat with Valerie (HO) and a couple of others . . . They were interested in what happens on ward rounds and what exactly it is that people don't like. A few of them had thought, 'Well that is how it is, what is the problem?', almost as if it hadn't occurred to them, but once you talk to them about it they are interested . . . There is a whole group of them who are very conscious about giving patients information and about patients' privacy. I noticed Valerie the other day, when one of the doctors was listening to a woman's chest and her breasts were just hanging out while she was being looked at. Valerie pulled the sheet up. It is just really nice for a doctor to do that. So, on the whole there is this nucleus of very aware doctors.* (Mike)

When the idea of doing ward rounds 'in teams' was introduced, Alison and other nurses explained to junior doctors how the system could work and asked for their co-operation and support. In particular, the doctors were asked, when a consultant did not announce his presence, to make sure that the ward secretary or one of the nurses was aware that a medical team had arrived to do a round. They were also asked to make it clear which patients were to be seen on the round, whether it was all the firm's patients or just their newly admitted patients. At introductory meetings for new doctors, the ward's approach to managing rounds was explained and the junior doctors' role in helping them run smoothly was reiterated, so that it was clear what was expected of newcomers from the start.

Being there for the patient

The strategies for helping nurses to organize and participate in ward rounds produced changes in their behaviour and their attitudes. Overall, nurses remained critical of the large traditional rounds as a means of planning and reviewing patients' management, but they became increasingly willing to acknowledge that they could serve their patients' interests best if they were present. They gradually learned not only to contribute effectively to the rounds, but also, in small but significant ways, to exert a favourable influence on the way they were conducted, making them a little more patient-centred. Doctors' responses to the nurses' active participation in ward rounds were generally very positive.

The system of organizing ward rounds 'in teams' did not always work perfectly. There were too many rounds, particularly during busy morning shifts, for nurses always to be able to free themselves without warning every time a group of doctors appeared. Furthermore, rounds done by doctors visiting only one or two 'outlying' patients could be very brief and these doctors were not always as familiar or willing to co-operate with the system as the doctors working in their home wards. Nurses' best efforts could thus sometimes be frustrated, as Angie noted:

> *Mark has been on the phone for at least half an hour. He sighed and I said, 'Having trouble?'*
>
> *'Yes. My German patient is being discharged tomorrow. He is going to spend a week in this country before returning to Germany. I have been given this information and nobody has thought about him needing oxygen at home. I am trying to contact the health centre near his daughter's now to arrange it, but I can't get through.'*
>
> *Mark said he was very cross that the doctors had not liaised with him until now – 'When they come to see him, they just wave and go, because he doesn't speak English, and they're gone before I can catch them.'* (AT – Fieldnote)

Overall, however, nurses began to be present on most of the ward rounds. This was a marked change which was noted and appreciated by the doctors.

> *My recollection very early on, and one of the things that stood out most was that nurses never came on ward rounds. But that has altered actually.* (Senior Registrar)

> *When there is a nurse there it is really good, because I don't have to repeat it all later. It is good when the nurses are there with the patients, or when they appear miraculously!* (HO)

No longer ignoring or 'boycotting' ward rounds, nurses began to talk of having a role to play as participants. They talked of wanting to 'be there for the patient' and saw themselves as being able to interpret ward round discussions to their patients. Gradually, evidence also emerged of their growing confidence on ward rounds.

> *I think that's improving actually. I think I'm more confident. I don't find them intimidating as much, I don't know why. It seemed like before I was worried because they were going to ask questions I couldn't answer. I don't seem to worry about it now . . . When I think there is something I need to discuss with the doctors, I do discuss it . . . I don't think I would stand in the background with my arms folded any more, because I don't think there's any point in being there if you are going to stand like that . . . If I'm going to be on the ward round, I stand within the group, definitely.* (Ruth)

Even Henrietta, who a year earlier had said that she hated ward rounds, was beginning to take them a little more in her stride.

Yeah, I suppose it is because I'm more confident . . . I still don't like doing ward rounds. I still go very red, but it's not as bad as it used to be. (Henrietta)

Nurses' stories about ward rounds late in the project show them no longer standing passively on the sidelines, but actively doing what they could, sometimes in difficult circumstances, to act on their patient's behalf.

'What did all that mean?'

I had managed to muscle my way into the group. I don't think I'd managed to get opposite him, as you're advised to do, but I'd managed to muscle my way into the semicircle. The doctors examined this chap and talked among themselves and turned round and said – I can't remember what they said, but it was a very fleeting comment. They didn't explain anything to him. I could see from his face, when they were talking, that he couldn't understand a word they were saying. So, at the end, as they were just about to go, I said to him, 'Have you got any questions? Did you understand that?'. And he actually said, 'Yes, what did all that mean?' So then they had to sit back down and explain it to him . . . and I was quite pleased. (Moira)

In Rosemary's account of working with her young primary patient Susan, she described in detail how she consciously acted in such a way as to reassure and comfort her during a ward round and to protect her in an intimidating situation.

'They're talking about me as if I'm not here'

I managed to catch them just as they were going in, so we went in together and the Professor welcomed me. I went to Susan's left-hand side and sat on the bed. The Professor walked round the other side and was level with me at the top and everybody else just remained gathered at the bottom of the bed. The Professor said hello to her, but he didn't introduce himself and just invited the medical students to start off in the usual way. Susan looked at me out of the side of her eyes and sort of raised her eyebrows and her eyes up towards me, and I interpreted that as, 'Here we go again, they're talking about me as if I'm not here.' I lent towards her and she looked up at me and said, 'I'm really frightened.' I sat facing her, with my back to the rest of the team and I held her hand. I wanted to be able to make eye contact with her and keep us together as a unit, if you like. I felt that if I sat the other way, I would be like the team, which was not what I wanted. She held my hand really tightly. I told her who the Professor was and he caught my eye when I did that and smiled . . . I wanted to be able to communicate with her and I guess I wanted to be able to interpret anything. As she was feeling frightened, I basically wanted to comfort her first of all, to show her that I was there for her and that's why I wanted to hold her hand. I also wanted to be able to tell her what was going on, to fill her in on anything that I felt she needed to know before they started interacting with her. We talked a little in quiet whispers while they were there. (Rosemary)

While nurses often felt that they had to act as a kind of buffer between their patients and the rather overpowering ward rounds, there were examples of nurses' sensitive, patient-centred behaviour at the bedside serving as a prompt to modify the way doctors interacted with patients. For example, nurses were observed sitting down at the bedside so as to encourage the leading doctor to sit at the patient's level too. Nurses were also observed responding to patients' non-verbal signals in such a way as to encourage doctors to acknowledge them or include them in the conversation. These were subtle but effective strategies that helped to soften and humanize the formal ritual of the traditional ward round.

When nurses began to participate actively in the ward rounds, bringing their thorough knowledge of their patients with them, they found that they could sometimes influence not only the conduct of the round, but also the decisions that were made. While nurses focussed on trying to achieve the best outcome for their patients, this could also lead to greater efficiency and more cost-effective use of resources. Alison had, for example, brought forward a patient's discharge by two days by speaking with the family before a ward round and being able to suggest a plan for home care, rather than the transfer to another hospital that the doctors had in mind. In a similar vein, Rachel told a story about her patient Bob Evans, who had come all the way from North Wales for special investigations, but while the professor in charge of his care had been away, things had progressed rather slowly.

'Excuse me'

He was miles away from home, so he had no visitors. He's a sociable person and he was basically fed up that he was only supposed to be coming in for four days, but he was still here . . . So it got round to Tuesday the following week and, meanwhile, for the last four days Bob had not seen a doctor, just had his blood pressure taken twice a day by us and that was it. He felt this was a total waste of time. On the ward round they said all the test results were normal . . . and they said, 'We think the next step is to have an angiogram, and goodbye Sir,' and started to walk off. Knowing how upset he was about being here and feeling, myself, that they had really messed him about quite a lot, as they turned their backs to go, I said, 'Excuse me, when will the angiogram be?' and they said, 'In the next couple of days.' And I said, 'Because Bob is a long way from home and he should be going home on Friday.' And they said, 'Well, I suppose so,' and went. After they had gone, Bob thanked me for pushing that. Otherwise they would have moseyed along and eventually phoned up and booked an angiogram. (Rachel)

Though ward rounds remained problematic throughout the project, doctors commented favourably on the new way that nurses were participating and some acknowledged the development work that had brought about this change.

I bumped into Prof. in the corridor. He said, 'Hello, how are you? I haven't seen much of you.' So little guilt bells went in my mind, thinking I'm not there enough, the doctors are noticing my absence. I said, 'Well, actually, I'm feeling rather tired and fed up, but I'm on holiday from tomorrow, so I'm sure I'll be better then.' He put his arm round me and said, 'I must tell you . . . ' – he'd done a ward round today. He said, 'You've done wonders with the nurses on this floor. They join the rounds, they look out for you, they're interested, they know what is going on.' He said, 'We haven't had it like that up here for a very long time.' So I just thought that was really nice. I felt reassured. I don't think he said it just to cheer me up. (AB)

Part Three

Chapter 9

Principles for practice development

INTRODUCTION

Looking back over the five 'journeys' during our final phase of analysis and interpretation, we identified common threads running through them. In drawing these threads together, we tried to abstract from the specific detail of the study the broad lessons that provided answers to our initial research questions. Thus, in this last chapter, we present, in general terms, what we have learned about how primary nursing can be used to develop a patient-centred nursing service in acute hospital wards. We propose a number of principles which we hope will be valuable to others engaged in practice development work.

Three overarching themes emerged from the final analysis. They concern the business of translating a new philosophy into practical reality, the management of this change process and, finally, the investment in professional development required to support the change.

CHANGING THE PRACTICE PHILOSOPHY

We began our work in wards where the style of nursing practice reflected many of the beliefs and values of the traditional system. However, the traditional system was no longer intact. The rigid ward routines and the formality in relationships had largely disappeared and the nurses no longer considered order, discipline, obedience and deference to medicine to be the hallmarks of good nursing. The ideals of individualized nursing had been influential in the classroom during the nurses' training, even if not particularly evident in the wards. So they accepted the existing organization and culture more because that was how things were, than because that was how they believed things ought to be. Similarly, in their practice, they adopted patterns of behaviour because they were the norm and because they knew nothing else, rather than from any real conviction that this was the best way to nurse their patients. It seemed that lack of commitment to the old order had eroded it, while the absence of a clear vision about what should replace it left a vacuum, so that the wards were in a kind of limbo. The old system was dying, but a new system was not yet springing up to replace it.

There were undercurrents of frustration and dissatisfaction caused by the dissonance the nurses experienced, at varying levels of consciousness, between their practice and their beliefs about nursing. This dissonance between what nurses do and what they believe they should do appears to be widespread across the United Kingdom. Even in a very traditional setting where nurses seemed quite happy with the status quo, Pearson (1992) reported the dissonance emerging once he helped them to question their own practice. As in Pearson's study and in work reported by Johns (1992), we exploited the tension between the nurses' ideals and the reality of their practice, raising awareness of this tension and using the discomfort it brought as a trigger for change.

There is nothing new in this strategy of opening people's eyes to the conflict between their work and their beliefs and of unsettling them so that they become open to change. It is recognized in formal change theory, for example, by Festinger (1957), who talked of creating 'cognitive dissonance' to stimulate change, and by Lewin (1958), who emphasized the need for the 'unfreezing' of an established situation before any movement could occur. Similarly, Argyris and Schon (1974) and Schon (1987) referred to the difference between 'espoused theory' and 'theory in use' and the value of exploring tensions that may exist between the two. In nursing, the idea of helping nurses to articulate their beliefs and values and making them explicit in a written ward philosophy statement is commonly advocated as an early step in the practice development process (FitzGerald, 1989b) and Pearson's (1992) study shows how valuable this exercise can be.

Before our project began, Alison had run workshops in the wards, similar to those described in the literature, and the nurses had produced a written philosophy, which made statements about their respect for patients as individual human beings, their valuing of nursing as a distinct therapy and their belief in patients' rights to information, choice and involvement. During the life of the project, in meetings and particularly at 'away days', nurses were similarly helped to explore and articulate the beliefs and values that they felt should be reflected in specific aspects of ward life and practice. However, a crucial lesson from the project was that, while this intellectual exercise of enabling nurses to clarify their philosophy was an important and necessary step in the process of developing a patient-centred style of care, it was nowhere near sufficient to bring about the fundamental changes in behaviour required to make the new philosophy a living reality, expressed in everyday practice. Furthermore, we discovered that formal education to support nurses wanting to work in new ways was again valuable, but not enough to bring about real change. As writers on primary nursing had suggested (e.g. Hegevary, 1982; Bowman and Thompson, 1986; FitzGerald, 1991), we enabled nurses to attend study days and courses about primary nursing or topics relevant to their work as primary nurses. We also encouraged them to read related literature. We found that this kind of educational input encouraged nurses to want to change and seemed to give them confidence to try new ways of working, but it was rarely what actually made things change at a fundamental level.

Educating the heart as well as the head

Our data show, time and again, that the *intellectual* grasp of a new idea or a new practice had to be reinforced at an *experiential* level before meaningful and lasting change was achieved. It was as if nurses had to understand with their hearts, as well as with their heads, what patient-centred practice really meant. Then, what had been just words and ideas came to life and they could live out their new philosophy. It was as if they had to learn at a feeling level, as well as at a thinking level, and this education of feeling was an experiential, rather than an intellectual, process.

The story 'Removing the Charts' (Chapter 5) provides an example of a nurse who, if questioned, would have said that she believed in working in partnership with her patients and whose education would have taught her that a nurse should be the patient's advocate. And yet, in practice, she fell back into the old pattern of following the doctor's instructions without question, even though she disagreed with what he proposed. Had her beliefs and her knowledge been internalized at a feeling level, she would have recognized that the doctor's instructions disempowered her patient by excluding him from the decision about his care. Similar examples occurred in relation to the nurses' development of primary and associate nurse roles. While they believed that primary nurses should form a special relationship with their patients and they knew, in theory, that primary nurses should take the initiative to manage their patients' care, their early performance in the role demonstrated little of this understanding and they were '*primary nurses in name only*'. Again, even after they had formally negotiated their new roles at 'away days', nurses still found themselves '*stepping on each other's toes*' and crossing boundaries which their experience of team nursing had not taught them to recognize. Familiar situations in practice triggered old responses and prompted familiar patterns of behaviour, quite undisturbed by the new ideas and theories in the nurses' heads.

Providing the experiential learning opportunities for nurses that touched them at the feeling level and enabled them to grasp an inner, personal understanding of what it meant to practise in a patient-centred way, became a major part of Alison's work as leader of the development. Her presence as a role model was pivotal because, through her own behaviour in the ward and her work with patients, she was able to provide a living image of a style of nursing that the staff had not seen before. In addition, by learning to articulate her expertise, by discovering practical strategies for coaching nurses in their new roles and by helping them to develop the skill and habit of reflection, she found other effective ways of confronting them with the *experience* of patient-centred nursing.

By demonstrating practices consistent with a patient-centred philosophy, Alison provided the nurses with a tangible model of actual behaviours that they could try out for themselves. The impact of this role modelling could be quite unconscious, for example in the way that the staff nurses gradually changed their body language and their style of interaction during bedside handovers. But when nurses became aware of the value of Alison as a role model, they also watched her consciously and tried to learn from her behaviour. For example, they noticed the way she spent time sitting down with her primary patients while they were constantly rushing about. Alison's role modelling had a powerful permission-giving function. In the example just given, it was as if nurses needed to see the ward sister actually living out her belief in the value of making time to listen to patients, before they could understand that it really was acceptable to sit with a patient, for a few minutes, in the midst of a busy shift. Similarly, Alison's explicit sharing of her own doubts, anxieties, frustrations and failures gave a clear message that openness about the emotional demands of patient-centred practice was not only acceptable, but also important.

By taking opportunities to talk with nurses about the fine detail of her own practice, Alison learned to make the art of patient-centred nursing more visible and accessible for them. The story 'Did you touch him?' (Chapter 6) illustrates this exposure of expertise in a situation where a nurse was involved, motivated and open to its impact at a feeling, as well as an intellectual, level. Similarly, because she practised alongside them, Alison could use the nurses' own clinical problems, while their impact was most immediate, as powerful learning experiences. The 'Removing the charts' story (Chapter 5) and the role boundary stories (Chapter 4) show Alison confronting nurses, in real situations, and alerting them to the contradictions between their old style behaviours and what they really wanted to achieve. In these everyday situations, the nurses were able to grasp what was wrong and how they might have behaved differently. The value of Alison's presence as coach, or supervisor, is shown in the story 'Saying the Word 'Cancer'' (Chapter 6), where she helped the nurse reflect on how to overcome the obstacle she had come up against. Through this kind of close contact with the nurses' practice, Alison was able to help them think deeply about the detail of their work. She was able to give them confidence and to nudge them forward as they experienced closer relationships with patients and families and as they experimented with more creative ways of caring.

Learning from experiences of practice enabled nurses to make sense of, and to apply more consciously, what they had learned theoretically. The excerpt from Barbara's diary (Chapter 5) shows this coming together of theory and practice through reflection on everyday experience. Barbara was surprised and shocked suddenly to realize that her behaviour in practice had contradicted everything she firmly believed. Little by little, the nurses were changed by the experiences they learned from; they came to see themselves, their patients and their practice differently. One nurse described this kind of learning as like a light going on, or like curtains being drawn away from in front of her eyes. She went on to say how difficult it was to explain what she had learned, because she could only use '*the same old words as before.*' The words had rich new meaning for her, but to someone else, who had not had a similar experience, the words conveyed nothing of her new insight and understanding. However, what the nurses learned at this deep, inner level was clearly evident in their practice. The sensitivity in 'The Lavender Story', the sophistication of 'The Reconciliation' and the subtlety of 'Making things familiar for Daphne' (Chapter 7) illustrate a style of practice quite different from nursing work perceived as a 'slog' or a 'chore'.

The crucial significance and the power of experiential learning are not emphasized in the general literature on change. Interestingly, however, although Pearson (1992) did not elaborate on its value, it is clear that experiential learning was critical to the success of his practice development work. He wrote little about his own influence as a clinical role model and supervisor, but we know from personal contact that he did practise regularly alongside the Burford staff. In addition, Pearson employed professional actors to engage nurses and other staff in simulated clinical situations, which were subsequently reflected upon from the perspectives of both the 'patients' and the professionals. From Pearson's account, these theatre sessions clearly provided powerful experiential learning, touching participants at the feeling level and stimulating deep insight. The theatre sessions reinforced the classroom learning provided earlier in the Burford education programme. As in our project, the experiential learning seems to have been the essential catalyst for change in the nurses' practice.

The ward sister as clinical leader

The second lesson about changing the practice philosophy that we have drawn from our work grows out of the first. Because the experiential learning factor is so important in changing the way nurses practise, so also is the presence of a senior practitioner who can demonstrate the living reality of patient-centred nursing and who can help nurses to learn from what they see, what they do and what they feel in their everyday work.

Starting from the uncertain state where the old system is in decline and the new still embryonic (a state which is likely to be the starting point for many hospital wards for years to come), developing the new patient-centred style of service is a complex process. Steering a ward team through this difficult transition, around the many obstacles that inevitably delay and confuse the journey, is a task for a clinical leader with maturity, confidence and experience, with a clear vision of what nursing should offer and with some expertise in patient-centred practice and clinical supervision, as well as in the management of change. Furthermore, our experience suggests that this practice leadership remains important even when the new style of nursing becomes established. It is not only as a change agent that the leader is required. Nurses continue to need support, for once they are genuinely open to their patients' needs for care, each day presents fresh clinical challenges. New nurses join the team and often their backgrounds have not prepared them to step easily into the new style of practice. External pressures, not least those of a financial nature, may threaten what has been achieved and need to be addressed. Demands like these remain and so there needs to be strong leadership, rooted in the reality of patient-centred practice, if the achievements of development work are not to be undermined and if the ward's practice is to continue to grow and flourish, as something living and responsive to the needs of those it serves.

The value of mature clinical leadership in hospital wards needs to be stressed. The idea of personalized nursing care, delivered by a responsible 'named' nurse, has been promoted from government level (DOH, 1991; NHSME, 1993) and education courses continue to promote the concept of patient-centred nursing. However, some changes occurring in the structure of practice life seem to run counter to this ethos. In particular, the role of the ward sister seems to be under threat. Our work strongly supports earlier evidence (e.g. McGhee, 1961; Pembrey, 1980; Runciman, 1983) that the ward sister is uniquely placed to exert to the most powerful influence, of anyone in the organization, upon the way hospital patients are cared for. And yet, this role remains poorly rewarded financially and therefore compares unfavourably, in terms of status, with senior roles in management and education. Indeed, in some centres, the most senior nurse in the ward has been downgraded and there is no senior clinical career structure at all. In many hospitals, the role of the sister as clinical leader and clinical expert is being further undermined by an apparent distortion and exaggeration of her management function, even to the extent of changing her title to 'ward manager'. This seems to greatly diminish the role, for management is only one part of the ward sister's function. Above all she is the *head nurse* in her ward. In this capacity, she needs to manage and to teach, but her greatest potential, as our work has shown, lies in her ability to lead nursing practice by being present as an expert nurse.

Management work has always been an important part of what the ward sister does and developing that function can be beneficial to practice. In the senior sister role that Alison and her colleagues have developed in Oxford, additional managerial responsibility has given them additional power and influence, but this is accompanied by additional status and reward, and so has attracted able, senior people who can handle an expanded role. Furthermore, the senior sisters are primarily committed to practice and, although there are tensions in their complex roles, the senior sisters aim to use their managerial authority to further the development of practice, rather than allowing it to distract them from nursing. The management agenda is heavier than it has ever been in the health service and it is easy to see how relatively junior sisters, with little or no administrative support, can become swamped by management business and see no alternative but to withdraw into a ward management function only, leaving the care of patients to junior staff. In this scenario, our study would suggest that the future for the development of patient-centred nursing is not promising.

Organizational support and leadership

This warning note leads on to the third lesson we learned about bringing the new philosophy into practice life, and it concerns the role of the wider hospital organization. Fundamental changes in the way ward nurses practise cannot occur in isolation from other disciplines or other parts of the hospital system. Conflict with, or obstruction from, others outside the nursing team could seriously damage, or halt altogether, the kind of development process we have described. It is crucial, therefore, that there are individuals, at the top of the organization, who are genuinely committed to the achievement of a patient-centred service. These individuals must trust and support the change agents charged with leading the development and create an organizational climate that is tolerant of experiment and risk-taking.

As we described in Chapter 2, the creation of the Oxfordshire nursing structure, in 1983, showed a major organizational commitment to the value of nursing practice. It gave senior nurses, practising as ward sisters, unprecedented status and authority in the organization and rewarded them with middle management level salaries. Investment in senior practice roles continued over the years, with support for higher education and a keen strategy of recruiting outstandingly able nurses to lead ward teams. Over a decade, the educational and professional profile of the nurses running wards was transformed to an exceptionally high level. In this way, the organization gave nursing practice strong leadership.

For Alison, being able to trust senior management to respond openly and fairly to initiatives that grew out of the development work was a crucial element of the organizational support she experienced. It was not a question of knowing that she could get anything she asked for, particularly when it came to finances; she lived in a cost-conscious health service like everyone else. It was more a matter of having the freedom to negotiate directly, at any level of the organization, and, while management could be expected to drive a hard bargain, it was in an atmosphere of respect for a senior sister's judgement and of general support for the development of nursing practice. Support for the controversial and potentially disruptive skill-mix project, which was an important antecedent of our work, was an example of the kind of organizational backing that practice development requires. During the life of our project, the willingness of senior managers to negotiate over the use of ward closure time for staff 'away days', without creating bureaucratic hoops for the sisters to jump through, was another important example of organizational support that had an enormously positive impact.

The Chief Nurse and the Director of Nursing, supported by Health Authority and hospital Chief Executives, created an organizational climate characterized by freedom from petty rules, freedom to experiment and freedom from any top-down attempt to control practice development. The medical sisters experienced this climate as tremendously encouraging and helpful. Attached to the considerable licence it offered was an obligation of responsibility and accountability that the sisters fully appreciated, but it left them scope to try out new ideas with their ward teams, in a manner and at a pace that was manageable for them. During the project, the unrestrictive atmosphere created by those at the top of the nursing hierarchy was exploited responsibly and to good effect. For example, when the nurses wanted to experiment with duty rotas, to try using three sets of drug keys or to change their care plan documents, they were able to take responsibility for these initiatives themselves, needing only Alison's support. Because there was no need to ask permission outside the ward, responsible innovation within the ward was a real possibility. Nurses were able to discuss problems in their meetings, propose solutions and then get on and initiate them. Learning to use this freedom, which would not have existed in a traditional, bureaucratic management structure, was empowering for the nurses and, ultimately, greatly enhanced what they could contribute to patient care.

Manthey (1980) wrote about the importance of the right kind of managerial support, above ward level, for primary nursing to flourish in a hospital. She emphasized that the decentralization of decision-making within wards should mirror the same process throughout the management structure. Moreover, she said that senior managers need to show the same trust and respect that sisters show their primary nurses, and need similarly to accept the risks associated with decentralization. Without this consistency of approach throughout the organiza-tion, the commitment to innovation and development within ward teams can falter and the creativity of primary nurses can be undermined. Manthey suggested that it is not impossible to implement primary nursing in a hostile management culture, but that '*it simply requires more courageous staff nurses*' (p. 71). Our development work took place within a nursing management structure that had been decentralized for some years and within an open, supportive, professional culture. The contribution of this management context to the overall success of our project should not be underestimated. In the absence of a hostile management culture, the staff nurses were free to reserve their courage for addressing openly the complex and sometimes distressing problems of their patients.

THE PROCESS OF CHANGE IN PRACTICE

We acknowledge the influence in our project of classical change theories, as presented in the works of Lewin (1958), Rogers (1962), Bennis *et al.* (1976) and Ottaway (1976; 1982). The ideas set out in this well-known literature formed part of our background theoretical repertoire as change agents. The informed reader will recognize, for example, that we avoided what Chin and Benne (in Bennis *et al.*, 1976) describe as a 'power-coercive' approach, because the kind of change we were seeking could not be imposed by edict. Instead, we opted for what the same authors call a 'normative-re-educative' strategy, which broadly means helping people to recognize the need for change and involving them fully in the change process. We reinforced this approach with formal educational input and rational discussion, which equates to the theorists' 'rational-empirical' strategy. However, it is not our intention to elaborate the value of these established theories in managing change in nursing, for this work has been done by others (e.g. Wright, 1989; Pearson, 1992). Rather, taking this general change theory as given, we add our own theorizing, drawn from our own data and applicable specifically to the business of managing the development of patient-centred nursing in acute hospital wards.

First, we address the issue of initiative and control in our project and emphasize, in the context of changing nursing practice, the importance of collaboration. Second, we consider our approach to managing change by describing the 'horticultural model', which emerged of its own volition during the course of our work and which seems particularly well suited to the conditions of hospital ward life. Finally, we draw together what we have learned about the nature of the change from a traditional to a patient-centred style of practice.

Initiative and control

Approaches to managing change are often described as being either 'top-down' or 'bottom-up', depending upon whether initiative and control in the change process emanate from the boardroom or the shop-floor. However, Beer (1980) shows how the success of both approaches is likely to be limited in terms of achieving a change that is fully internalized by people throughout the organization and in terms of achieving long-term results. Where these outcomes are important, as was the case in our project, he advocates a 'shared responsibility' approach to change,

> '. . . in which those at the top and those at lower levels are jointly involved in identifying problems and/or solutions. Top management does not decide everything nor do they abdicate authority and responsibility for the change to lower levels. There is almost continual interaction between top and bottom levels and a process of mutual influence.' (p. 55)

The disadvantage of this approach is that it takes time, but, according to Beer, as well as being the most effective way to achieve a genuine and lasting change, it has the additional benefit of causing less anxiety and frustration than the other approaches and it produces fewer unanticipated dysfunctional effects within the organization. Beer's 'shared responsibility' approach is broadly the same as our 'collaborative change strategy' (Chapter 2) and it served us well in delivering the results that Beer predicted.

It is interesting to note, looking back over our project, that collaborative change was occurring simultaneously at three levels within the service. At ward level, we set out to initiate, to support and broadly to steer a major change, while at the same time involving staff – responding to their ideas, stimulating their creativity and embracing their contributions. In this way, we set in motion the 'process of mutual influence' that enabled us to share responsibility for change with the staff nurses. Though we were less conscious of it at the time, the same approach was being taken towards us by senior management. The collaboration at this level was less intense and less detailed, but the principles of both parties being involved and being committed to the change and sharing responsibility for it, applied equally. Finally, the same approach to change was being developed by the nurses in their work with patients, for therapeutic work is about helping patients achieve positive change. As nurses became more patient-centred in their practice, they abandoned the traditional top-down approach of 'nurse knows best' and began to work collaboratively with their patients, sharing responsibility with them for decisions about their care.

The congruence between the approach to change at these three levels was important. The freedom and support that came with a collaborative change strategy were passed down the organization, manifesting finally in the individual nurse–patient relationship.

A 'horticultural model' of change

A 'horticultural model' of change fits well with the collaborative approach, because it assumes that both the leader of the change and other participants have a degree of initiative and control. It also fits well where organizational conditions tend to be unstable and unpredictable, as in a busy hospital ward where the nature, intensity and amount of nursing work cannot be easily anticipated. Both scenarios happen to mirror life in a garden. While the gardener may have green fingers, he will be the first to acknowledge that the creation of a garden is a collaborative venture between himself and nature and, of course, he is constantly confronted with the vagaries of the weather. Parallels between gardening and our change management process emerged gradually and at first unconsciously. Then, one day, it struck Angie that Alison was always using horticultural terms when she talked about her work in the wards. For example, she spoke of '*identifying fertile ground for a new project*', of '*sowing ideas*' and of '*nurturing staff*'. When we examined the idea of gardening as a metaphor for the process of developing patient-centred practice in a hospital ward, we found that it captured very helpfully the essence of our approach to managing this particular change.

A central notion in the horticultural analogy is the recognition that, in dealing with change in nursing practice, one is dealing with something living and dynamic. Approaching ward life much as we would approach life in a garden helped us to avoid being too mechanistic in our handling of change. We appreciated the value of the careful planning that is emphasized in formal change theory, and this is shown in the conduct of our action cycles, but, like a garden design, most of our plans related more to the general shape, colour and style of what we were trying to create, than to the precise details of what we hoped would emerge. We focussed on careful tending and nurturing, encouraging the nurses' practice to grow and blossom in its own way and in its own time. Rather than forcing the ward's development to follow a rigid, predetermined timetable, we tried to be sensitive to prevailing conditions and to adapt our plans accordingly. For example, much as the gardener would wait for the last frost before putting out his delicate plants, we waited for staffing levels to stabilize before we formalized primary nursing.

Our work involved striking a balance between following an overall plan and, from day to day, working opportunistically – waiting for the right moment to take a nurse aside to discuss her patient; waiting for a very busy spell to pass before pushing the nurses on with some new project; watching out for nurses who were stressed, struggling or bored and giving them extra time and help. This is the same work pattern as the gardener's. He uses the opportunity of a fine day to further some new scheme, then watches out for harsh conditions or failing plants and responds appropriately. The attitudes of the gardener were useful to us too. We found that it was wise to remember that not every seed germinates and not every plant produces the finest fruit. Thus, we learned to be tolerant and realistic and, on the positive side, we learned to be open to the unexpected and to accommodate, as it were, the seedlings that sprung up in unexpected places and the fine plants that flourished beyond expectation.

The 'horticultural model' provides a lively image, capturing aspects of the reality of managing change in nursing practice that are missing in the orthodox organizational change theories. It emphasizes the creativity, sensitivity and flexibility, which we learned were crucial attributes for a change agent to cultivate in a nursing practice context. The relationship between horticulturalist and nature also reflects the kind of respect, love and care, which we learned were so important to foster real growth in nursing practice.

The change as a series of 'journeys'

Our final comments about the process of changing practice concern the nature of the specific transition from a traditional style of nursing to a style that is genuinely patient-centred. We have conceptualized this transition as a complex, difficult and time-consuming series of journeys. Here, we consider the relationship of the journeys to each other and the place of each journey in the context of the whole transition.

In relation to managing practice development in a ward, we suggest that there are five journeys to be undertaken simultaneously. Issues of ward organization, culture and leadership are intimately related to each other, as well as to the actual practice of nursing, and all in turn effect the relationship between nursing and medicine. Embarking upon one of the journeys throws up challenges in other aspects of ward life and makes the other journeys necessary, if some sort of equilibrium is to be restored. For example, beginning to make organizational changes by decentralizing decision-making had enormous repercussions. It demanded a more open, participative culture, challenged the traditional leadership of the sister, disrupted interdisciplinary communications and gave the nurses unaccustomed freedom in their clinical practice. We learned that developing patient-centred practice means being prepared to review, and possibly to change, virtually every aspect of ward life. One change triggers others, and so the process continues over a period of a few years, until finally there is degree of harmony again, with the different elements of ward life all supporting and complementing the new style of practice.

The five journeys relating to ward practice need to be thought of as running in parallel, so that one might think of managing different layers of change. As progress is made with one layer, the others need to be nudged along, or sometimes held back, so that the different aspects of the change roughly keep pace with each other and the development grows as a whole. For example, we found that it was inappropriate to give nurses too much clinical freedom before they had learned to be part of a culture that was both challenging and supportive. Similarly, Alison, as the ward sister, saw that it was unwise to abdicate responsibility for taking ward rounds (as she progressed along her 'leadership journey') until the staff nurses were becoming established in their primary and associate nurse roles ('organizational journey') and becoming confident enough to represent their patients and their nursing perspective in a multidisciplinary forum ('practice journey'). In a simple diagrammatic form, the development process could be depicted as shown in Figure 9.1.

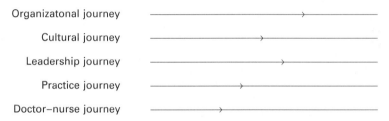

Organizatonal journey

Cultural journey

Leadership journey

Practice journey

Doctor–nurse journey

Figure 9.1 *The development of practice as a series of parallel journeys*

Managing this process well meant trying to keep all the arrows moving forward approximately in line with each other. As we saw, for example with the false starts at introducing primary nursing, practice development tends to follow something of a 'snakes and ladders' course, and so an additional challenge in managing the process is the fact that the arrows on the diagram can move backwards as well as forwards. Managed this way, the pace of change was halting and uneven, but our approach did address the complexity of both the process itself and the context in which it occurred.

Looking back at the project, it is possible to differentiate the relative contributions of the different journeys and to see their place in relation to the whole development. While it was true that we needed to pay attention to five journeys at once, or at least to keep shifting our focus between them, they did not all require equal emphasis all the time. For at least the first half of the project, it was organizational, cultural and leadership issues that dominated the development agenda. There was also the early background practice work of helping nurses to see the potential of 'basic' care and of encouraging them to take advantage of the team system to get to know their patients better, but the major investment in the practice of individual nurses came towards the end of the project, when conditions (i.e. the structure, culture and leadership) could support patient-centred practice. We have presented the change in the doctor–nurse relationship as a journey in its own right, because it emerged as a strong theme in our data and because we have found that it is often a major concern for other nurses. However, though important, this journey was somewhat peripheral to the others and it could have been subsumed within the organizational, cultural and leadership journeys (changing the pattern of communication with doctors was an organizational change; nurses developing a collaborative rather than subordinate relationship with doctors was a cultural change; changing doctors' perception of the ward sister role was connected with the leadership journey).

The organizational, cultural and leadership journeys together (embracing the doctor–nurse journey) can be seen as representing the development of the *infrastructure* for patient-centred nursing. In each of these journeys, the overall task to be addressed was that of dismantling the remnants of an old system, which was hostile to the practice of patient-centred nursing, and building a new system, which made logical, practical sense in relation to the modern philosophy of nursing. Returning to the gardening analogy, it made sense to anticipate that a decentralized primary nursing structure, an open, supportive culture and democratic, clinically based leadership would provide the conditions within which patient-centred nursing was likely to flourish. Developing this new infrastructure for ward life involved, initially, a great upheaval which required careful management, but eventually the system stabilized in its new form. Then, only light 'maintenance' work was required to keep it vital and responsive to the continuing flow of ward life.

The practice journey had a different place in the overall development. Nursing practice is the product of individuals working within the ward system. The infrastructure of ward life plays a crucial role in shaping nurses' practice by creating or denying opportunities for them to work in particular ways, by sanctioning certain attitudes and by establishing norms of behaviour. However, the style and quality of the care patients receive are ultimately determined by individual nurses at the bedside. For this reason, investment in developing the full professional potential of each nurse has to be of paramount concern to the ward sister. We say more about professional development in the next section, but here we simply wish to point out that professional development strategies are the sister's tools for enabling individual nurses to make the most of what the system offers and to give of their best in their practice. This work of the ward sister does not diminish greatly once the major thrust of the development is complete, because new nurses join the team and established staff continue to need stretching and challenging as their expertise grows. However, this work may be shared with team leaders if they, in particular, are helped to develop and mature.

The relationship between the key aspects of ward life in a balanced, stable system can be depicted as a 'diamond' structure (Figure 9.2). If a patient-centred philosophy is the guiding principle behind the development of the organization, culture and leadership in the ward, then an 'infrastructure' emerges that promotes and supports the 'right' kind of practice. Within this context, investment in the professional development of individual nurses is the final catalyst, transforming the nurses' daily work with patients and producing a style of practice that reflects the underlying philosophy.

If there is a fundamental change in the philosophy of nursing, as has been the case with the decline of traditional beliefs and values and the rise of the patient-centred ideal, then, from our analysis, it follows that all the other elements of the 'diamond' will need to be changed before a coherent, stable, new form of practice emerges.

A final word about the 'medical sisters' journey', which has been omitted from the discussion so far. The main focus of our project was the process of developing

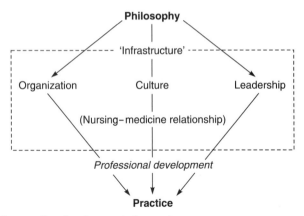

Figure 9.2 *The practice development diamond*

a patient-centred style of practice within one ward and the five 'journeys' that we have reported form a theorized account of that work. The 'medical sisters' journey', which is not included in this publication, traced the way that Alison was able to stimulate and indirectly support the same practice development process in other wards in the Medical Unit. Alison made this contribution to the development of the other medical wards largely by forming, facilitating and participating within the Medical Sisters' Group. She functioned as a change agent within her peer group, a change strategy that appears to be rare in clinical nursing. Angie's research and facilitation skills and the opportunity to participate in the action research process also helped the group in its early development. As the peer group became established, cohesive and comfortable working together, its dependence upon Alison's contribution diminished. The group developed a strong identity and became an influential force within the Medical Unit, as well as a source of inspiration and support for its members.

INVESTING IN PROFESSIONAL DEVELOPMENT

In the traditional nursing system, investment in professional development was minimal because it was not really needed. Initial training taught nurses the rules and procedures they required for a practice life that was not expected to change greatly. Expertise was gained through experience. Additional skills for promotion were acquired from senior colleagues, in a haphazard fashion, through 'sitting by Nellie'. Within practice, the scope of what nurses did was narrowly confined to a series of practical tasks and opportunities for them to use their judgement, their creativity or their personal presence were limited. Thus, nurses could continue through their careers with little or no conscious, focussed professional development.

As we saw throughout the project, patient-centred nursing and the kind of ward life that supports it, make much greater demands on nurses, as individuals and as members of a team. Recognition that modern nursing gives nurses greater autonomy and wider professional discretion, and that it occurs in a world where knowledge and skills frequently need updating, has brought a change of attitude in the profession to continuing education. The UKCC (1994) has formalized this change in its PREP framework, which commits registered nurses to continuous learning throughout their careers. Our concern was to mirror this commitment within the fabric of ward life in such a way as to create, and latterly to support, a patient-centred style of practice.

We use the term professional development in a broad sense, meaning a growth in competence and maturity of nurses as professional practitioners. Reviewing the strategies that we found helpful for facilitating progress on the various 'journeys' in our project, many of them were in fact, by this definition, strategies that promoted professional development. An important lesson that we learned, in managing these strategies, was the value of creating a balance between development opportunities provided within the ward and outside it and, also, between opportunities provided for individuals and for groups.

In Chapter 4, we discussed the 'time out' theme in some detail. The first 'away days' highlighted the value of addressing the development needs of the ward team as a whole and of giving the nurses time together, away from the pressures of everyday work, to listen to each other and to think, reflect and make plans. As the project continued, we observed how nurses, as individuals and as groups, were refreshed by time out and brought back new energy and enthusiasm to the ward. Alison learned to sense when nurses needed the variety and stimulation of time out and tried to be creative in making opportunities more varied than just the usual study days. When possible, she also tried to link what nurses learned outside the ward with experiences in practice, and vice versa, so that each was enriched by the other.

In relation to each 'journey', Alison learned to use her own presence in the ward to foster the growth of nurses as practitioners and as team members. Indeed, this conscious, focussed use of her own time in the ward became one of Alison's key functions in her 'new style' ward sister role. Keeping in touch with the nurses' practice, using opportunities to help them learn from experiences in the ward and using her own clinical work as a model and as a rich source of material for discussion were all strategies that Alison used to stimulate reflection and growth. In Chapter 6, we showed how specific supervision strategies were developed for use in an opportunistic fashion, amid the hurly-burly of ward life. Essentially, the supervision strategies involved the conscious, purposeful use of specific clinical situations as learning opportunities. These strategies tapped the rich educational potential of everyday practice and helped nurses to gain insight, confidence and practical know-how.

The high priority that we both gave to learning from and within practice influenced the ward's 'cultural journey'. In Chapter 5, we showed how attitudes to criticism, enquiry and professional debate gradually shifted and how, eventually, a new ethos emerged which supported the professional development of the nurses as a group. They learned to challenge each other, to explore clinical problems together and to enjoy lively, critical discussions about their work. In this atmosphere, the nurses were able to learn from each other, as well as from us and from more conventional outside sources. We found that promoting and supporting a climate, in which work was experienced as intellectually stimulating and as providing rich learning opportunities, was a way of releasing energy and enthusiasm in the nursing team and of sustaining the momentum of the development process.

Investment in the nurses' professional development was a vital element in the creation of a patient-centred nursing service. It was important for helping nurses to adapt to new roles, for encouraging them to embrace a more open culture, for enabling them to respond to more challenging leadership and for giving them confidence to work as colleagues with doctors. Promoting the professional development of the nurses thus enabled us to establish what we have called the 'infrastructure' for patient-centred nursing. However, even more crucially, it was the development of individual nurses as 'skilled companions' to their patients that finally transformed the style of nursing in the ward. The continued nurturing of each nurse's practice was, as it were, the spark that ultimately brought the new ward system to life.

Focussing upon the professional development of the nurses meant taking an interest in each one as an individual, being alert and sensitive to their particular strengths and weaknesses, valuing their special contributions to the ward and addressing their specific educational needs. In this way, the nurses were recognized and cared for, as people and as professionals. They received the kind of individual attention and support that they were expected to give their patients.

SOME REFLECTIONS ON ACTION RESEARCH

Finally, we return to our methodology and present some reflections on the experience of engaging in an ambitious action research venture. Action research provided us with a strategy for pursuing our aims both to achieve and to study a major change in nursing practice. We began with a rather naive understanding of action research and, only as the project developed, did we come to appreciate what a complex and demanding methodology it can be. Here, we consider our experience of action research as a means of stimulating and directing change and as a means of promoting the professional development of participants, and we comment on its value as a method for generating theory.

The action research process provided a discipline which made us more thoughtful, sensitive and rigorous than we might otherwise have been as change agents. The steady flow of rich data, from different sources, constantly challenged and broadened our perspective on what was happening in the wards and kept us alert to problems and priorities that we might have preferred to ignore. Being able to use raw data to help other participants to confront difficult issues and to inform their decisions about how the development should proceed was also enormously helpful and, in many instances, speeded up the change process. The practice of regularly and systematically reviewing progress in relation to each of the action spirals committed us to seeking feedback on every aspect of the development work and ensured that we were critical of our achievements.

In these specific ways, action research proved to be an effective change strategy, but it also presented us with some serious challenges. At a practical level, it generated a vast amount of data and keeping track of the data, giving them sufficient attention and making timely use of them were quite onerous tasks, given the many other demands of the development work. Less tangible, but at times equally problematic, were tensions inherent within the action research process. We had to struggle to maintain a balance between the commitment to openness that allowed participants genuinely to influence the course of change, and the need to impose some order on the change process, so that we could understand what was happening and provide effective leadership and facilitation. Similarly, we had to live with the unpredictability of action research, while also recognizing the reasonable managerial expectations existing within a hospital context and the inevitable time and funding limitations associated with the project.

Returning to the benefits of the methodology, we were impressed by the way that involvement in the action research process enhanced the professional development of participants, including ourselves. Furthermore, we noted how the professional development experiences that came with engaging in action research were particularly appropriate for nurses learning to practise in a patient-centred way. As we have shown, sharing project data with staff was a valuable way of stimulating reflection and creative thinking. In the action planning that followed, we were able to involve nurses in negotiation and decision-making. The skills that nurses acquired through this process were readily transferable to their increasingly independent practice and their more active roles in ward life. For us, participation in the action research process challenged and helped to refine our understanding of ward life, the nature of patient-centred practice and the relationship between the two. The insights we gained made us more sensitive and more discriminating in steering the development and in supporting the nurses' practice. Our particular way of handling the action research process, through a partnership, was also valuable from a professional development point of view. The constant clash of our different perspectives, Alison's predominantly that of the practitioner and Angie's that of the researcher, was productive not only for the research, but also for each of us in our own practice. Alison's demands for accessible, common-sense interpretations of theoretical and methodological issues helped Angie to achieve greater depth and clarity in her research thinking. Similarly, Angie's analytical probing helped Alison to explore taken for granted aspects of her practice and helped her to develop a habit of rigorous reflection.

Critics of our intensive approach to professional development and our investment in one particular clinical setting may argue that this kind of practice development is not sustainable in the long term and that it could produce nurses who are not able to work comfortably in 'ordinary' hospital wards. The problem of where to go next did arise for a number of nurses involved in the project. Junior nurses were particularly concerned that they would not easily find another position in which they had a similar balance of freedom, responsibility and support. Many of them stayed longer than staff nurses would traditionally have done 'to gain medical nursing experience'. Some sought promotion within their own ward or within another ward in the Medical Unit, where practice was developing along similar lines. Many nurses recognized that moving on from one specialty to another, in the traditional manner, was not necessarily the best way to develop professionally and, instead, they chose to stay within the Medical Unit, taking advantage of the development opportunities it offered, often combining them with part-time higher educational study. When experienced nurses were ready to move on, they took with them a strong grounding in the practice of patient-centred nursing and many were able to seek positions where they would have authority to lead or contribute to the development of the same style of nursing in another ward. For example, in the three years after the completion of the project, five of the nurses from Oriel Ward alone took up ward sister posts, three within the Medical Unit and two in a neighbouring hospital. These nurses, and other 'second generation' ward sisters appointed from the Medical Unit, are playing a substantial role in consolidating the development work within the Medical Unit and in exporting it to other hospital settings.

Those who have moved on to senior clinical roles have taken with them a conscious, articulated understanding of patient-centred nursing and of the process required to develop it in a hospital ward. Much of this knowledge will have been acquired from participating in a project which, as an action research project, sought not only to achieve a change in nursing practice, but also to generate theory about that change. Like us, throughout the project nurses were constantly challenged to reflect upon their experiences and upon data that presented them with a range of perspectives. This process forced us all to explore and to articulate what had previously been hidden or taken for granted. As a result, new concepts of ward life and practice emerged and relationships between them became apparent, forming the beginnings of a theoretical understanding of the change we were experiencing. At the end of the fieldwork, we took the theory development further by immersing ourselves again in all the data, refining the initial conceptualization and clarifying the relationships between concepts, until we produced the theoretical framework that has provided the structure for our account of the development of patient-centred nursing. We hope that this final exercise in theorizing has left those nurses who worked with us a more substantial picture of what we all learned together. We hope too that many other nurses will find in our theorized account a framework for analysing and steering their own practice development work.

Nursing practice remains misunderstood and undervalued within the health service and within society generally. The task of realizing the true potential of nursing practice within the sphere of health care and healing presents an enormous challenge to the profession. If our work offers, in some small way, encouragement and practical help to nurses who have the vision and the courage to respond to this challenge, then our efforts will have been worthwhile.

SUMMARY OF PRINCIPLES FOR PRACTICE DEVELOPMENT

- The *intellectual* grasp of a new idea or a new practice has to be reinforced at an *experiential* level before meaningful and lasting change can be achieved.

- Experiential learning in a ward is facilitated by the presence of a senior practitioner who can demonstrate the living reality of patient-centred nursing and who can help nurses to learn from what they see, what they do and what they feel in their everyday work.

- It is crucial that there are individuals at the top of the hospital organization who are genuinely committed to the achievement of a patient-centred service. These individuals must trust and support the change agents charged with leading the development and create an organizational climate that is tolerant of experiment and risk-taking.

- The freedom and support inherent in a collaborative change strategy can be passed down the organization, manifesting finally in the individual nurse–patient relationship.

- The 'horticultural model' of change emphasizes creativity, sensitivity and flexibility as crucial attributes for a change agent to cultivate in a nursing practice context. The relationship between the horticulturalist and nature also reflects the kind of respect, love and care that can foster real growth in nursing practice.

- Developing patient-centred practice means being prepared to review, and possibly to change, virtually every aspect of ward life.

- The process of developing practice in a ward can be conceptualized as a series of parallel 'journeys'.

- The organizational, cultural and leadership journeys together (embracing the doctor–nurse journey) can be seen as representing the development of the *infrastructure* for patient-centred nursing.

- If a patient-centred philosophy guides the development of the organization, culture and leadership in a ward, then an infrastructure emerges that promotes and supports the 'right' kind of practice. Within this context, investment in the professional development of individual nurses is the final catalyst, transforming the nurses' daily work with patients and producing a style of practice that reflects the underlying philosophy.

- It is helpful to create a balance between professional development opportunities provided within the ward and outside it and, also, between opportunities provided for individuals and for groups.

- Supervision strategies can be developed from the conscious, purposeful use of specific clinical situations. These strategies can be used to tap the rich educational potential of everyday practice, enabling nurses to gain insight, confidence and practical know-how.

- Promoting and supporting a climate in which work is experienced as intellectually stimulating and as providing valuable learning opportunities, releases energy and enthusiasm in a nursing team and sustains the momentum of the development process.

- The continued nurturing of each nurse's practice is, as it were, the spark that ultimately brings patient-centred practice to life.

References

Abdellah, F.G., Beland, I.L., Martin, A. and Matheney, R.V. (1960). *Patient Centred Approaches to Nursing*. New York: Macmillan.

Alderman, C. (1983). Individual care in action, Burford: a model for nursing. *Nursing Times*, **79** (3), 15–17.

Anderson, E.R. (1973). *The Role of the Nurse*. London: Royal College of Nursing.

Appleton, C. (1993). The art of nursing: the experience of patients and nurses. *Journal of Advanced Nursing*, **18**, 892–899.

Argyris, C. and Schon, D. (1974). *Theory in Practice: Increasing Professional Effectiveness*. London: Jossey-Bass.

Armitage, P., Champney-Smith, J. and Andrews, K. (1991). Primary nursing and the role of the nurse preceptor in changing long-term mental health care: an evaluation. *Journal of Advanced Nursing*, **16** (4), 413–422.

Audit Commission (1992). *Making Time for Patients: A Handbook for Ward Sisters*. London: HMSO.

Ausubel, D.P., Novak, J.S. and Hanesian, H. (1978). *Educational Psychology: A Cognitive View*. New York: Holt, Rinehart and Winston.

Baly, M. (1980). *Nursing and Social Change*. London: Heinemann.

Batehup, L. (1991). *Personal Reflections*. Action Research Workshop, 18 April, Department of Nursing, King's College, London.

Beer, M. (1980). *Organization Change and Development: A Systems View*. Santa Monica: Goodyear Publishing Company.

Benner, P. (1984). *From Novice to Expert: Excellence and Power in Clinical Nursing Practice*. London: Addison-Wesley.

Benner, P. (1985). Quality of life: a phenomenological perspective on explanation, prediction and understanding in nursing science. *Advances in Nursing Science*, **8** (1), 1–14.

Benner, P. and Wrubel, J. (1989). *The Primacy of Caring*. California: Addison-Wesley Publishing Company.

Bennis, W.G., Benne, K.D.R. and Corey, K.E. (1976). *The Planning of Change*. London: Holt, Rinehart and Winston.

Berry, A.J. and Metcalf, C.L. (1986). Paradigms and practices: the organization of the delivery of nursing care. *Journal of Advanced Nursing*, **11**, 589–597.

Binnie, A.J. (1987). Primary nursing – structural changes. *Nursing Times*, **83** (39), 36–37.

Binnie, A.J. (1988). *The Working Lives of Staff Nurses – A Sociological Perspective*. MA Dissertation, Warwick University.

Binnie, A.J. (1989). Primary nursing – where to start. *Nursing Times*, **85** (24), 43–44.

Binnie, A. and Titchen, A. (1998). *Patient-Centred Nursing. An Action Research Study of Practice Development in an Acute Medical Unit*. Report No. 18. Oxford: RCN Institute.

Bond, S., Bond, J., Fowler, P. and Fall, M. (1991). Evaluating primary nursing. *Nursing Standard*: Part 1, **5** (36), 35–39; Part 2, **5** (37), 37–39; Part 3, **5** (38), 36–39.

Boud, D., Keogh, R. and Walker, D., eds (1985). Promoting reflection in learning: a model, in *Reflection: Turning Experience into Learning*. London: Kogan Page.

Bowman, G. and Carter, E. (1990). Making sense of primary nursing. *Nursing Times*, **86** (27), 39–41.

Bowman, G. and Thompson, D. (1986). Curbing routine and ritual. *Nursing Times*, July 30th, 43–45.

Bradshaw, A. (1994). *Lighting the Lamp, The Spiritual Dimension of Nursing Care*. Middlesex: Scutari Press.

Bredemeier, H.C. and Stephenson, R.M. (1962). *The Analysis of Social Systems*. London: Holt, Rinehart and Winston.

Brown, E.L. (1966). Nursing and patient care, in *The Nursing Profession: Five Sociological Essays* (F. Davis, ed.). New York: John Wiley and Sons.

Brown, S. and McIntyre, D. (1981). An action research approach to innovation in centralised educational systems. *European Journal of Science Education*, **3** (3), 243–258.

Burgess, R.G. (1984). *In the Field*. London: Allen and Unwin.

Busby, A. and Gilchrist, B. (1992). The role of the nurse in the medical ward round. *Journal of Advanced Nursing*, **17**, 339–346.

Butterworth, T. and Faugier, J. (1992). *Clinical Supervision and Mentorship in Nursing*. London: Chapman and Hall.

Campbell, A.V. (1984). *Moderated Love: A Theology of Professional Care*. London: SPCK.

Campen, Y. (1988). Breaking new ground. *Nursing Times*, **84** (22), 38–40.

Carpenter, M. (1977). The new managerialism and professionalism in nursing, in *Health and the Division of Labour* (M. Stacey, ed.). London: Croom Helm.

Carr, W. and Kemmis, S. (1986). *Becoming Critical: Education, Knowledge and Action Research*. London: Falmer Press.

Carr-Hill, R., Dixon, P., Gibbs, I., Griffiths, M., Higgins, M., Mccaughan, D. and Wright, K. (1992). *Skill Mix and the Effectiveness of Nursing Care*. University of York: Centre for Health Economics.

Chapman, G.E. (1983). Ritual and rational action in hospitals. *Journal of Advanced Nursing*, **8**, 13–20.

Chilton, S. (1991). A change in the right direction. *Nursing Times*, **87** (25), 44–46.

Clarke, M. (1978). Getting through the work, in *Readings in the Sociology of Nursing* (R. Dingwall and J. McIntosh, eds). Edinburgh: Churchill Livingstone.

Collier, J. (1945). United States Indian administration as a laboratory of ethnic relations. *Social Research*, **12**, 275–276.

de la Cuesta, C. (1983). The nursing process: from development to implementation. *Journal of Advanced Nursing*, **8**, 365–371.

Davies, C. (1980). *Rewriting Nursing History.* London: Croom Helm.

Denzin, N.K. (1978). *The Research Act: A Theoretical Introduction to Sociological Methods.* New York: McGraw-Hill.

Department of Health (1991). *The Patient's Charter.* London: HMSO.

Department of Health and Social Security (1972). *Report of the Committee on Nursing (Briggs).* London: HMSO.

Department of Health and Social Security (1977). *Patients First. Consultation paper on the structure and management of the National Health Service in England and Wales.* London: HMSO.

Dewing, J. (1991). Primary nursing – implications for the nurse, in *Primary Nursing in Perspective* (S. Ersser and E. Tutton, eds). London: Scutari Press.

Dingwall, R. and McIntosh, J. (1978). *Readings in the Sociology of Nursing.* Edinburgh: Churchill Livingstone.

Dingwall, R., Rafferty, A.M. and Webster, C. (1988). *An Introduction to the Social History of Nursing.* London: Routledge.

Eldridge, J.E.T. and Crombie, A.D. (1974). *A Sociology of Organisations.* London: Allen and Unwin.

Elpern, E. (1977). Structural and organisational supports for primary nursing. *Nursing Clinics of North America*, **12** (2), 205–219.

English National Board for Nursing, Midwifery and Health Visiting (1994). *Lifelong Learners: Partnerships for Care.* London: ENB.

Ersser, S.J. (1991). A search for the therapeutic dimensions of nurse–patient interaction, in *Nursing as Therapy* (R. McMahon and A. Pearson, eds). London: Chapman and Hall.

Ersser, S.J. (1992). *An Account of the Work Role of a Clinical Lecturer in Nursing Based in the Department of Dermatology, Oxford, 1990–1992.* Oxford: National Institute for Nursing.

Ersser, S.J. (1995). *An Ethnographic Study of the Therapeutic Effect of Nursing.* PhD Thesis, King's College, University of London.

Ersser, S.J. and Tutton, E. (1991). *Primary Nursing in Perspective.* Harrow: Scutari Press.

Estabrooks, C.A. and Morse, J.M. (1992). Towards a theory of touch: the touching process and acquiring a touching style. *Journal of Advanced Nursing*, **17**, 448–456.

Faulkner, A. (1979). Monitoring nurse–patient conversation in a ward. *Nursing Times*, **75**, Occasional Paper No. 23, 95–96.

Ferrin, T. (1981). One hospital's successful implementation of primary nursing, *Nursing Administration Quarterly*, Summer, 1–12.

Festinger, L. (1957). *A Theory of Cognitive Dissonance.* Illinois: Row Perteson, Evanston.

FitzGerald, M. (1989a). *Lecturer-practitioner: Action-researcher.* Master of Nursing Dissertation, University of Wales, Cardiff.

FitzGerald, M. (1989b). A unit profile, in *Managing Nursing Work* (B. Vaughan and M. Pillmoor, eds). London: Scutari Press.

FitzGerald, M. (1991). Educational preparation for primary nursing, in *Primary Nursing in Perspective* (S. Ersser and E. Tutton, eds). London: Scutari Press.

Fradd, E. (1988). Achieving new roles. *Nursing Times*, **84** (50), 39–41.

Fretwell, J.E. (1980). Hospital ward routine – friend or foe? *Journal of Advanced Nursing*, **5**, 625–636.

Fretwell, J.E. (1982). *Ward Teaching and Learning*. London: Royal College of Nursing.

Fretwell, J.E. (1985). *Freedom to Change: The Creation of a Ward Learning Environment*. London: Royal College of Nursing.

Gadamer, H.-G. (1979). The problem of historical consciousness, in *Interpretive Social Science: A Reader* (P. Rabinow and W.M. Sullivan, eds). London: University of California Press.

Gamarnikow, E. (1978). Sexual division of labour: the case of nursing, in *Feminism and Materialism* (A. Kuhn and A. Wolfe, eds). London: Routledge.

General Nursing Council for England and Wales (1977). *Training Syllabus, Register of Nurses, General Nursing*. London: GNC.

Giovannetti, P. (1986). Evaluation of primary nursing, in *Annual Review of Nursing Research* (H. Werley, J. Fitzpatrick and R. Taunton, eds). New York: Springer.

Glaser, W.A. (1966). Nursing leadership and policy: some cross-national comparisons, in *The Nursing Profession: Five Sociological Essays* (F. Davis, ed.). New York: John Wiley.

Goddard, H.A. (1953). *The Work of Nurses in Hospital Wards: Report of a Job Analysis*. Leeds: Nuffield Provincial Hospitals Trust.

Goulding, J. and Hunt, J. (1991). Accountability and legal issues in primary nursing, in *Primary Nursing in Perspective* (S. Ersser and E. Tutton, eds). Scutari Press, London.

Graham, H. (1986). *The Human Face of Psychology*. Milton Keynes: Open University Press.

Hart, E. and Bond, M. (1995). *Action Research for Health and Social Care*. Buckingham: Open University Press.

Hedges, J. (1993). Into new life: a reflective account. *Journal of Clinical Nursing*, **2** (4), 194–195.

Hegevary, S.T. (1982). *The Change to Primary Nursing*. St Louis: C.V. Mosby Company.

Heidegger, M. (1962). *Being and Time*. New York: Harper and Row.

Henderson, V. (1966). *The Nature of Nursing*. London: Collier-Macmillan.

Henderson, V. (1982). The nursing process – is the title right? *Journal of Advanced Nursing*, **7**, 103–109.

Heron, J. (1989). *The Facilitators' Handbook*. London: Kogan Page.

High, D.M. (1989). Truthtelling, confidentiality and the dying patient: new dilemmas for the nurse. *Nursing Forum*, **24** (1), 5–11 [cited in Whale, Z. (1993). The participation of hospital nurses in the multidisciplinary ward round on a cancer-therapy ward. *Journal of Clinical Nursing*, **2**, 155–163].

Holmes, C.A. (1990). Alternatives to natural science foundations for nursing. *International Journal of Nursing Studies*, **27** (3), 187–198.

Hughes, D. (1988). When nurse knows best: some aspects of nurse–doctor interaction in a casualty department. *Sociology of Health and Illness*, **10** (1), 1–22.

Hunt, M. (1987). The process of translating research findings into nursing practice. *Journal of Advanced Nursing*, **12**, 101–110.

Jenkinson, V. (1958). Group or team nursing: report on a five year experiment at St George's Hospital, London. *Nursing Times*, **54**, 62–64, 92–93.

Johns, C. (1989). *The Impact of Introducing Primary Nursing on the Culture of a Community Hospital*. Master of Nursing Dissertation, University of Wales, Cardiff.

Johns, C. (1990). Autonomy of primary nurses: the need to both facilitate and limit autonomy in practice. *Journal of Advanced Nursing*, **15**, 886–894.

Johns, C. (1992). Ownership and the harmonious team: barriers to developing the therapeutic nursing team in primary nursing. *Journal of Clinical Nursing*, **1** (2), 89–94.

Johns, C. (1993a). Professional supervision. *Journal of Nursing Management*, **1**, 9–18.

Johns, C. (1993b). On becoming effective in taking ethical action. *Journal of Clinical Nursing*, **2**, 307–312.

Johns, C. (1994). Guided reflection, in *Reflective Practice: The Growth of the Professional Practitioner* (A. Palmer, S. Burns and C. Bullman, eds). Oxford: Blackwell Scientific Publications.

Jones, D.C. (1975). *Food for Thought*. London: Royal College of Nursing.

Jourard, S.M. (1971). *The Transparent Self*. New York: Van Nostrand Reinhold Company.

Keddy, B., Jones Gillis, M., Jacobs, P., Burton, H. and Rogers, M. (1986). The doctor–nurse relationship: an historical perspective. *Journal of Advanced Nursing*, **11**, 745–753.

Kemmis, S. and McTaggart, R. (1988). *The Action Research Planner*. Victoria: Deakin University Press.

Kidd, P. and Morrison, E.F. (1988). The progression of knowledge in nursing: a search for meaning. *Image: Journal of Nursing Scholarship*, **20** (4), 222–224.

Kohner, N. (1994). *Clinical Supervision in Practice*. London: King's Fund Centre.

Kramer, M. (1968) Nurse role deprivation – a symptom of needed change. *Social Science and Medicine*, **2** (4), 461–474.

Kron, T. (1987). *The Management of Patient Care: Putting Leadership Skills to Work*. Philadelphia: W.B. Saunders.

Lathlean, J. (1988). Viable reality or pipe dream? *Nursing Times*, **84** (49), 39–40.

Lathlean, J. (1997). *Lecturer Practitioners in Action*. Oxford: Butterworth-Heinemann.

Lathlean, J. and Farnish, S. (1984). *The Ward Sister Training Project: An Evaluation of a Training Scheme for Ward Sisters*. Report No. 3, University of London Nursing Education Research Unit, Department of Nursing Studies, Chelsea College.

Lathlean, J., Smith, G. and Bradley, S. (1986). *Post-Registration Development Schemes Evaluation*. University of London Nursing Education Research Unit, King's College.

Lawler, J. (1991). *Behind the Screens: Nursing, Somology, and the Problem of the Body*. Edinburgh: Churchill Livingstone.

Lelean, S.R. (1973). *Ready for Report Nurse? – A Study of Nursing Communication in Hospital Wards*. London: Royal College of Nursing.

Levine, M.E. (1991). Introduction to patient-centred nursing, in *Levine's Conservation Model: A Framework for Nursing Practice* (K.M. Schaefer and J.B. Pond, eds). Philadelphia: F.A. Davis Company.

Lewin, K. (1946). Action research and minority problems. *Journal of Social Issues*, **2**, 34–46.

Lewin, K. (1958). The group reason and social change, in *Readings in Social Psychology* (E. MacCoby, ed.). London: Holt, Rinehart and Winston.

Lewis, T. (1990). The hospital ward sister: professional gatekeeper. *Journal of Advanced Nursing*, **15**, 808–818.

Lewis, P.H. and Brykczynski, K.A. (1994). Practical knowledge and the competencies of the healing role of the nurse practitioner. *Journal of the American Academy of Nurse Practitioners*, **6** (5), 207–213.

Lukes, S. (1986). *Power: A Radical View.* London: Macmillan.

Macdonald, M. (1988). Primary nursing: is it worth it? *Journal of Advanced Nursing*, **13**, 797–806.

MacGuire, J. (1961). *From Student to Nurse. Part 1: The Induction Period.* Oxford Area Nurse Training Committee.

MacGuire, J. (1989a). An approach to evaluating the introduction of primary nursing in an acute medical unit for the elderly – I. Principles and practice. *International Journal of Nursing Studies*, **26** (3), 243–251.

MacGuire, J. (1989b). An approach to evaluating the introduction of primary nursing in an acute medical unit for the elderly – II. Operationalizing the principles. *International Journal of Nursing Studies*, **26** (3), 253–260.

MacGuire, J. (1989c). Primary nursing – A way to better care? *Nursing Times*, **85** (46), 50–53.

MacGuire, J. (1991). Quality of care assessed: using the Senior Monitor index in three wards for the elderly before and after a change to primary nursing. *Journal of Advanced Nursing*, **16**, 511–520.

MacGuire, J. and Botting, D.A. (1990). The use of the Ethnograph program to identify the perceptions of nursing staff following the introduction of primary nursing in an acute medical ward for elderly people. *Journal of Advanced Nursing*, **15**, 1120–1127.

Mackay, L. (1993). *Conflicts in Care: Medicine and Nursing.* London: Chapman and Hall.

MacLeod, M. (1994). It's the little things that count: the hidden complexity of everyday clinical nursing practice. *Journal of Clinical Nursing*, **3**, 361–368.

Macleod Clark, J. (1984). Verbal communication in nursing, in *Recent Advances in Nursing, 7: Communication* (A. Faulkner, ed.). Edinburgh: Churchill Livingstone.

Manley, K. (1989). *Primary Nursing in Intensive Care.* London: Scutari Press.

Manthey, M. (1980). *The Practice of Primary Nursing.* Oxford: Blackwell Scientific Publications.

Manthey, M., Ciske, K., Robertson, P. and Harris, I. (1970). Primary nursing, a return to the concept of "my nurse" and "my patient". *Nursing Forum*, **9** (1), 65–83.

Manthey, M. and Kramer, M. (1970). A dialogue on primary nursing. *Nursing Forum*, **9** (4), 356–379.

Marson, S.N. (1982). Ward sister – teacher or facilitator? An investigation into the behavioural characteristics of effective ward teachers. *Journal of Advanced Nursing*, **7**, 347–357.

May, C. (1991). Affective neutrality and involvement in nurse–patient relationships: perceptions of appropriate behaviour among nurses in acute medical and surgical wards. *Journal of Advanced Nursing*, **16**, 552–558.

Mayeroff, M. (1971). *On Caring.* New York: Perennial Library, Harper and Row.

McFarlane, J. (1977). Developing a Theory of Nursing. *Journal of Advanced Nursing,* **2** (3), 261–270.

McGhee, A. (1961). *The Patient's Attitude to Nursing Care.* Edinburgh: E. and S. Livingstone Ltd.

McMahon, R. (1991). Power and communication issues in primary nursing, in *Primary Nursing in Perspective* (S. Ersser and E. Tutton, eds). London: Scutari Press.

McMahon, R. and Pearson, A. (1991). *Nursing as Therapy.* London: Chapman and Hall.

McNiff, J. (1988). *Action Research Principles and Practice.* London: Macmillan Education.

McPhail, A., Pikula, H., Roberts, J., Browne, G. and Harper, D. (1990). Primary nursing. A randomized crossover trial. *Western Journal of Nursing Research,* **12** (2), 188–200.

Menzies, I.E.P. (1960). A case study in the functioning of social systems as a defence against anxiety. *Human Relations,* **13**, 95–121.

Menzies, I.E.P. (1970). *The Functioning of Social Systems as a Defence Against Anxiety.* London: The Tavistock Institute of Human Relations.

Merton, R.K. (1968). *Social Theory and Social Structure.* New York: Free Press.

Meyer, J. (1993). New paradigm research in practice. *Journal of Advanced Nursing,* **18**, 1066–1072.

Morgenbesser, S. (1987). The American Pragmatists, in *The Great Philosophers* (B. Magee, ed.). London: BBC Books.

Morse, J.M. (1991). Negotiating commitment and involvement in the nurse–patient relationship. *Journal of Advanced Nursing,* **16** (4), 455–468.

Muetzel, P.A. (1988). Therapeutic nursing, in *Primary Nursing – Nursing in the Burford and Oxford Nursing Development Units* (A. Pearson, ed.). London: Croom Helm.

National Health Service Management Executive (1993). *A Vision for the Future: The Nursing, Midwifery and Health Visiting Contribution to Health Care.* London: NHS Executive, Department of Health.

Nightingale, F. (1859). *Notes on Nursing: What It Is and What It Is Not.* London: Harrison [facsimile published by J.B. Lippincott Company, Philadelphia].

Nolan, M. and Grant, G. (1993). Action research and quality of care: a mechanism for agreeing basic values as a precursor to change. *Journal of Advanced Nursing,* **18**, 305–311.

Norton, D. (1981). The nursing process in action – 1. The quiet revolution: introduction of the nursing process in a region. *Nursing Times,* **77**, 1067–1069.

Nursing Times (1989). NT News. *Nursing Times,* **85** (10), 5.

Ogier, M.E. (1982). *An Ideal Sister.* London: Royal College of Nursing.

Ogier, M.E. (1989). *Working and Learning.* London: Scutari Press.

Orton, H.D. (1981). *Ward Learning Climate.* London: Royal College of Nursing.

Ottaway, R.N. (1976). A change strategy to implement new norms, new style and new environments in the work organization. *Personnel Review,* **5** (1), 13–15.

Ottaway, R.N. (1982). Defining the change agent, in *Changing Design* (B. Evans, J.A. Powell and R. Talbot, eds). London: Wiley.

Owen, S. (1993). Identifying a role for the nurse teacher in the clinical area. *Journal of Advanced Nursing*, **18**, 816–825.

Paterson, J. and Zderad, L. (1976). *Humanistic Nursing*. New York: John Wiley and Sons.

Pearce, E.C. (1937). *A General Textbook of Nursing*. London: Faber and Faber Limited.

Pearson, A. (1985). *The Effects of Introducing New Norms in a Nursing Unit and an Analysis of the Process of Change*. Doctoral Thesis, University of London, Goldsmith's College, Department of Social Science and Administration.

Pearson, A. (1988). *Primary Nursing: Nursing in the Burford and Oxford Nursing Development Units*. London: Croom Helm.

Pearson, A. (1992). *Nursing at Burford: A Story of Change*. London: Scutari Press.

Pembrey, S.M. (1975). From work routines to patient assignment: an experiment in ward organization. *Nursing Times*, **71**, 1768–1772.

Pembrey, S.M. (1980). *The Ward Sister – Key to Nursing*. London: Royal College of Nursing.

Pembrey, S.M. (1995). Of no fixed abode: homeless house officers. *British Medical Journal*, **311**, 1706–1707.

Pondy, L.R., Frost, P., Morgan, G. and Dandridge, T. (1983). *Organizational Symbolism*. Greenwich, CT: JAI.

Porter, S. (1991). A participant observation study of power relations between nurses and doctors in a general hospital. *Journal of Advanced Nursing*, **16**, 728–735.

Reed, S. (1988). A comparison of nurse related behaviour, philosophy of care and job satisfaction in team and primary nursing. *Journal of Advanced Nursing*, **13** (3), 383–395.

Revans, R. (1964). *Standards for Morale, Cause and Effect in Hospital*. Oxford: Nuffield Provincial Hospitals Trust, Oxford University Press.

Rogers, C.R. (1967). *On Becoming a Person*. London: Constable.

Rogers, C.R. (1983). *Freedom to Learn for the '80s*. London: Charles E. Merrill.

Rogers, E.M. (1962). *Diffusion of Innovations*. New York: Free Press.

Roper, N., Logan, W. and Tierney, A. (1980). *The Elements of Nursing*. Edinburgh: Churchill Livingstone.

Royal College of Nursing (1956). *Observations and Objectives: A Statement on Nursing Policy*. London: RCN.

Royal College of Nursing (1981). *Towards Standards. A Discussion Document*. RCN, London.

Runciman, P.J. (1983). *Ward Sisters at Work*. Edinburgh: Churchill Livingstone.

Savage, J. (1995). *Nursing Intimacy, An Ethnographic Approach to Nurse–Patient Interaction*. London: Scutari Press.

Schon, D.A. (1983). *The Reflective Practitioner: How Professionals Think in Action*. London: Temple Smith.

Schon, D. (1987). *Educating the Reflective Practitioner*. London: Jossey-Bass.

Schutz, A. (1962). *Collected Papers: Volumes 1–3*. Dordrecht: Kluwer Academic.

Schutz, A. (1967). *The Phenomenology of the Social World*. Evanston: Northwestern University Press.

Shea, H. (1984). Communication among nurses: the nursing care plan, in *Communication, Recent Advances in Nursing – 7* (A. Faulkner, ed.). Edinburgh: Churchill Livingstone.

Shukla, R.K. (1981). Structures vs. people in primary nursing: an inquiry. *Nursing Research*, **30** (4), 236–241.

Shukla, R.K. (1982). Primary or team nursing? Two conditions determine the choice. *Journal of Nursing Administration*, **11**, 12–15.

Singleton, P. and Gamblin, R. (1989). A primary change-over. *Nursing Times*, **85** (40), 39–41.

Smith, G. (1986). Resistance to change in geriatric care. *International Journal of Nursing Studies*, **23** (1), 61–70.

Stein, L.I. (1978). The doctor–nurse game, in *Readings in the Sociology of Nursing* (R. Dingwall and J. McIntosh, eds). Edinburgh: Churchill Livingstone.

Stein, L.I., Watts, D.T. and Howell, T. (1990). The doctor–nurse game revisited. *The New England Journal of Medicine*, **322** (8), 546–549.

Stockwell, F. (1972). *The Unpopular Patient*. London: Royal College of Nursing.

Strauss, A. (1966). The structure and ideology of American nursing: an interpretation, in *The Nursing Profession: Five Sociological Essays* (F. Davis, ed.). New York: John Wiley and Sons.

Street, A.F. (1992). *Inside Nursing: A Critical Ethnography of Clinical Nursing Practice*. Albany: State University of New York Press.

Susman, G. and Evered, R. (1978). An assessment of the scientific merits of action research. *Administrative Science Quarterly*, **23**, 582–603.

Sweet, S.J. and Norman, I.J. (1995). The nurse–doctor relationship: a selective review. *Journal of Advanced Nursing*, **22**, 165–170.

Tanner, C.A., Benner, P., Chelsa, C. and Gordon, D.R. (1993). The phenomenology of knowing the patient. Image: *Journal of Nursing Scholarship*, **25** (4), 273–280.

Taylor, B.J. (1992). Relieving pain through ordinariness in nursing: a phenomenologic account of a comforting nurse–patient encounter. *Advances in Nursing Science*, **15** (1), 33–43.

Thomas, L.H. and Bond, S. (1990). Towards defining the organization of nursing care in hospital wards: an empirical study. *Journal of Advanced Nursing*, **15**, 1106–1112.

Thomas, L.H. and Bond, S. (1991). Outcomes of nursing care: the case of primary nursing. *International Journal of Nursing Studies*, **28** (4), 291–314.

Titchen, A. (1987a). The design and implementation of a problem-based, continuing education programme: a guide for clinical physiotherapists. *Physiotherapy*, **73**, 318–323.

Titchen, A. (1987b). Problem-based learning: the rationale for a new approach to physiotherapy continuing education. *Physiotherapy*, **73**, 324–327.

Titchen, A. (1993). Action research as a research strategy: finding our way through a philosophical and methodological maze, in *Changing Nursing Practice Through Action Research* (A. Titchen, ed.). Oxford: National Institute for Nursing.

Titchen, A. (1994). Roles and relationships in collaborative action research. *Surgical Nurse*, **7** (5), 15–19.

Titchen, A. (1995a). Issues of validity in action research. *Nurse Researcher*, **2** (3), 38–48.

Titchen, A. (1995b). A case study of a patient-centred nurse, in *Essential Practice in Patient-Centred Care* (K.W.M. Fulford, S. Ersser and T. Hope, eds). Oxford: Blackwell Science.

Titchen, A. (1998a). *Professional Craft Knowledge in Patient-Centred Nursing and the Facilitation of its Development.* Unpublished DPhil Thesis, University of Oxford.

Titchen, A. (1998b). *A conceptual framework for facilitating learning in clinical practice.* Occasional Paper No. 2, Centre for Professional Education Advancement, Lidcombe, Australia.

Titchen, A. and Binnie, A. (1993a). Changing power relationships between nurses: a case study of early changes towards patient-centred nursing. *Journal of Clinical Nursing*, **2** (4), 219–229.

Titchen, A. and Binnie, A. (1993b). What am I meant to be doing? Putting practice into theory and back again. *Journal of Advanced Nursing*, **18**,1054–1065.

Titchen, A. and Binnie, A. (1993c). A unified action research strategy in nursing. *Educational Action Research*, **1**(1), 25–33.

Titchen, A. and Binnie, A. (1993d). Research partnerships: collaborative action research in nursing. *Journal of Advanced Nursing*, **18**, 858–865.

Titchen, A. and Binnie, A. (1993e). A 'double-act': co-action researcher roles in an acute hospital setting, in *Changing Nursing Through Action Research* (A. Titchen, ed.). Oxford: National Institute for Nursing.

Titchen, A. and Binnie, A. (1994). Action research: a strategy for theory generation and testing. *International Journal of Nursing Studies*, **31** (1), 1–12.

Titchen, A. and Higgs, J. (1995). Facilitating the use and generation of knowledge in clinical reasoning, in *Clinical Reasoning in the Health Professions* (J. Higgs and M. Jones, eds). Oxford: Butterworth-Heinemann.

Titchen, A. and McIntyre, D. (1993). A phenomenological approach to qualitative data analysis in nursing research, in *Changing Nursing Practice Through Action Research* (A. Titchen, ed.). Oxford: National Institute for Nursing.

Travelbee, J. (1971). *Interpersonal Aspects of Nursing.* Philadelphia: F.A. Davis Company.

United Kingdom Central Council for Nursing, Midwifery and Health Visiting (1994). *The Future of Professional Practice – The Council's Standards for Education and Practice Following Registration (PREP).* London: UKCC.

Wallace, C.L. and Appleton, C. (1995). Nursing as the promotion of well-being: the client's experience. *Journal of Advanced Nursing*, **22**, 285–289.

Walsh, M. and Ford, P. (1989). *Nursing Rituals, Research and Rational Actions.* Oxford: Butterworth-Heinemann.

Warnock, M. (1970). *Existentialism.* Oxford: Oxford University Press [cited in Graham (1986). *The Human Face of Psychology.* Milton Keynes: Open University Press].

Waters, K. (1985). Team nursing. *Nursing Practice*, **1**, 7–15.

Watson, J. (1985). *The Philosophy and Science of Caring.* Colorado: Colorado Associated University Press.

Webb, C. (1986). *Women's Health: Midwifery and Gynaecological Nursing.* London: Hodder and Stoughton.

Webb, C. (1989). Action research: philosophy, methods and personal experiences. *Journal of Advanced Nursing*, **14**, 403–410.

Whale, Z. (1993). The participation of hospital nurses in the multidisciplinary ward round on a cancer-therapy ward. *Journal of Clinical Nursing*, **2**, 155–163.

White, E., Davies, S., Twinn, S. and Riley, E. (1993). *A detailed study of the relationship between teaching, support, supervision and role modelling for students in clinical areas, within the context of Project 2000 courses.* English National Board for Nursing, Midwifery and Health Visiting Research Highlights, October.

Wilson, N. and Dawson, P. (1989). A comparison of primary nursing and team nursing in a geriatric long-term care setting. *International Journal of Nursing Studies*, **26** (1), 1–13.

Wilson-Barnett, J., Corner, J. and De Carle, B. (1990). Integrating nursing research and practice – the role of the researcher as teacher. *Journal of Advanced Nursing*, **15**, 621–625.

Wilton, L. (1994). *Audit of accounts 1992/93: a review of the management and utilization of ward nursing resources* (unpublished paper). John Radcliffe Hospital, Oxford.

Wright, L. (1974). *Bowel Function in Hospital Patients.* London: Royal College of Nursing.

Wright, S.G. (1989). *Changing Nursing Practice.* London: Edward Arnold.

Wright, S.G. (1990). *My Patient, My Nurse.* London: Scutari Press.

Yura, H. and Walsh, M. (1967). *The Nursing Process.* New York: Appleton-Century-Crofts.

Zander, K.S. (1977). Primary nursing won't work…unless the head nurse lets it. *Journal of Nursing Administration*, October, 19–23.

Index

Accountability:
  calling nurses to account, 141, 145
Action research, 31–6, 56, 231–3
  action spirals, 40–6
  design of, 37–9
Activities of living model, 14
Associate nurse role, 43, 83–6
Attention to detail, 186–7
Authority, 20, 28
  decentralization, 20, 59–60, 61–2
  See also Decision-making
Auxiliaries, 60
Away days, 43, 82, 86–9, 230

Basic care, 151–2
  uncovering the potential of, 153–6
Bed scatter problem, 205
Bedford-Fenwick, Mrs, 10
Bereaved relatives, 161
Bias, 53
Burford Nursing Development Unit, 27, 29

Campbell, Alistair, 150–1
Care Plan Project, 44, 52, 115
Caring relationship, 150
Caring team, 120–2
Caseload size, 61
Change in practice, 223–9, 233–4
  change as a series of journeys, 226–9
  horticultural model of change, 225–6
  initiative and control, 224–5
  See also Organizational culture; Practice
    issues; Work organization
Co-ordinator role, 72–4
Collaboration with doctors, promotion of,
    195–201
  informing doctors about changes in nursing,
    198–200
  practical communication strategies, 200–1
  role modelling and coaching, 196–8

Communication issues, 44, 194–5
  co-ordinator role and, 73–4
  practical communication strategies, 200–1
  restructuring communication channels,
    69–70
Concern and support, 118–20
Concurrent data analysis, 53–4
Confidence building, 96–8, 162–3
Confidentiality issues, 52, 179
Consultants, *See* Doctor–nurse relationship;
    Ward rounds
Continuity of care, 15, 19
  establishment of, 65–6
Creative team, 104–5
Critical community, 114–16
Critical friendships, 113–14
Critical theory, 32, 34
Criticism as reprimand, 111
Curiosity, promotion of, 111–14

D grade nurses, 79–80
Data analysis, 53–6
  exploratory case study, 53
  main study, 53–6
Data collection methods, 47–8
  depth interviews, 49–50
  documentary evidence, 50–1
  participant observation, 48–9
  reflective conversations, 50
Debate, promotion of, 111–14
Decentralization of, 7–8, 44, 59–62, 66–9,
    223
  authority, 20, 59–60, 61–2
  clinical decision-making, 67–8
  managerial decision-making, 68–9, 81–2,
    223
  responses to organizational change, 71–2
  results of, 81–2
  teething troubles, 75–81
  ward sister role and, 123–5

Decision-making, 28
  decentralization of, 7–8, 44, 59–60, 61–2,
    66–9, 223
    clinical decision-making, 67–8
    managerial decision-making, 68–9, 81–2,
      223
    teething troubles, 75–6
Delegation, 133
Depth interviews, 49–50
Doctor–nurse relationship, 44, 189–90, 227–8
  communication difficulties, 74, 194–5
  earning respect, 190–1
  promotion of collaborative work, 195–201
    informing doctors about changes in
      nursing, 198–200
    practical communication strategies, 200–1
    role modelling and coaching, 196–8
  reluctant handmaidens, 191–5
  working as colleagues, 201–4
  See also Ward rounds
Documentary evidence, 50–1

Education issues, 12–14, 21, 27
  investment in professional development,
    229–31, 232
  traditional ward teaching, 137–9
  See also Learning
Ends system, 62–4
  being in charge, 63–4
  doing the baths, 62–3
Existentialism, 16–17
Experiential learning, 218–21
Experimental research, 21–2
Experimentation, encouragement of, 103–4

Families, relationships with, 160–1, 165,
    178–82
  bereaved relatives, 161
  of terminally ill patients, 182
Focussed attention, 168

Goodrich, Annie, 12

Handover system, 69–70, 104–5, 153, 155, 164
  bedside handover, 70, 153, 164, 171, 188
Healthcare Assistants, *See* Auxiliaries
Health Service reforms, 30
Helping relationship, 17, 150
Higher education, 12–14, 21
  See also Learning
Horticultural model of change, 225–6
Humanistic psychology, 16–17
Hypothesis formulation, 53–6
  action hypothesis, 54–5

Individualized care, 7, 12–16, 18

Junior doctors, 204
  enlisting the help of, 210

Leadership role, 123, 125–36, 221–3
  new style supervision, 141–8
  See also Ward sister
Learning:
  at work, 109–16, 230
    critical community, 114–16
    missed learning opportunities, 110–11
    promotion of curiosity, openness and
      debate, 111–14
  from experience, 91–3, 218–21
  from practice, 139–41
    enhancing role modelling, 139–40
    guiding reflection and independent
      thinking/action, 140–1
  from patients, 173–5
  role model, importance of, 92–3, 119, 138,
    154, 163–4, 219
    in doctor–nurse relationships, 196–8
    in ward rounds, 209–10
  to work professionally, 105–9
    getting through the work, 105–6
    professional commitment, 108–9
    professional work ethos, development of,
      106–7
  See also Education issues

Management structures, 6, 28, 222–3
Manthey, Marie, 20, 24–25
Meetings, 68–9
Menzies, Isobel, 11
Models of nursing, 11, 14
Month on/month off system, 130–1, 132
Mutual concern and support, 118–20

Nightingale, Florence, 10, 21
Nurse–patient relationship, 17–19, 154,
    159–60, 165
  addressing the patient's experience, 167–75
  therapeutic relationships, 166–7
  unpopular patients, 175–8
Nurses, 60–1
  associate nurse role, 43, 83–6
  being in charge, 63–4
  calling to account, 141, 145
  co-ordinator role, 72–4
  D grade nurses, 79–80
  investment in professional development,
    229–31, 232
  primary nurse role, 43, 78–80, 83–6, 94–7
  registered nurses, 28, 60–1
  role development, 43, 45
  skill-mix, 60–1
  See also Doctor–nurse relationship;
    Nurse–patient relationship

Nursing, 151–8
    basic care, 151–2
        uncovering the potential of, 153–6
    daily grind, 152
    excitement of, 156–8
    styles of,
        individualized, 12–16
        patient-centred, 16–21
        traditional, 9–12
Nursing process, 7, 13–15

Observational study, 40
Openness, promotion of, 111–14
Organization, *See* Work organization
Organizational culture, 99
    caring for each other, 116–22
        concern and support, 118–20
        the caring team, 120–2
        the sociable team, 116–18
    changing practice philosophy, 217–23
        experiential learning, 218–21
        organizational support and leadership,
            222–3
        ward sister as clinical leader, 221–2
    learning at work, 109–16
        critical community development, 114–16
        missed learning opportunities, 110–11
        promotion of curiosity, openness and
            debate, 111–14
    learning to work professionally, 105–9
        getting through the work, 105–6
        professional commitment, 108–9
        professional work ethos development,
            106–7
    shaping ward life, 100–5
        encouraging experimentation, 103–4
        facilitating participation, 102–3
        the creative team, 104–5
        using initiative, 100–3
    See also Change in practice

Participant observation, 48–9
Participation, facilitation of, 102–3
Patient-centred nursing, 7, 16–21, 149–50,
        158–88
    making a difference, 185–8
        attention to detail, 186–7
        patients' experiences of, 185–6
    personal cost of, 182–5
        endless demand, 183–4
        interrupted relationships, 183
        letting go, 184–5
    role development for, 45, 162–5
        confidence building, 162–3
        planning ahead, 164–5
        role modelling and articulating practice,
            163–4
    See also Primary nursing; Skilled
        companions

Patients:
    allocation of, 14–15
    having time for, 171
    nurse–patient relationship, 17–19, 154,
        159–60, 165
        addressing the patient's experience, 167–75
        therapeutic relationships, 166–7
        unpopular patients, 175–8
    phenomenal field, 169–70
    receiving and learning from, 173–5
    terminally ill patients, 182
    working with, 171–3
Pearson, Alan, 25–6
Pembrey, Susan, 14–15
Permission-giving, 107, 119, 155, 219
Personalized care, 6–8
Phenomenal field, 169–70
Phenomenology, 33, 37
Planning, 41, 164–5
Practical knowledge, 142–3
Practice issues, 9–21
    individualized nursing, 12–16
    patient-centred nursing, 16–21
    traditional nursing, 9–12
    See also Change in practice; Organizational
        culture; Work organization
Practice philosophy, *See* Organizational culture
Practice development, 27, 29–30, 33, 217–18,
        226–9
Primary nursing, 6–8, 19–21
    definitions of, 19
    establishment of, 29, 67–8
    move to, 42
    primary nurse role, 43, 78–80, 83–6
    research issues, 22–6
    See also Patient-centred nursing
Professional commitment, 108–9
Professional development, investment in,
        229–31, 232
Professional work ethos, development of, 106–8
Psychotherapy, 17

Reflective conversations, 50
Registered nurses, 28, 60–1
Relationships, 150
    caring relationship, 150
    doctor–nurse relationship, 44, 189–90, 227–8
        earning respect, 190–1
        promotion of collaborative work, 195–201
        reluctant handmaidens, 191–5
        working as colleagues, 201–4
        See also Ward rounds
    helping relationship, 17, 150
    interrupted relationships, 183
    letting go, 184–5
    nurse–patient relationship, 17–19, 154,
        159–60, 165
        addressing the patient's experience, 167–75
        therapeutic relationships, 166–7
        unpopular patients, 175–8
    See also Relatives, relationships with

Relatives, relationships with, 160–1, 165, 178–82
  bereaved relatives, 161
  terminally ill patients, 182
Research issues, 21–6, 30–1
  access, 51
  action research strategy, 33–6, 37–9, 231–3
  action spirals, 40–6
  bias, 53
  confidentiality, 52
  data analysis, 53–6
    exploratory case study, 53
    main study, 53–6
  data collection methods, 47–51
    depth interviews, 49–50
    documentary evidence, 50–1
    participant observation, 48–9
    reflective conversations, 50
  exploratory work, 39–40
  generalization from study, 56
  methodology, 31–2
  observational study, 40
  participation, 51–2
  research partnership, 46–7
Retrospective data analysis, 54, 55
Rogers, Carl, 150
Role development, 45, 82–98
  co-ordinator role, 72–4
  confidence building, 96–8
  knowing what is expected, 93–8
  patient-centred nursing, 45, 162–5
    confidence building, 162–3
    planning ahead, 164–5
    role modelling and articulating practice, 163–4
  primary nurse role, 78–80, 94–7
  role ambiguity, 83–6
  role clarification strategies, 86–93
    facilitating learning from experience, 91–3
    time out, 86–90
  ward clerk role, 74
  ward sister, 42–3, 45–6
Role modelling:
  enhancement by articulation of expert clinical knowledge, 139–40
  importance of, 92–3, 119, 134, 138, 154, 163–4, 219
  in doctor–nurse relationships, 196–8
  in ward rounds, 209–10

Senior sister, 28
Service delivery units (SDUs), 30
Shared clinical experience, 146–8
Skill mix, 60–1
Skilled companions, 150–1, 165–88
  addressing the patient's experience, 167–75
  family care, 178–82
  therapeutic relationships, 166–7
  unpopular patients, 175–8
  See also Patient-centred nursing

Sociable team, 116–18
Socialization, 99
Staff nurse support group, 46
Supervision strategies, 141–8
  See also Ward sister

Task allocation, 13, 14
Team days, 89–90
Team leaders, 67
  meetings, 69
Team nursing, 8, 13–15
  creating effective teams, 64–70
    devolving decision-making, 66–9
    establishing predictable continuity, 65–6
    restructuring communication channels, 69–70
  doctor-nurse relationship and, 191–5
  establishment of, 100
    co-ordinator role, 72–4
    responses to organizational change, 71–2
    teething troubles, 75–7
  move to primary nursing, 42
  ward sister team attachment, 131–2
Team rota system, 66
Terminally ill patients, 182
Theorists, 12–13, 17
Theory generation, 53–5
Therapeutic nursing, 16
  See also Patient-centred nursing
Time management, ward sister, 130–1
Time out, 86–90, 230
  away days, 86–9, 230
  team days, 89–90
  variety and refreshment, 90
Traditional nursing, 9–12, 151

University education, 12–14, 21
Unpopular patients, 175–8

Visiting hours, 160–1

Ward clerk, 74, 133, 135
Ward meetings, 68–9, 104
Ward rounds, 44, 204–13
  being there for the patient, 210–13
  influencing ward round behaviour, 207–10
    creating incentives, 207–8
    enlisting the help of junior doctors, 210
    organizational strategies, 208–9
    role modelling and articulating practical strategies, 209–10
  nurses' views of, 205–7
  See also Doctor–nurse relationship
Ward secretary, 133, 135, 209
Ward sister, 28, 123–5
  absence of, 126–7
  as role model, 92–3, 119, 134, 138, 154, 163–4, 219

in doctor–nurse relationships, 196–8
in ward rounds, 209–10
clinical role of, 42–3, 45–6, 131–3
  leadership, 123, 125–36, 221–3
facilitating learning from practice, 139–41
  calling nurses to account, 141
  enhancing role modelling, 139–40
  guiding reflection and independent
    thinking/action, 140–1
influencing and supervising practice,
  137–48, 162–5
  confidence building, 162–3
  planning ahead, 164–5
  role modelling and articulating practice,
    163–4
  traditional ward teaching, 137–9

new style, 133–6
  supervision, 141–8
outside commitments, 135–6
redesigning the role of, 128–33, 221–2
  delegation, 133
  reshaping expectations, 128–30
  structuring the clinical role of, 131–3
  time management, 130–1
Work organization, 7–8, 9, 16, 29, 59–60
  changes in, 14, 71–82
    responses to organizational change, 71–2
    teething troubles, 75–81
  resource implications, 60–1
  See also Change in practice; Organizational
    culture
Working models, 11, 14